TO DO NO HARM

TO DO NO HARM

Ensuring Patient Safety in Health Care Organizations

Julianne M. Morath
Joanne E. Turnbull

Foreword by Lucian L. Leape

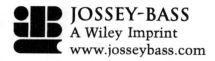

JOSSEY-BASS
A Wiley Imprint
www.josseybass.com

Published by Jossey-Bass
A Wiley Imprint
989 Market Street, San Francisco, CA 94103-1741   www.josseybass.com

Jossey-Bass books and products are available through most bookstores. To contact Jossey-Bass directly
call our Customer Care Department within the U.S. at 800-956-7739, outside the U.S. at
317-572-3986, or fax 317-572-4002.

Jossey-Bass also publishes its books in a variety of electronic formats. Some content that appears in print
may not be available in electronic books.

The WalkRounds questions listed on p. 19 are © Joint Commission Resources: *Jt Comm J Qual Safe.*
Oakbrook Terrace, IL: Joint Commission on Accreditation of Healthcare Organizations, 2003, 18.
Reprinted with permission.

The excerpt on pp. 186–187 by Donald Berwick is copyright 1996, BMJ Publishing Group. Reprinted
with permission.

The excerpt on p. 198 by Valerie Reitman is copyright 2003, *Los Angeles Times.* Reprinted with
permission.

Library of Congress Cataloging-in-Publication Data

Morath, Julianne M.
    To do no harm : ensuring patient safety in health care organizations / Julianne M. Morath,
Joanne E. Turnbull ; foreword by Lucian L. Leape. — 1st ed.
        p. ; cm.
    Includes bibliographical references.
    ISBN 0-7879-6770-X (alk. paper)
    1. Medical errors—Prevention.   2. Health facilities.   [DNLM: 1. Medical Errors—prevention &
control.   2. Safety Management—organization & administration.   3. Health Facilities—organization
& administration.   4. Organizational Innovation.   5. Truth Disclosure.   WX 185 M831t 2004]
I. Turnbull, Joanne E.   II. Title.
    R729.8.M665   2004
    362.1—dc22   2004002758

FIRST EDITION
HB Printing   10 9 8 7 6 5 4 3 2 1

CONTENTS

FOREWORD

Lucian L. Leape

In the aftermath of public and political reaction to the Institute of Medicine (IOM) report *To Err Is Human* (Kohn, Corrigan, and Donaldson, 1999), and despite the initial fixation on mandatory reporting, two of the report's key lessons seemed to have caught hold: "It's a systems problem" and "We need to create a culture of safety." Although both phrases were widely mouthed by politicians and health care leaders alike, it was quickly apparent that few who spoke them had much understanding of the profound implications of either mantra.

Moving to Systems Thinking

Of the two lessons, the one concerning systems theory has had the better time of it. A host of mechanisms have been flowering in the ensuing five years to stimulate, encourage, and goad hospitals into revamping their systems to reduce the likelihood of errors. The field was fertile for change. Hospital systems, designed for an era when care was far simpler, have not successfully changed to cope with dramatic advances in technology, divergent professions, and the variety and complexity of health care methods. For example, the number of prescription drugs now available is fifteen to twenty times greater than the number a doctor could prescribe fifty years ago, and yet in many hospitals the basic structure of the medication system is not very much different from that of fifty years ago. Doctors still rely on their memories to select drugs, and they write prescriptions by hand, whereas pharmacists and nurses still struggle to read doctors' handwriting and correct their mistakes.

But this is changing. Well before the IOM report, with the 1996 Institute for Healthcare Improvement (IHI) Breakthrough Series collaborative on reducing adverse drug events, hospitals began to be provided with a plethora of tools and instructions for analyzing systems, detecting failures, and redesigning systems to reduce errors. The implementation of "rapid cycle change," using plan-do-study-act cycles, has proved especially effective, and examples of success abound. Several hospitals, such as Luther-Midelfort in Eau Claire, Wisconsin, have made amazing changes. Like other participants in the IHI collaborative, Luther-Midelfort's initial learning and improvements focused on the hospital's medication system, but Luther-Midelfort has taken on other systems as well. Systems change theory clearly works in practice.

Major players have now entered the systems game. The Joint Commission on Accreditation of Healthcare Organizations (JCAHO) has required hospitals to establish systems for identifying quality and safety problems and to develop strategies for dealing with them. In 2002, JCAHO announced six new safe practices (which actually embed eleven new practices) that it was requiring hospitals to develop and implement, and on January 1, 2003, JCAHO began inspecting for them.

The Business Roundtable's health care purchasing collaborative, the Leapfrog Group, has also weighed in, indicating that major companies associated with the Business Roundtable will contract only with health care organizations that have implemented computerized physician order entry, that meet minimum volume levels for several specified surgical procedures, and that have full-time intensivists in their ICUs. These requirements were greeted with little enthusiasm, but hospitals are now beginning, grudgingly, to comply; more purchasers have been signing on as time goes by, and more practices are scheduled to be implemented.

The Agency for Healthcare Research and Quality (AHRQ), in addition to performing its primary role of supporting research, has taken the lead in promoting the identification and implementation of safe practices. To do this, AHRQ commissioned the National Quality Forum (NQF) to develop a list of thirty safe practices, published in May 2003. NQF's expert committee found sufficient evidence of impact to recommend these thirty practices to all hospitals. Both JCAHO and the Leapfrog Group will probably look to this list for additional practices to be recommended.

Another player in systems change is the Accreditation Council for Graduate Medical Education (ACGME), which has required specialty residency programs to observe an eighty-hour work week for doctors in training. This requirement, which went into effect on July 1, 2003, has caused great consternation among program directors who have long relied on residents to perform myriad tasks that now, presumably, will be found appropriate for lesser-trained (and lesser-paid) personnel. ACGME has also partnered with the American Board of Medical Specialties in an extensive project to define competencies for each specialty. These are a blend of general competencies that every physician should have and those specific to each specialty. Safety measures are now being included as well.

Creating a Culture of Safety

The second IOM lesson, regarding the need to create a culture of safety, has not fared as well. Although system redesign requires some change in culture—it can't be done without the formation of multidisciplinary teams, in itself a significant culture change for most organizations—these efforts are often focal and limited to a few enthusiasts and units within an organization. Even at this level, however, the sad fact is that most doctors are not involved in the planning and rollout of such changes; they are merely passive recipients (some would even say "victims") of these changes when they occur. Systems changes at the micro level (for example, removing concentrated potassium chloride from nursing units, implementing a "sign your site" policy, establishing a heparin protocol) are important, indeed crucial, but they do not in themselves constitute a culture of safety, nor do they rapidly lead to one; they are but a start.

Sadly, the predominating culture of most health care organizations is not one of safety but of fear. Doctors fear malpractice suits if they foul up, nurses fear loss of their licenses if they make serious mistakes, and patients fear becoming victims of mistakes made in their care. Doctors, because of the persistent myth of their infallibility—or, more to the point, the belief that they *should* be infallible—are smitten with guilt when serious injuries occur as a result of their mistakes, and they may be unable to admit their errors to their patients and others or to participate in meaningful efforts to understand the underlying systemic causes of errors.

This cult of perfectionism is enforced by punishment, overt or covert, which further aggravates the baseline level of fear. Not surprisingly, when injuries caused by errors do occur, nurses and physicians are loath to report them: studies show that 90 to 95 percent of serious errors are not reported. It should come as no surprise, then, that hospital leaders are often blissfully unaware of the true extent of the accidents and errors occurring in their own institutions. It is not uncommon for a CEO to state that although the national numbers are a cause for alarm, "we don't see that in our hospital."

The dysfunctional nature of hospitals is also manifest in the lack of clear definitions of accountability for key personnel. Although every actor—doctor, nurse, pharmacist, therapist, technician—has a sense of personal responsibility for patients, none feels responsible for overall care or even for care outside narrowly defined areas of competence. This "silo" mentality leads to miscommunication and friction between professions and individuals. Changing that culture is a formidable task, indeed.

Despite the shocking numbers and the entreaties from the IOM, CEOs seem unwilling to make safety a corporate priority. The combination of a dysfunctional culture, fear, ignorance, and blurred lines of responsibility leads most hospital executives to avoid playing an active role in advancing safety, and to deny the need to do so. Indeed, most CEOs, like physicians, are skeptical of the whole safety movement. For anyone seeking to create a culture of safety, the inability to engage hospital and health care system leaders is one of the most frustrating barriers. This book confronts that problem head-on.

Fortunately, an occasional leader has recognized the gravity of the situation and the need to take responsibility for changing this type of culture. The authors of this book not only found support from such individuals but also knew what to do with it. They had two very different experiences, as chronicled in the Introduction, but both authors made impressive changes in the cultures of their institutions. Each has been on the front line, and each has experience in implementing the techniques recommended in this volume. The lessons they learned from their experiences form the core around which this remarkable book is constructed. This book is not the outcome of a theoretical exercise. Its skeleton comes from the Harvard Executive Session on Medical Error and Patient Safety manifesto for leaders, but the knowledge and advice it offers come from practical, front-line experience.

The book rings with clarion calls to assume executive responsibility, install a blameless reporting system, assign accountability, accelerate change. And action is what this book is all about. Theory, yes—right up front for those who don't already know, and as a refresher for those who do: the extent of the problem, lessons from cognitive psychology and human factors engineering, the epidemiology of errors, the concept of latent errors, and organizational theories of coupling and normalized deviance. All are here—a distillate of decades of studies from industries that have succeeded in becoming safe—but then on to what to do, and how to do it.

The "Concept to Action" vignettes in almost every chapter are one of the novel and most useful features of this volume. In these sections, the authors take a real-world safety problem and demonstrate how the concepts being described apply to its solution. The problems span a gamut that encompasses teaching safety, improving the use of information technology, teaching teamwork, and the practical and ethical considerations of fully informing the patient when things go wrong. Chapter Seven, which deals substantially with disclosure, is itself a "must" reference for those who are working to break down the barriers of fear and guilt that inhibit honest relations with patients.

Most important, the authors take on the tough issues involved in changing organizational culture, bringing insights from a broad range of literature that are heavily sprinkled with the teachings of Don Berwick, the acknowledged guru of quality improvement. Learnings from his Institute for Healthcare Improvement are found throughout this volume, as well they should be, for these are the building blocks for the new pathbreaking collaborative and patient-affirming approach to improvement called for in *Crossing the Quality Chasm* (Institute of Medicine, 2001).

Above all, this is an optimistic book. Julianne Morath and Joanne Turnbull have no doubt that we can indeed create the new culture of safety that is so desperately needed in health care. And they know how to do it. Fortunately, they share both their conviction and their wisdom with us.

We dedicate this book to victims of medical accidents: patients, their families, and those health care professionals who struggle valiantly to create safety at the sharp end.

PREFACE

In the past decades, we have seen medical miracles become routine treatments. Organ transplantation and open-heart surgery are expected. Chemotherapeutic agents take people to the brink of death and back. Dramatic increases in ultrasensitive tests uncover underlying disease and create earlier opportunities for diagnosis and treatment (Fisher and Welch, 1999). More than a thousand new prescription drugs have been approved in the United States since 1975 (Cohen, 1999). All these advances are taking place in the framework of a care delivery system that is operated and managed in much the same way as it was decades ago. While the complexity of the system has been skyrocketing, so have risks to the patients who receive care and the professionals who provide it. As Sir Cyril Chantler has stated, "Medicine used to be simple, ineffective and relatively safe. Now it is complex, effective, and potentially dangerous" (Chantler, 1999, p. 1181).

Complex systems are inherently risk-prone, and health care is no exception. The job of today's health care leader is to design and operate systems that provide safe care—systems that, in the words of Hippocrates, do no harm.

Health care leaders—executives, medical directors, nurse executives, pharmacy leaders, patient care managers, quality and risk professionals, and front-line workers—are deeply concerned about the relationship between their organizations and the communities they serve. Given the growing body of evidence about the number of people harmed annually by the health care system, and in view of a public that has digested thousands of media headlines about medical errors, leaders are acutely aware that patients believe their lives to be at risk when they seek help from "healing" institutions. Health care leaders are distressed that their public no longer trusts them. Worse, they are painfully aware that good intentions and vigilance, in the face of the overwhelming complexity that characterizes the delivery of medical services, are inadequate strategies that fall woefully short in their ability to prevent harm. As one chief operating officer put it, "I feel like I'm always racing against time. I know that another accident will occur. It's just a matter of time. I don't know where or when, and I'm always hoping that someone won't be killed or seriously hurt."

Creating patient safety requires more than hoping. It requires leadership, new knowledge and skills, and the willingness to recommit oneself every day to the difficult and time-consuming work necessary to changing the culture of health care to one that learns from medical error and uses the knowledge to keep future errors from creating harm to patients.

Even knowledgeable health care leaders are vulnerable to the error-prone health care delivery system. Dr. Don Berwick experienced the vital importance of patient safety—the foundation of quality—through a personal ordeal: his wife, a former runner, developed an elusive, debilitating illness and was unable to walk. Physicians were unable to find a diagnosis, even though Berwick had arranged care in some of the best hospitals in the United States.

Berwick, founder and president of the Institute for Healthcare Improvement (IHI), began his career as a pediatrician. IHI, a not-for-profit organization, offers resources and services to health care organizations seeking to improve clinical outcomes and reduce costs. Berwick's passion is improving the quality of health care through safe, effective, patient-centered, timely, efficient, and equitable health care delivery. Commenting on his wife's illness in a speech delivered in 1999, Berwick said that the experience had left him more impressed than he had ever been before "with the good will, kindness, generosity, commitment, and dignity of the people who work in health care. The people work well, by and large," he continued. "But the system often does not."

Berwick watched as his own and other health professionals' interventions prevented one medical accident after another.

"The errors were not rare," he said. "They were the norm. The neurologist in one admission told us in the morning, 'By no means should you be getting anticholinergic agents,' and a medication with profound anticholinergic side effects was given that afternoon. The attending neurologist in another admission told us by phone that a crucial and potentially toxic drug should be begun immediately. He said, 'Time is of the essence.' That was on Thursday morning at 10:00 A.M. The first dose was given 60 hours later.

"Nothing I could do, nothing I did, nothing I could think of made any difference. It nearly drove me mad. Colace was discontinued by a physician's order on Day 1, and was nonetheless brought by the nurse every single evening throughout a 14-day admission. Ann was supposed to receive five intravenous doses of a very toxic chemotherapy agent, and the nurse labeled dose #3 as dose #2. For half a day, no record could be found that dose #2 had ever been given, even though I had watched it drip in myself.

"I tell you from my personal knowledge, no day passed—not one—without a medication error. Most weren't serious, but they scared us.

"The experience did not actually surprise me, but it did shock me. If what happened to Ann could happen in our best institutions I wonder more than ever before what the average must be like.

"Put in other terms, before this, I was concerned. Now I am radicalized" (Berwick, 2003).

As health care leaders, many of us may have had similar experiences. Family members and loved ones assume our expertise can help make sure they receive the best possible quality of care. Yet we know that sometimes our expertise isn't enough. The complexity of the health care system can overwhelm even an insider. The statistics and stories we've heard in professional meetings can suddenly play out in front of us.

No health care leader practicing today has received adequate training in safety science, medical-error reduction, or patient safety, but anyone who has worked in health care realizes that we can and should do better. Nevertheless, acknowledging failure is a painful experience for the entire health care industry, and especially for those who lead it. We are leaders in a culture that has a long history of pretending to be infallible, a culture that has placed physicians on a pedestal. Rarely has our judgment been questioned, and when it was, we did not welcome the questions. Yet acknowledgment of failure is the first step toward success; acknowledging failure is an act of strength, not weakness.

The devastating problem of medical error has forever changed the lives of too many patients and providers. Creating a culture of safety, a culture of harm-free care delivery, is the only course of action for the health care leaders of today and tomorrow. Its achievement rests on a profound change, and its creation is the duty of today's health care leaders. As leaders, we have learned and continue to learn from those we have served and failed and from providers who were giving care when systems failed them.

The existing health care culture is so entrenched that there is danger of patient safety becoming marginalized as health care organizations attempt to reduce the number of errors artificially by manipulating statistics, or by blaming and removing individuals. That is, not only can the goal of patient safety be co-opted by the existing blame-oriented culture, it can also be made to sustain that culture instead of being allowed to change it. For example, a typical response to the new standards being put forth by accrediting bodies is the trend to create a new position: the patient safety officer. The danger here is that the patient safety officer, instead of serving as a knowledge resource, a catalyst for culture change, and a developer of a system that learns from error, may focus on quick fixes. In this scenario, the goal of patient safety is absorbed into the existing dysfunctional culture and organizational structure instead of serving as a force for cultural and structural change. Periodic assessments of patient safety create a veneer of safer care, but in the long run the culture does not change; patient safety becomes the subject of one more report to the governing board, and this reporting activity disguises the fact that patient safety itself is suffering in the actual environments of care.

By contrast, an organization that is serious about adopting a culture of safety may opt not to have a patient safety officer, using the rationale that safety is everyone's business, and that safety must be integrated into all work processes throughout the organization. In this scenario, the chief executive officer or other senior leaders oversee the integration of safety into work processes and are directly accountable to the board for the changes needed to advance safety. The accounts produced by these leaders will include not just measures of actual harm but also the number of errors reported, and the goal will be to observe an increase in reports and a decrease in harm. In the safety culture, individual accountability is the norm; blame is not.

Most leaders are acutely aware of working in a stressful environment, but they are often oblivious to the pathological elements that make up their environment. This lack of awareness renders leaders unable to change the conditions operating in the organizational culture. They are caught in the unfortunate situation described by Edgar Schein (1997, p. 15): "The bottom line for leaders is that if they do not become conscious of the culture in which they are embedded, those cultures will manage them."

The Need for This Book

Our goal in writing this book is to equip you with the knowledge, insights, strategies, and tools that will enable you to create and lead a culture of safety. Certain characteristics of health care culture are setups for error. For example, a primary barrier to safety in health care settings is the hierarchical nature of relationships between executives and clinicians, between physicians and nurses, and between all clinicians and their patients. Another is the fact that most health care practice today takes place in "silos"; that is, each discipline practices its craft with little or no awareness of what other disciplines are doing, and yet the practices of pharmacists, nurses, and physicians are highly interdependent. Silo practice is error-prone practice. To transform hierarchies into partnerships and tear down silos, we wrote this book for health care leadership as a whole, not just for one discipline.

To Our Audience

To Do No Harm is relevant to leaders in all health care disciplines today: senior health care executives, medical directors, nurse executives, pharmacy leaders, patient care managers, quality and risk professionals, and leaders of clinical disciplines as well as board members. The content is applicable to any health care setting: hospital inpatient services, emergency services, acute care, rehabilitation services, nursing homes, home health services, and ambulatory services ranging from physicians' offices to infusion and surgery centers. The wide applicability of the book's content is in keeping with the principle that care is provided through a complex system of sites, services, and relationships, and that we can create safety only by understanding relationships, communicating effectively, anticipating gaps in patient safety, and acting collectively to close or bridge them. This book is also for the leaders of tomorrow: graduate-level students in the disciplines just mentioned, and those who have embraced the vision embodied in these pages and plan to make the field of patient safety their career focus.

Description of Contents

The chapters in this book are structured around the patient safety manifesto developed at the Harvard Executive Session on Medical Error and Patient Safety. The Executive Session brought together senior leaders in health care from around the nation to examine the failures in current health care models and to develop models of health care delivery that do no harm (see the Introduction and Chapter Nine for further information on the Harvard Executive Session). Leaders emerged with a seven-point manifesto for creating a system of harm-free care. With the exception of Chapters Two and Three, which provide basic information about the science of patient safety, and Chapter Ten, which recaps the lessons offered by the book as a whole, the titles of the chapters are the same as the seven commitments of the manifesto:

- Chapter One, "Declare Patient Safety Urgent and a Priority," explores the patient safety manifesto's first challenge to leadership. The chapter discusses how and why to develop and create a vision and a platform for patient safety in your organization.

- Chapter Two, "Error and Harm in Health Care," departs momentarily from the patient safety manifesto, as already mentioned, to provide background knowledge on current research in patient safety, the patient safety movement to date, and the reasons why today's health care system is so error-prone.
- Chapter Three, "Understanding the Basics of Patient Safety," provides an overview of basic concepts and terms in the science of patient safety. These concepts and terms form the foundational touchpoints of the book.
- Chapter Four, "Assume Executive Responsibility," returns to the commitments embodied in the patient safety manifesto. It hones in on the leader's role in making the commitment to create harm-free care, outlines the specific characteristics of the leader's role in safety, and discusses the leader's responses to error.
- Chapter Five, "Import New Knowledge and Skills," translates concepts from safety science and lessons from high-reliability organizations into practical applications for health care.
- Chapter Six, "Install a Blameless Reporting System," is devoted to the design and implementation of voluntary reporting systems, an indispensable feature of the safety culture. The chapter presents the rationale for developing an internal voluntary reporting system, and it offers an overview of the successful use of such a system in the field of aviation and beginning efforts in health care. Chapter Six also discusses the voluntary reporting system as a management decision-support tool and a tool for culture change, and it addresses legal concerns and other barriers to a blameless reporting system.
- Chapter Seven, "Assign Accountability," addresses issues of management and front-line responsibility in the context of safety, and within a systems perspective.
- Chapter Eight, "Align External Controls and Reform Education," focuses on the need to bring such external forces as academic, legal, and regulatory systems into alignment, since external forces can help or hinder a systems approach to health care safety.
- Chapter Nine, "Accelerate Change," discusses methods and techniques for accelerating and sustaining change.
- Chapter Ten, "The End of the Beginning," concludes the book with a review of lessons learned and challenges for advancing the work of patient safety.

The book also includes a glossary of terms used frequently in patient safety science. Starting in the Introduction, the first time we use one of these terms, it appears in boldface type. A list of references is provided along with resources intended to encourage and guide further education in patient safety. Finally, the glossary is followed by a series of appendixes containing examples of policies, projects, tools, and other items helpful in beginning and sustaining a patient safety initiative.

The book follows a logical sequence, moving from general information (research, background, safety science) about patient safety in health care to more specific and practical aspects of implementation (the safety culture, voluntary reporting systems, the leader's role, and training). Accordingly, reading the book in a linear fashion will offer the most comprehensive picture of patient safety, but each chapter also stands on its own, so a particular topic can be selected for reference.

This primer is a succinct yet comprehensive resource on patient safety for today's busy health care leader. It summarizes key research, with an emphasis on what the findings mean for practice. It translates the concepts of safety science into practical applications, and it captures learning from failures as well as from "best practices" that are emerging from the work of leaders who are testing new models for patient safety. Action strategies are presented along with precepts of safety science so that both can be integrated into health care operations, and so that leaders can develop the necessary skills to lead a culture of safety. Throughout the book, we strive to be mindful of the demands on our readers' time, summarizing existing knowledge and mapping lessons from other fields in a succinct, practical way. Case studies, labeled "Concept to Action," provide examples of good practice and contribute to our effort to make the material relevant.

The goals of this practical guide are to teach the science of safety, introduce the lessons that other high risk industries can teach us, present ways to learn from health care's failures and successes, and examine the growing body of better practices and achievable, effective initiatives that can help transform the concepts of patient safety into action.

Research and new applications of safety science in health care are increasing exponentially. To meet our publication deadlines, we concluded our own research in April 2003. Had we not done so we would still be writing, as new lessons emerge daily. We encourage you to keep abreast of new activities in the field by using the organizations and Web sites listed in the Resources section.

Changing the culture of the organization is the key to creating and sustaining patient safety, and the leader's role is the crucial feature. Therefore, the heart of the effort represented by this book is the effort to help leaders move their organizational cultures from blame, shame, and cover-up to vigilance, transparency, and learning. Only culture change will create an environment devoted to and equipped for harm-free care. Health care leaders need a new competency for this challenge—knowledge of patient safety—together with deep integrity and unflappable vision. Taken together, these attributes will enable a leader to call the existing culture into question and expose the myths that operate within it. The goal is to empower the health care leader to create, lead, and sustain a new culture—a culture of safety.

ACKNOWLEDGMENTS

The journey toward a culture of safety is in no way a solitary one. Rather, many minds and hearts have joined in numerous efforts over the past two decades to face the enormous challenge of keeping patients from harm. This book is no exception to that pattern. We have been fortunate to have the eager contributions of many people.

First, we make a general acknowledgment to major contributors to the field of patient safety whose work we have drawn on for this book. Among them are James Reason, Karl Weick, Jens Rasmussen, Richard Cook, David Woods, and Karlene Roberts. Special thanks to Lucian Leape for writing the Foreword; he has been not only a pioneer in the field but also a mentor. Don Berwick, president of the Center for Healthcare Improvement, and Jim Conway, chief operating officer of the Dana-Farber Cancer Institute, both in Boston, have made substantial contributions through their work, which appears in this book.

We also recognize the following individuals, most of whom serve at the "sharp end," who participated in case study preparation either by giving us interviews or by writing material: Allan Frankel, M.D., director of Patient Safety, Partners Health Care, and senior fellow for the Institute for Healthcare Improvement, Boston; Caryl Lee, R.N., M.S.N., program director, Veterans Administration Center for Patient Safety, Ann Arbor, Michigan; Katharine Luther, R.N., M.P.A., director of performance improvement, and Ann-Claire France, Ph.D., former director for the center of healthcare improvement at Memorial Hermann Healthcare System,

Houston; Paul Uhlig, M.D., Valerie Cote, R.N., Elisa Kendall, Pharm. D., and the rest of the team at Concord Hospital, Concord, New Hampshire; Todd Miller, M.D., director of medical affairs and quality improvement (retired), Abbott Northwestern Hospital, Minneapolis; Ginger Malone, R.N., M.S.N., director of patient care and care innovation, Judith Napier, R.N., M.S.N., director of patient safety and risk management, Tom Hellmich, M.D., pediatric emergency room physician and medical director for patient safety, Glenn Galloway, chief information officer, Theresa Duffy, R.N., M.S.N, patient care manager, Casey Hooke, R.N., M.S.N., clinical nurse specialist, Mark Thomas, R.Ph., Ph.D., director of pharmacy services, Kelly Fredrickson, R.N., and Linda Hamilton, R.N., clinical staff nurses, Chris Robison, M.D., senior director of clinical services and vice chief medical officer, Ginny Hustead, M.D., neonatologist and director of ECMO services, and Pam Graves, N.N.P., patient safety coordinator, all of Children's Hospitals and Clinics, Minneapolis/St. Paul, Minnesota. Special thanks go to the following people for particular contributions: Brock Nelson, former CEO of Children's Hospitals and Clinics for his trust and courage to start the journey; Jim Levin, M.D., Ph.D., director of medical informatics of Children's Hospitals and Clinics, Minneapolis/St. Paul, Minnesota, for his reporting-system case study; Beth Lanham, R.N., B.S.N., Froedert Hospital, Milwaukee, for her Six Sigma case study; Boris Kalanj, M.S.W., Tim Culbert, M.D., and Mursal Khalif, R.N., of Children's Hospitals and Clinics for their contributions to the material on cultural competence; Susan Weicker, marketing analyst, also of Children's, who was the architect for the focus groups for the content on cultural care included in Chapter Eight.

The contributions of the following reviewers vastly improved the content of the book: Roger Rezar, M.D., Luther-Midelfort Hospital, Eau Claire, Wisconsin; Della Lin, M.D., the Queen's Medical Center, Honolulu, Hawaii; Richard Cook, M.D., Cognitive Technologies Laboratories, University of Chicago; Peter Provonost, M.D., Ph.D., critical care medicine, Johns Hopkins University; Jim Conway, Dana-Farber Cancer Institute; Linda Connell, M.A., R.N., the NASA Ames Research Center; and Anne-Claire France, Ph.D., the Center for Healthcare Improvement, Memorial Hermann Healthcare System, Houston.

For information, support, and assistance, we thank Pamela M. Barnard, A.H.I.P., M.L.S., Allina Health Systems Library Services; Holly Ann Burt, M.L.S., Information Resource Center, National Patient Safety Foundation; Sara Tompson, Packer Engineering Library; John R. Combes, M.D., Hospital and Healthsystem Association of Pennsylvania; Diane Cousins, U.S. Pharmacopeia; and Linda Williams, R.N., Veterans Administration National Center for Patient Safety. We also thank the editorial team from Jossey-Bass, Andy Pasternack, Seth Schwartz, and Gigi Mark, who made the project flow smoothly.

We extend our gratitude to Linda Zespy, Lorri Zipperer, and Margaret Teele for their editorial and project management assistance as well as for their insights, great questions, and humor. Finally, our generous and understanding families have supported our work by tolerating our consuming passion with this topic, which often takes time from them. We recognize this and appreciate it.

THE AUTHORS

Julianne M. Morath is chief operating officer and chief nurse executive for Children's Hospitals and Clinics, Minneapolis/St. Paul, Minnesota. She has been a participant-observer at the Harvard Executive Sessions on Medical Error and Patient Safety and an appointed fellow to the Salzburg International Seminar on Patient Safety and Medical Accident. Morath is also serving a second term as an elected board member of the National Patient Safety Foundation, where she served as a member of the executive committee. In addition, she is a board member of the Healthcare Evaluation and Research Foundation, past chair of Best Practices of the Minnesota Alliance in Patient Safety, and current co-facilitator of the Minnesota Executive Sessions. She has held faculty appointments in the College of Medicine and Biology at Brown University; in the College of Nursing, and in medicine and psychiatry in the College of Medicine, at the University of Cincinnati; in the College of Nursing at the University of Rhode Island; and in the College of Nursing at Rhode Island College.

Among a variety of rewards recognizing her work in patient safety is the Patient Safety Initiative Award for Patient-Provider Communication Solutions, presented to Morath in 2000 by the National Patient Safety Foundation and the Joint Commission on Accreditation of Healthcare Organizations. She was the inaugural recipient, in 2002, of the John M. Eisenberg Patient Safety Award for Individual Lifetime Achievement. Before she joined the staff at Children's, Morath's experience in health care included clinical practice, consultation, academic work, and over twenty years as a health care executive at major medical centers. She is the author, among many other publications, of *The Quality Advantage: A Strategic Guide for Health Care Leaders*. Her work as a leader in patient safety was featured in the July 17, 2000, issue *of U.S. News & World Report* and is the subject of a Harvard Business School case study that was published in November 2001. Morath is a frequent speaker and consultant in the fields of quality and patient safety and has worked in Norway, Sweden, and Denmark as well as throughout the United States.

Joanne E. Turnbull, Ph.D., served as the second executive director of the National Patient Safety Foundation. In that role, she began a program to develop a Web-based patient safety education program, implemented the Minnesota Executive Session in partnership with the Minnesota Hospital Association, and established the Patient and Family Advisory Council. In collaboration with the American Hospital Association's Health Forum, she developed the Patient Safety Fellowship, a program that trains forty to fifty health care executives each year in methods of leadership in the area of creating safety for patients. In April 2002 she was appointed a fellow of the Salzburg International Seminar on Patient Safety and Medical Accident and has worked with colleagues in Japan, Denmark, and Sweden to advance patient safety initiatives in those countries. Turnbull was co-chair of the National Advisory Council on Patient Safety for the American Society of Healthcare Risk Management and served on the Steering Committee on Safe Practices for the National Quality Forum.

Turnbull received a doctorate in psychology and social work from the University of Michigan and spent more than twenty-five years as a clinician, researcher, teacher, and senior health care administrator at several major teaching centers, specializing in patient safety, performance improvement, population management, and resource utilization. She has held faculty appointments in psychiatry at Duke University, in psychiatry and physical therapy at the University of Pittsburgh, in medicine and nursing at the University of Texas Health Sciences Center in Houston, and in social work at Columbia University. Her academic work includes more than thirty research and clinical publications that address such topics as reduction of medical error, health care quality, patient satisfaction, and mental health.

TO DO NO HARM

INTRODUCTION

The most important transformation in health care in the last twenty years is not managed care, minimally invasive surgery, or diagnostic-related groups (DRG)s. It is the transformational knowledge about **safety science**, how **medical accident** occurs, and how we can prevent **harm** from reaching patients through **accidents**. To prevent patients from being harmed, our health care leaders—executives, medical directors, nurse executives, pharmacy leaders, patient care managers, quality and risk professionals, and front-line staff providers— need critical knowledge and skills, but the skills crucial to designing care that *does no harm* have not been part of the educational process in health care. The health care professional has been educated and acculturated in individual responsibility and personal failure, shame, blame, and embarrassment, often with the accompanying threat of litigation, when things go wrong. A **transforming concept** of safety science is that the **system**, not individuals acting alone, creates safety. The **patient safety** movement is about building a culture and systems that do no harm. Although the safe care of patients is a primary **accountability** of health care leaders, it is the least understood. This book is for leaders who need a strategic, practical guide based on safety science so that they can answer such fundamental questions as *Is this a safe place to give and receive care?* and *How can we prevent medical accident from ever harming a patient?*.

We wrote this book so we could gather in one place the knowledge, resources, and tools needed to understand and create a patient safety culture. Our aim, as explained in the Preface, is to help health care executives, medical directors, nurse executives, pharmacy leaders, patient care managers, quality and risk professionals, and front-line workers face the clear-cut and urgent challenge of launching and maintaining a **culture of safety**. We would like you to think of this book as a "primer" (Zimmerman, Lindberg, and Plsek, 1998). It is intended to help you take the first steps in understanding safety science and its applications to creating a culture of safety in health care. Just as the primer, in painting a house, is not the finished surface, the primer you hold in your hands is not the finished product. Rather, the finished product will be a culture of safety for patients, and this book is intended to help you think more strategically, to create the conditions for your continuous inquiry and learning, and to help you develop a solid, coherent base of patient safety, where the "finish" reflects what is unique to your organization. Because the achievement of patient safety is always a work in progress, we, as the authors of this book, owe it to those who receive and provide care to offer this "first coat" of lessons.

Building a culture of safety requires threshold change, that is, a magnitude of change that moves the entire organization to a new and higher level of performance, and as usual with such efforts, the work is informed by profound personal experiences. Our journeys in the realm of patient safety have given us much that we want to share, and each of us has a unique story to tell. The first author's story offers an example of how one individual, after twenty-five years in health care **leadership**, moved from a focus on people and **continuous quality improvement** to a focus on creating systems that do no harm. It is the story of discovering a different theory base from which to lead and making an unflinching commitment to find strategies for improving health care delivery. The second author's story describes a disorienting dilemma, that is, a learning experience in which her perspective was transformed as a result of her confronting a new and unfamiliar reality (Meziroff, 2000). The experience provoked and inspired her to challenge preconceived notions, and it led her to a new level of awareness and to a more **complex** understanding of the **causation** and management of medical harm. This mandatory growth experience, undergone in the heat of tragedy, forced an about-face for leadership. The second author's story also shows how fragile and transient a safety culture is in the absence of support from top leadership. Both stories demonstrate the strong and direct relationship between leaders' response to medical **error** and the culture change that can ensue from leaders' response.

Julianne Morath: Moving from Theory to Practice

An intensive care nurse with nineteen years of experience appeared in my office one day, tremulous and tearful, to tell me about an accident involving a child in her care the previous day. She hadn't slept all night, reliving the event in her memory: a misplaced decimal point had caused the child to receive a potentially lethal overdose. A reversal drug was nearby, and the child recovered, but the nurse had not. If this could happen to her, she realized, with all her years of experience, then it could happen to anyone. She believed that if she let hospital leaders and her co-workers know about the incident, they would all take action to prevent that type of error from reaching a child again. Together, the nurse and I discussed plans for a review of the many factors and systemic issues that could have contributed to the accident. When she left, I realized how far I had come in my patient safety journey.

My reaction to medical accident, both as a clinician and later as an executive, wasn't always system-focused. Today's health care professionals, who have trained in a culture of unremitting, uncompromising personal responsibility, know the long-accepted reaction to a medical accident: a hard, solitary look in the mirror, inspired by the belief that if one could only have been better prepared or more perfect, one could have prevented the accident.

The culture of absolute personal responsibility, sometimes referred to as the "blame and shame" culture, is pervasive in health care—and, as I would grow to learn, it has never been effective in preventing accidents. This nurse's experience was enlightening, showing both the opportunity for improving systems and the relief that sharing knowledge about an error or a **near miss** might bring to the burdened work life of front-line staff.

From 1997 to 2000, I had the opportunity to attend the Harvard Executive Session on Medical Error and Patient Safety, where health care leaders from around the nation gathered to learn about the growing epidemic of medical error and consider actions to restore public confidence and achieve greater safety in care delivery. The method of these executive sessions, which have been used for years to create breakthrough change in industries other than health care, was to create a forum in which leaders learn from leaders—removed from their normal work environments, so they can be helped to recognize how organizational culture influences and shapes their work. Refer to Chapter Nine for greater detail of the Executive Session.

At the executive sessions, distinguished experts and mentors in the science of accident causation, **human factors** research, and **patient safety science** challenged health care leaders to consider that harm-free care is possible, and that the leader's job is to create systems that do no harm. Once I started reading and learning, I developed the belief that harm-free care was possible. Information I learned and later applied to health care included the work of James Reason, whose **Swiss Cheese Model of Accident Causation** illustrates how faulty systems and multiple aligned errors, rather than the error of a single individual, create the conditions for accidents to reach patients. **Hindsight bias** was another new concept, and it gave me insights into how to examine events when things go wrong. A scientific validation of the old adage "Hindsight is 20/20 vision," hindsight bias explains why human beings are wired to attribute accidents to **simple** and immediate causes, and usually to human error. I learned about the concept of **normalization of deviance**—the phenomenon whereby human beings, over a period of time in highly risk-prone conditions, tend to develop "work-arounds" (Norman, 1988) to compensate for problems but then lose **situational awareness** and begin to view these work-arounds as normal practice—that is, they normalize this deviance as a defense against working in conditions of unmitigated risk. In this way, perilous situations—such as the use of only partially functional equipment, the diminishing of safety issues to maintenance problems, or the use of fatigued medical residents who are expected to work dangerously long hours—come to be minimized by the culture. Lessons were available from **high-reliability organizations (HROs)** that, like health care organizations, perform complex, dangerous work that must be carried out with absolute precision; unlike health care organizations, however, these HROs have achieved remarkably low accident rates by transforming their work environments into safety-oriented cultures.

Study of the 1949 Mann Gulch disaster also provided lessons, this time on the collapse of **sensemaking** and on **teamwork** in unexpectedly hazardous situations. The analysis of this disaster emphasized the importance of trust, communication, and innovation in creating conditions of safety and resilience. It was sobering information, detailing how both reliance on methods of the past and failures in teamwork can create hazardous conditions that place lives in danger, but it contained the seeds of a transforming thought: I had been worrying all along about patient safety, but my approach, although heartfelt, disciplined, and well-intended, had been naive and at the wrong level of intervention to affect the delivery of care. I carefully reconsidered approaches to errors and failures that I had confronted throughout my years of health care leadership and was convinced that more effective approaches needed to be applied. As demonstrated by experience in other industries, and by the safety science they had developed, local efforts and isolated improvements could not produce the widespread, sustainable change needed to create greater patient safety. The entire culture of health care needed to change in order for harm-free care to be achieved.

In the summer of 1999, I was presented with the opportunity to become the chief operating officer for a pediatric health care system. The work gave me the opportunity to apply what I had learned about the organizational elements required for an effective, patient safety–oriented culture:

- Leadership and **reciprocal accountability** between front-line staff and management
- A **blameless reporting** system
- **Transparency** (openness) about error, and learning from error

- Partnership with and **disclosure** to families when things go wrong
- Design and engineering of systems of care that are purposely created to reduce reliance on human memory and performance alone, and to prevent harm from reaching patients
- Complex conversations around how care is provided, and anticipation of gaps in care so they can be closed or proactively bridged
- Teamwork between and among disciplines and levels based on principles of **crew resource management**
- Application of lessons from HROs
- Identification of sources of organizational success and resilience

Now here was the test. Could theory and lessons learned from settings outside health care be effectively applied to patient safety? All of us—myself, the CEO, vice presidents, medical directors, nurse leaders, and front-line providers of care—worked together to craft a comprehensive patient safety initiative.

We began by learning how to have productive, blame-free conversations about error and accidents, and by considering new knowledge from patient safety science. This effort matured into developing partnerships with families, partnerships that included our disclosure of medical accidents and near misses. Organizational leaders considered the question of how we would want a health care organization to respond to us if we or our loved ones ever faced the tragedy of a medical accident. A policy of full disclosure was developed—a collaborative effort on the part of executives, families, caregivers, board members, and professional medical staff members—and this policy served as a **culture carrier** for patient safety throughout the organization. Next, the creation of a blameless reporting system formed the foundation of transparency and learning within the developing culture. As staff members began to focus on learning instead of blaming, lessons were shared about how to improve our systems and reduce the probability of accidents.

Eventually our thinking about patient safety evolved to the deeper understanding that a safety culture requires patients and families to become part of the safety system, not passive consumers of the system of care. Our model of family-centered care expanded to a promise made to patients and their families: "Nothing about me without me" (Delbanco and others, 2001). They would be partners in informed decision making and full participants in care, to the extent of their willingness and ability, and their participation would also be welcomed when failures in safety occurred. Our approach of integrating families into the culture of safety included respect for their knowledge and expertise in judging whether things looked wrong. We codified this attitude in a **stop-the-line** policy that obligates all caregivers to halt a procedure and reassess safety issues if a family member questioned the level of safety or the appropriateness of care. Family members became involved in our **patient safety steering committee** and were architects of the strategies for patient safety.

Patient safety has become a key value for our entire organization and the foundation of our operations. Patient safety is everyone's job. High-risk processes and procedures are analyzed to detect vulnerabilities and failure points that could contribute to an accident. Employees are engaged in anticipating where the next failure or accident may occur and are empowered to act in the interest of restoring safety if they perceive that we are moving into conditions of intolerable risk. Local teams operate with simple rules: "Fix what you can. Tell what you fixed. Find someone to fix what you cannot."

Multicausal analysis is focused on learning from near misses before the occurrence of an event that causes harm. Slowly, our culture is evolving into one explicitly devoted to safety. Our evolution began with one-to-one encounters. As time went on, more providers, such as intensive care nurses, began to talk, first to each other and then in small groups, about near misses or errors—sometimes going back a decade—that had haunted them. Together, we worked to reframe our perspectives, learn from errors, and create resilient systems in the face of risk. The concept of "forgive and remember" (Bosk, 1981) became real and liberating. As clinicians forgive themselves and move away from shame to harness the lessons learned from medical error and accident, the opportunity to create harm-free care is within our grasp. We need to apply the same discipline, rigor, and resources to creating patient safety as we do to understanding and eradicating cancer, AIDS, heart disease, and other conditions that prematurely rob people of their lives.

Our work to change our culture continues today. Patient safety is a fragile and transient state that requires constant attention and vigilance. Most important to the culture change has been the acknowledgment of full responsibility for patient safety by the executive staff of our organization. We now understand that we hold a collective obligation to design and operate safe systems, and that the decisions we make have a direct effect on the ability of front-line staff to provide care. We now acknowledge that communication and trust between and among all the people in the health care environment are imperatives in creating safety. We now declare that our job as leaders is to keep the promise made by those who work in health care: to *first, do no harm*. We do this through building and operating systems that advance harm-free care.

Joanne Turnbull: A Cautionary Tale

The phone call that changed my life came around ten o'clock on a Saturday morning in early August of 1995. "I'm calling to let you know about an incident that happened last night," the overnight administrator said impassively. Nothing in her tone hinted at the gravity of the call's purpose.

On a personal level, that "incident" changed the course of my career and consumed my work and personal life for the next six years. On a broader level, it transformed an organization with a fixed culture—behaving the way most health care organizations do, by expending enormous energy in attempts to bury **mistakes** and placing blame on the unfortunate soul who happened to be in the wrong place at the wrong time when an accident occurred—into an organization with a culture where people began to openly report and discuss mistakes. For its efforts, the organization was later rewarded with a significant reduction in serious medication errors and found itself well on the way to addressing the underlying issues whose resolution would bring a culture of safety into being.

But back to that phone call. The "incident" it announced was the accidental death of a six-week-old infant. The child had been admitted to our hospital for an initial "loading" dose of digoxin, a powerful medication that was expected to control his symptoms of early congestive heart failure, but a conversion error from micrograms to milligrams, and a misplaced decimal point written by a distracted medical resident, produced an order for ten times the prescribed amount. That order set in motion a chain of events that transformed a healing medication into a lethal overdose.

After getting the call, as chief quality and utilization officer, I had to phone the medical director and tell him the bad news. The backup system—other physicians, along with nurses and pharmacists—had failed to keep the deadly drug from reaching the infant. The medical director began by recalling mistakes that he had made during his years of training and practice, many of which could have resulted in harm to patients. He was sure that none of the professionals involved in this event had gone to work planning to kill a baby. We both realized that the tragedy also had victims besides the baby and his family: the resident, the attending physician, the nurse, and the pharmacist were probably all suffering. The medical director and I eventually concluded that human beings make mistakes, and that it was the system that had failed to protect both the patient and these professionals. Thus, during our long conversation, our anger toward the resident, the nurse, and the pharmacist evolved into a joint commitment: we would refuse to engage in blaming these individuals.

We agreed to form a partnership. Together, we would model collaboration between administrator and physician and would push to redesign the care delivery system in our organization. This must never happen again, we agreed; not only patients but also doctors, nurses, and pharmacists had to be protected. The system had allowed this tragedy to happen, and a system had to be designed to prevent it from happening again.

The timing of the incident created a "burning platform"—a powerful reason for change, a reason that could not be ignored. The event had occurred two weeks before the triennial survey by the Joint Commission on Accreditation of

Healthcare Organizations (JCAHO). In the language of JCAHO, the baby's death was a **sentinel event**, an incident of such magnitude that it warranted reporting, examination, and perhaps sanction. The hospital leadership disclosed the death to the surveyors during the opening interview.

The baby's death occurred at a pivotal time in JCAHO's history as well. JCAHO was then making the transition from issuing the sanction of "Conditional Accreditation," for organizations experiencing sentinel events, to designating a new status, "Accreditation Watch." The intent of the new designation, which does not affect an organization's accreditation status, was and continues to be non-punitive. Its purpose is to notify the public that an organization is working in partnership with JCAHO to correct systemic problems that have led to an event. What JCAHO's watchfulness meant for our organization was that the issue of error reduction would not only be sustained in the collective organizational consciousness over a long period but would also remain a top priority.

The centerpiece of JCAHO's new approach to sentinel events under Accreditation Watch was **root cause analysis (RCA)**—the process of continually asking "why" questions to uncover hidden, underlying causes of harm and near misses. At that point, a final procedure had not yet been developed for conducting RCAs, so the RCA on the baby's death was undertaken in close collaboration with JCAHO. The hospital leadership set the tone and supported a system-oriented, blame-free approach as the analysis was conducted in a two-month multi-step iterative process. The analysis was long, tedious, and worthwhile.

For the first time, the administration and the participating health care disciplines—medicine, pharmacy, and nursing—came together to formulate terms and definitions related to the management of error. A common language emerged. Previously, the hospital culture had been bifurcated, with administration on one side and medical staff on the other; worse, physicians were patronized by the administration and viewed as an entity to be "managed." As a result of the RCA process, these groups began to interact, tentatively but earnestly.

The final phase of the RCA replaced the organization's Accreditation Watch status with the highest status given: Accreditation with Commendation. The majority of the contributing factors identified in the RCA revolved around communication:

- *Lack of a callback system to signal when a physician went off duty.* The callback system was needed for order clarification.
- *Duplicate order delivery to the pharmacy.* Nonemergent orders were first faxed—against hospital policy, which allowed only emergent orders to be faxed—and were then followed up with a courier-delivered order. In this case, the pharmacist recognized the danger in the faxed order, but she missed it in the hand-delivered order because she was paying attention to other details of the dispensing process.

- *An order ambiguously written.* Trailing zero and the infant's weight were not used in calculating the dose.
- *Lack of clear accountability in relationships among multiple physicians and caregivers.*
- *Delays in returning a page.*
- *Inability to resist the **authority gradient**.* What this means is unwillingness or inability to "tell truth to power" for fear of the response. In this situation, the pharmacist and the nurse were both concerned about the order, but neither felt empowered to halt it.

The hospital's **performance improvement** department began to conduct RCAs on a routine basis, and as we went along, we worked out the RCA protocol. All front-line staff who had been involved in an accident would be required to participate. The RCA sessions themselves would be conducted by a trained facilitator, assisted by a scribe, who would help the participants adhere to two simple rules: there would be no blaming, and the focus would be on systems rather than on people.

After some initial hesitation, due to fear, all staff, irrespective of discipline, expressed what a positive experience it was to participate in the RCA process. Word spread throughout the organization, and very soon the performance improvement department became deluged with requests for RCAs, for problems other than non-sentinel events.

Staff reaction to this early experience taught us that root cause analysis served at least two purposes in addition to its intended diagnostic one. First, staff welcomed the opportunity to talk in a safe place about a shared traumatic experience. We became aware that front-line staff had been carrying an enormous psychological burden—unexpressed guilt and remorse when accidents occurred, and the daily fear of making a mistake—and that root cause analysis had a healing effect, serving as a debriefing that allowed those involved to share perceptions and emotions. Second, we realized that the requests for root cause analyses for nonemergent problems were coming because staff desperately needed problem-solving skills for carrying out their daily work functions. By participating in the RCA process, staff began to glimpse the possibility of solving problems in a multidisciplinary, collaborative fashion.

Soon we established a multidisciplinary panel composed of senior leaders who met quarterly to review all analyses and reach consensus on **root causes**. As findings grew from our collection of analyses, we learned that the most frequent root cause of sentinel events was the same as the one found in the infant's death: impaired communication among staff. This information provided the foundation of our performance improvement plan for the coming year.

Given the high-profile nature of the initial case, we could not wait for technological solutions like a **computerized provider order entry (CPOE)** system.

Interventions were simple and low-cost, but all were based on empirical evidence or sound safety principles, and all targeted communication. To reduce faulty orders, physicians were provided with strong incentives to write their orders according to a standardized method. Nurses and pharmacists were trained to communicate assertively in their interactions with physicians, and they received strong support from the medical leadership for doing so.

These interventions, along with supporting policies and an infrastructure for conducting root cause analyses, began to transform the culture significantly. Serious medication errors were reduced by 50 percent over a year and a half. Nonnumerical indicators also spoke powerfully of cultural transformation. For example, the physician leadership, initially resistant to complying with the order-writing policy, felt that the 97 percent compliance that was achieved in the first year was not good enough; without sanctions or incentives, the leadership set the target at 100 percent for the upcoming year.

Another example of transformation was evident at a board meeting. During the first report of **adverse events** and near misses to the board, the following exchange took place between a board member and an administrator:

Board member: The number of errors reported sure seems low, given the **complexity** of the system.

Administrator: I am so glad you said that. We want to create an environment that encourages reporting of errors so that we can study them and improve the system.

Upon hearing this nonjudgmental comment by the board member and witnessing the commitment of the administrative leader, a pediatric surgeon strode across the room to the administrator, mentioned a medication overdose that had occurred during a **complicated** surgical procedure, and asked why it had not been included in the report. This exchange reinforced the lessons we were learning about our staff's enthusiastic response to root cause analysis: front-line providers are willing, even eager, to report and discuss errors if the environment is perceived to be safe.

Then came the merger. Two organizations—one an academic medical center, the other a group of community hospitals—came together to forge a strong presence in the local marketplace. The CEO position did not go to the leader of our organization, and the new CEO did not share our former CEO's commitment to patient safety; in fact, he was afraid of making such a commitment. He showed this fear by challenging speakers who had come to town to provide education about patient safety. In matters of accreditation, he seemed to rely on his friendship with the head of JCAHO, perhaps hoping that surveys revealing problems could be dealt with through networking instead of through changes to the system. The final nail in the coffin of our budding, fragile safety culture was set in place after the suicide of an inpatient. In a weekly administrative newsletter sent to board members and senior management, the CEO included a statement that the suicide had occurred because two nurses failed to follow policy, and in conversation he said that the incident was an unfortunate but unavoidable by-product of caring for psychiatric patients. This CEO partook of the myths plaguing medical culture. He avoided the unfamiliar. Like most of us, his training and experience as a leader had given him neither knowledge about the problem, harm in health care, nor any skill in dealing with it.

Many of the lessons I have touched on in this story address the possibilities for creating a culture of safety, but the primary lessons are these: without commitment and energy, patient safety is a fragile and transient state, and leaders who do not believe that harm-free care is achievable will not be able to achieve a culture of safety for patients.

Moving Forward

The journey to a culture of safety begins with the belief that health care workers go about their daily work wanting the best for their patients and do not intend to harm them. The truth is professionals are devastated by error when it occurs, and they create safety every day by anticipating, compensating for, and recovering from risk. But people are imperfect instruments and cannot create safety alone. The work of patient safety is certainly not about cautioning people to be more careful. It is about changing the medical culture and changing our personal responses to error and unintended events. As Zimmerman, Lindberg, and Plsek have stated (1998, p. iv), referring to complexity, "This is not a program that you roll out in the organization with banners and coffee mugs. It's a new way of thinking and seeing the world—and hence, a new way of working with real organizational and health care issues." The work of patient safety is about transforming and fundamentally changing how care delivery is designed, organized, and managed, and that is the leader's job.

CHAPTER ONE

DECLARE PATIENT SAFETY URGENT AND A PRIORITY

Where to Begin

To create a solid platform from which to build safety and resilience in an organization, leaders must declare patient safety to be urgent and a priority. A first strategy is to convene influential clinicians. They are readily identifiable. They are the individuals whom peers seek out for new information, opinions, and consultations. They can help explore three important questions:

1. Is this a safe place to receive and give care?
2. How do you know?
3. What is your experience?

Asking these questions invites and legitimizes conversations about accidents, near misses, barriers, and sources of safety. The answers to these questions are not typically shared but rather are individually experienced. In dialogue, collective consciousness regarding safety in the organization is raised. Recognition of the experience of risk leads quickly to conversations about what actions need to be taken to understand errors and prevent accidents from occurring. Dialogue creates a safe place to nurture and encourage a willingness to expand the conversation throughout the organization in the quest for improvement and harm-free care.

These nonjudgmental questions begin to build a culture committed to learning from errors and mistakes. Joseph Campbell has been quoted as saying, "Dig where you stumble, for that is where the treasure is" (Osbon, 1995). Just as in finding an archeological treasure under uneven ground, deeper stories of medical error and accidents uncover treasures of knowledge and opportunities for improvement when the conditions in which we fail or stumble are understood.

Assessing the State of Your Organization

The perceptions and commitment of thought leaders are vital, but the next step for leaders committed to deep systemic change is to look inward and gain a fuller picture of the state of safety in the organization.

Embracing patient safety means committing to a habit of excellence and to the creation of the same experience for patients that you would want for your child, parent, spouse, friend, loved one, and yourself. It takes courage to accept responsibility for the state of things today, to declare an intent to do better, to listen to the lessons in the system and the wisdom of those on the front line, and to take informed action for the changes that need to be made. If this were easy, it would have been done already. It is uncomfortable to objectively assess your own leadership practices and the state of safety in your organization.

One of the first steps taken in connection with the comprehensive patient safety agenda at Children's Hospitals and Clinics, Minneapolis/St. Paul, Minnesota, was to invite randomly selected employees, residents, students, physicians, and families to participate in focus groups. The following case study illustrates how focus groups were used to gather information and to create awareness of patient safety.

Concept to Action

Using Focus Groups to Assess Current State of Patient Safety

A Children's executive explained, "We wanted to understand directly from clinicians and families whether this was a safe place to give and receive care, based on their experience and to learn what they perceived to be barriers in patient safety. The goal was to gain a portrait of the actual safety experience within the organization as a starting point to understand the culture. The focus group methodology was used to create a locally relevant view of safety rather than extrapolate from published studies."

An outside consultant with a background as a registered nurse, Ginger Malone, R.N., M.S.N., was engaged to work with Children's market researchers to organize and conduct the focus groups. Seventeen focus groups from across the care delivery system were conducted. A focus group was conducted with each of the following stakeholder groups:

- Nurses
- Advanced-practice nurses, a group that included clinical nurse specialists, nurse practitioners, neonatal nurse practitioners, and certified registered nurse anesthetists
- Practicing clinical nurses
- Respiratory care practitioners
- Pharmacists
- Practicing physicians
- Social workers, chaplains, and child life specialists
- Medical directors
- Medical students and residents
- Directors and managers
- Families

Involving families was a controversial and much debated decision. "The concern was that it would frighten families to talk with them about safety issues," said the executive. "However, we found that families knew everything, and they worried about safety all the time."

The invitation to participate in a focus group included a note that employees would be paid if groups were scheduled during their time off and that their work responsibilities would be covered by a qualified colleague if groups were conducted during their scheduled shifts. This compensation for participating re-emphasized management's support as well as the importance assigned to this work. Five to eleven employees participated in each focus group. Conversations about safety were framed by the use of eight questions based on the work of Dr. Nancy Wilson, who developed some of the patient safety culture tools for a 1998 Department of Veterans Affairs cooperative study.

1. When you hear the term *patient safety*, what comes to mind?
2. Give some examples of events that have a negative effect on a patient's medical outcome.
3. Is patient safety a priority of the leadership team?
4. What are some of the barriers to patient safety?
5. What influences free and open communication for patient safety?
6. Suppose that an error occurs, resulting in serious injury to a patient. What happens?
7. Do you believe that reporting an error or a near miss will ultimately improve patient care? Why or why not?
8. What are some of the things done in this organization that contribute to patient safety?

The group members provided a rich source of ideas and concerns, according to Ginger Malone. "They provided the information needed to shape a safety culture and provided a baseline from which to start. That is, we are safe but we can be safer. Most people expressed a genuine interest in being the safest clinician they could be, but they reported needing the entire operations of the system to support them. We all learned about ways to strengthen the culture and safety infrastructure, how to improve reporting, how to promote safe prescribing practices, how to build a more reliable medication system, how to better work with families, and how to improve teamwork. The focus group findings informed the design of the patient safety initiative."

For example, through the focus groups, leaders discovered pervasive anxiety among residents and students about disclosing errors or mistakes, for fear of receiving a poor grade or a poor recommendation. "We realized our culture was enabling the next generation to repeat and sustain a culture of silence and cover up," said the executive who commissioned the focus groups. Those findings helped to inform a variety of initiatives. For example, key clinical leaders began working with the academic health sciences faculty of the local university to introduce patient safety and reduction of medical accidents as areas of study in the core curriculum of clinical disciplines. In the hospital itself, the medical director of the pediatric ICU has created "safety rounds" or dialogues where students join him periodically to discuss risks, mistakes, and strategies for detection and recovery in the clinical practice environment. In a confidential setting, the medical director talks about his personal experiences with medical error, thereby modeling transparency and teaching about how to keep an error from reaching a patient.

In addition to gaining information, the focus group methodology was a deep cultural intervention. By creating a safe and supportive environment for talking about medical error and patient safety, the focus groups began to model the way to break the code of silence and talk about making health care safer.

The compelling consistency of the responses from clinicians and families challenged the organization. "Everyone who participated had been touched by error in some way," says Malone. "It was a privilege to listen to the personal stories. Hearing them was very powerful, and a challenge to the organization to eliminate the barriers and become even safer."

"The focus groups provided a toehold to begin to advance a very aggressive patient safety agenda. By reflecting the results back to the organization, we created the portrait that we can and will do better," added the executive.

The Kübler-Ross Phenomenon

Examining patient safety in your organization can evoke what Don Berwick characterized as a "Kübler-Ross response" (Berwick, 2002a). In her classic work on the study of death and dying, Kübler-Ross (1969) formulated five stages that an individual works through when facing death: denial, anger, bargaining, depression, and acceptance. The death-and-dying analogy, applied to patient safety, points to mourning for an idealized culture of health care that has shown to have a dark side of harm; it is no longer believable or viable and is being replaced by a culture of safety and reliability.

When safety performance begins to be measured, the first response is often denial. "The data are wrong," leaders might say, "or the research is flawed. This can't be." Typically, this initial denial evolves into rationalization, signaled by comments like "The data are good enough, but this is not a problem" or "We are within control limits."

A stage of anger follows, with indignation and justifications: "My patients are sicker or different." The messenger is often shot.

The third stage is bargaining. In health care this stage is translated into perhaps its most dangerous manifestation, that of blame. "I will accept the validity of the data," the administrative leader acknowledges, "and, yes, I will accept that there is a problem, but it is not my problem. The problem rests with the clinicians. They need to be more careful."

In the next stage, leaders may experience depression as they accept responsibility but feel overwhelmed by the enormity of the issue and paralyzed because they do not know what to do.

Finally, as they hear the experiences of others and realize they are not alone, leaders become educated and move into the last phase, of acceptance. With acceptance comes hope and action. "It is our problem," leaders declare. "We can do better. We will do something about this." Berwick (2002a) suggests that health care leaders experience these stages when confronted with the realities of patient safety work. He urges rapid movement through these stages so that the work of improving patient safety can begin.

Recognizing the Power of the Patient and the Sharp-End Staff

Safety is created in knowing, anticipating, and closing or bridging the gaps that allow risks to reach a patient to create harm. Our traditional methods of health care management have tolerated and at times encouraged divisions among health care disciplines, and between health professionals and patients and their families, that create and exacerbate gaps. We have encouraged fragmentation by siloed departmental functions and touted business theories that reduce complex, highly intimate care processes to transactional industrial production schemata. As risks appear in the workplace, front-line staff compensate for inadequate system support on a daily basis, fearing what could happen when factors outside their control slip through their carefully constructed personal defenses. Meanwhile, the gaps in the system of care delivery continue to grow.

The current health care culture demeans, confines, silences, and dismisses the contributions for safety and improved care that staff, patients, and families offer to us (Berwick, 2002a). Leaders have the opportunity to recognize and accept the gifts that patients' families and sharp-end health professionals bring to the health care encounter. A clear choice rests with leadership: to amplify and choreograph these gifts into a web of safety that protects patients, or to overlook them, undermining the engagement and teamwork of people in caregiving relationships by making demands related to production and cost cutting rather than focusing on relationships and improvement. The links between safety and service are strong.

Health care professionals are privileged to enter people's lives at a time of vulnerability and need. Along with hope, trust, and belief in us, patients and their families bring their knowledge and experience, their expertise, their natural capacities to heal, and their love of each other. Accepting these strengths and sources of resilience means abandoning the traditional health care systems that create fragmentation, **hierarchy**, confusion, and gaps in communication, knowledge, and processes. These are the gaps that promote the conditions for medical error and accidents to occur. To be truly patient- and family-centered requires the design of care delivery through a detailed understanding of **process flow** and patients' experience rather than a focus on professional disciplines and departmental functions and convenience.

Believing in Harm-Free Care

We are on the cusp of a patient safety movement, a movement that demands a discipline of transparency, collaboration, learning, and striving for excellence in all we do. As leaders, we regularly face detractors in our workplace who tell us nothing can be done. In the case of patient safety, it is especially important that leaders know and believe harm-free care to be achievable. According to Leape and others (1991), 72 percent of medical accidents are recurrent. Hospitals across the nation make the same mistakes over and over, altering families' and patients' lives forever and traumatizing health professionals, who usually assume they are the only ones who make mistakes. Meanwhile, the conditions that combined to cause an accident lie in wait for the next individual or event to set the chain reaction in motion. The examples are numerous and include errors in prescribing and administering medication as well as errors in surgical procedures and even surgical sites. For example, orthopedic surgeons, working with fragmented surgical teams and efficiency-oriented preoperative procedures, have a 1 in 4 chance of performing wrong-site surgery in their careers (Canale and others, 1998). No matter how careful and engaged one person is, there are forces at play in the system that no single individual can overcome.

If medical accidents are recurrent, then they are predictable and therefore preventable. It is the job of leadership to change the culture of health care so that shame does not revolve around the fact that error exists but instead revolves around the fact that the rich potential of error as a teacher has remained unmined for so long. The individuals who give, receive, and support care are intrinsically linked within the common purpose of discovering these conditions and preventing them from ever causing harm to a patient again. Until leaders believe in patient safety and create the conditions for seeking knowledge and improvement, rhetoric about harm-free care will be meaningless. Cultural change in the direction of patient safety cascades from the attitudes and responses of leaders who clearly articulate harm-free care as the aim that will be achieved.

Getting to Work

Unfortunately, it is the atypical executive leader who takes a long, unflinching look at the real work on the front line. Nevertheless, that act is a prerequisite of a culture of safety. The following two case studies demonstrate how leaders can directly access unedited, unprocessed data about the experience of patient safety in their organizations. Leaders' visibility and personal engagement make patient safety visible as a value and a priority. The first case study is from health care; the second is from industry.

Concept to Action

Making Patient Safety Rounds: Linking Management and the Front Line

As patient safety director for Partners Healthcare, Dr. Allan Frankel has worked intensively with front-line clinicians who had ideas for patient safety initiatives. Even when ideas were well developed and sound, says Frankel, some of them still failed. The difference between the successful and unsuccessful projects often was related to support of leadership. "If you wanted safety as a concept, and the safety project itself to take hold," he says, "you need[ed] leadership insight and support."

His insights led Frankel to develop WalkRounds™, a specific process of joining **sharp-end** and **blunt-end** workers in content-rich, nonthreatening, productive dialogues around patient safety. WalkRounds begins with senior executives visiting a preselected unit for one hour, to ask staff members questions about potential risks in the workplace. Staff members' comments are harnessed to create and prioritize patient safety projects. Then the leaders report back to the front line about how staff comments have resulted in improvements, a practice that further encourages dialogues around patient safety.

The WalkRounds process was piloted at Brigham and Women's Hospital (BWH), Boston. The team, consisting of one senior leader (the president, chief operating officer, chief medical officer, or chief nursing officer), the patient safety manager, a senior director for quality/safety, the pharmacist assigned to the unit being visited, the hospital vice president with responsibility for the unit being visited, and a research assistant, met to conduct the rounds for one hour in one unit per week. Nurse managers were contacted twenty-four hours in advance so they could notify staff members of the visit and, it was hoped, prompt a more thoughtful, robust discussion when the WalkRounds team arrived.

Upon arrival on the unit, the WalkRounds team invites attending and resident physicians, the nurse manager, patient care assistants, pharmacists, and others from the unit to join the group. The team asks the nurse manager to identify one or two nurses to answer the following questions (Frankel and others, 2003, p. 18):

1. Were you able to care for your patients this week as safely as possible? If not, why not?
2. Can you describe how communication between caregivers either enhances or inhibits safe care on your unit?
3. Can you describe the unit's ability to work as a team?
4. Have there been any "near misses" that almost caused patient harm but didn't?
5. Is there anything we could do to prevent the next adverse event?
6. What do you think this unit could do on a regular basis to improve safety? For example, would it be feasible to discuss safety concerns, e.g., patients with same name, near misses that happened, etc., during report?
7. When you make an error, do you always report it?
8. If you prevent/intercept an error, do you always report it?
9. If you make or report an error, are you concerned about personal consequences?
10. Do you know what happens to the information that you report?
11. Have you developed any personal practices that you do to specifically prevent making errors (memory aids, double-checking, forcing functions, etc.)? [See Chapter Three for a discussion of forcing functions.]
12. Have you discussed patient safety issues with your patients or their families?
13. Do patients and families voice any safety concerns?
14. What specific intervention from leadership would make the work you do safer for patients?
15. What would make these executive WalkRounds more effective?

Comments gathered during WalkRounds are entered into a database, and each comment is assigned to one of four main categories based on Charles Vincent's framework for analyzing risk: teamwork, hardware (equipment), the individual, and the patient (Vincent, 1998). Comments are subclassified into such categories as concerns related to inadequate staffing or poor communication between providers. Then the aggregated comments are given "priority scores," based on the potential or actual impact of risk-prone situations and the frequency of their occurrence. Priority scores determine pilot projects and help make the best use of limited hospital resources. The patient safety manager or another patient safety staff member stays in touch with unit managers about the patient safety concerns raised during WalkRounds and about how the concerns are being addressed.

A frequent WalkRounds comment at BWH concerned the inability of staff members to find supply items needed for patient care. Some nurses thought they spent up to 30 percent of their time searching for equipment, a process that delayed patient care. Because the comment was frequent, and because there was some potential for harm to a patient, the problem was given a high priority score, and hospital resources were designated for an initiative around this problem.

A key to the success of WalkRounds is that staff members feel safe sharing information. At BWH, discussion and analysis from WalkRounds are tied in with the hospital's peer review committee and therefore protected by the state's peer review statutes. A blameless reporting system also helps staff members feel safe discussing their experiences.

The WalkRounds have resulted in many changes in how BWH's system functions, ranging from the purchase of a mechanical lift for obese patients (reducing the likelihood of patient or staff injuries) to changes in the orientation of new nurses and pharmacists (resulting in fewer delays in the receiving and administering of medications). Staff members report increased discussions of safety issues on the units and a desire for more communication from leaders about how their comments are used and about and what is happening with patient safety initiatives.

Sharp-end staff members are helping to shape the patient safety agenda, but they are also changing their perceptions of leadership. Through WalkRounds, leaders listen, educate others about patient safety concepts, model a systems perspective, and show the front line that they are responsive and action-oriented. Sharp-end providers, in turn, are more likely to report concerns and problems. The WalkRounds concept, says Frankel, has evolved over time from a process for engaging leaders to a process that has changed how the organization perceives and reacts to safety issues. "Initially it was just to get leadership involved," he says. "Then we realized it was a tool for changing culture."

Concept to Action

Leadership Through Declaring Safety as a Priority in the Work Place

Another example of bringing the principles of safety into leadership practice is that offered by Paul O'Neill, former CEO of Alcoa and former secretary of the treasury. O'Neill became CEO of Alcoa in June 1987 and was reported to have immediately stunned corporate directors, industry analysts, and competitors when he announced his top priority: safety. He believed that the names of employees killed or injured should not be turned into numbers and rates. He did not believe that productivity goals necessitated increased risk, or that accidents and injuries were inevitable costs of doing business. Rather, he believed that focusing on safety required understanding processes and systems in exquisite detail, and that this type of understanding would lead to higher productivity. Although Alcoa had an industry record for safety, O'Neill raised the bar and demanded that management eradicate accidents and injuries. This goal required a recalibration of Alcoa's operational approach, from measuring what had caused accidents to learning how to prevent them in the first place. For example, if a worker fell off a machine, O'Neill asked what the worker had been doing on the machine and whether the machine's design included control mechanisms that actually increased risk.

O'Neill recognized that an explicit focus on safety could be a rallying point for the workforce. By focusing on safety and pursuing the root causes of accidents, the company prioritized an improved process flow, which led to increased productivity and reduced cost of accidents and errors. The results at Alcoa are legendary. Alcoa's profits soared. The same focus, discipline, and commitment can be executed in health care (Margolis and Clark, 1991).

The experience at Alcoa shows that the foundation for work in patient safety is nurturing a culture, or "people system," that sees, lives, and breathes safety. This is not about cautioning people to be more careful. This is a call to action. It is about improving the systems in which people operate and increasing their ability to perceive, identify, and close the gaps in the system that create vulnerability. With time and commitment, this improvement is wholly achievable.

Summary Points

1. Leaders must believe that harm-free care is achievable. Leaders create the conditions for seeking knowledge and improvement. The cultural shift toward safety cascades from the attitudes and responses of leaders who clearly state that harm-free care is an aim that the organization will achieve.

2. Leaders must declare patient safety urgent and a priority and must embrace safety as an integral part of the health care environment. Leaders need to lead with courage and take an unflinching look at their own leadership, accepting responsibility for the current state and declaring the intention to do better. Leaders must be visible to the front line and must understand the technical work of the front line, both from the perspective of process flow and from the patient-family experience.

3. Leaders must listen to the lessons in the system and the wisdom of those on the front line by asking, "Is this a safe place to give and receive care?" This approach allows leaders to take informed action toward the changes that need

to be made. Ascertaining a portrait of the actual safety experience in the organization is a starting point to develop a safety culture.

4. Leaders should expect to go through stages of denial, anger, bargaining, depression, and acceptance as they mourn the loss of an idealized culture and face reality. Leaders must face these stages head-on and move through them quickly in order to get on with the work at hand.

5. The job of leadership is to move a culture from shame and silence to a culture that views error as a rich, untapped source of knowledge that can be used to define the boundaries of safety and to inform improvement.

ERROR AND HARM IN HEALTH CARE

Chapter Two provides a historical overview of the patient safety movement. There are two parts to this. One is the epidemiologic error studies that have dominated the medical literature. The second part describes the early organized efforts in patient safety. Researchers and theorists in the safety field have moved beyond a limited conceptualization of safety that focuses solely on counting errors. It is now understood that a focus on hazard and harm is more meaningful. This focus will be introduced in Chapter Three.

As early as the 1960s, researchers began tracking the disease of medical accident that afflicts the health care system. This medical literature is often motivated by experiences with health care accidents and has produced a variety of unrelated attempts to gauge the nature and scope of the "error" in health care. Such investigations are largely exploratory and not grounded in any theoretical base. Describing **epidemiology** as "the sum of factors that influence the incidence and distribution of a disease," Dr. Lucian Leap summarizes the evolution in thought regarding medical accident: "That medical errors are caused by bad systems is a transforming concept. It relieves the burden of guilt and shame that occurs when error is focused on the individual. The epidemiology of medical error about ten years ago was simple: Error is due to carelessness. Blame and punishment is the response" (Leape, 2001). The focus on error in the research was a reflection of the medical culture's flawed, entrenched belief that the actions of individuals, "bad apples," were responsible for harm to patients. Two guiding principles have emerged to frame patient safety research:

1. ERROR IS BEST VIEWED AS A SYMPTOM OF A LARGER PROBLEM—A BROKEN HEALTH CARE SYSTEM.

Like bacteria in the human system, errors are a normal part of life. Errors need not create harm. Just as distribution of bacteria and existing physiological conditions determine whether a human being can be harmed by the bacteria, a system's design, conditions, and responses to failure will determine whether or not errors concatenate to reach and harm a patient. Medical injury is now studied with the same rigor that is applied to a disease state. Evaluating accidents involves viewing them not as individual acts that deserve blame and punishment but as variables that allow us to learn about, diagnose, and treat a larger problem—the design and operation of the health care system.

This approach is beginning to make some inroads into the traditions of blame and denial that burden the health care culture. Medical accidents are still laden with seemingly intractable connotations of fault finding, mistake making, or carelessness, and the associated responses of shame and blame. However, research now reveals recurring elements in accidents and near misses: culture- and system-based failures in teamwork, communication, and transitions.

2. ERRORS WILL ALWAYS EXIST AND ARE USEFUL ONLY AS A DATA SOURCE TO HELP US AVOID HARM.

"Error is all around us like the air we breathe. Error is ever present, and attempts to eliminate it are fruitless. Error itself is neutral and boring; it is how we understand and respond to it that shapes whether harm may later result" (Reason, 2001). There are tens of millions of unsafe events and faulty work processes in the aviation industry but relatively few plane crashes. Most perils are intercepted or are insufficient by themselves to create conditions for a crash. Because the airline industry studies near misses, it can use the information to create systems that are designed to prevent potentially dangerous situations from lining up to create the trajectory for an accident (crash) to occur. This process of making hazardous conditions transparent and learning from them is explored in the upcoming chapters of this book.

The goal is not to eradicate all risk but rather to make it transparent and learn from it, mitigate it, in order to prevent harm in the delivery of care. As National Patient Safety Foundation leaders state, "Fundamental misunderstandings about medical accidents (harm to patients) are among the barriers to making progress on patient safety. Most accidents do not happen because of one mistake or error, but rather [are] due to multiple small causes, each insufficient to create an accident, but potentially deadly when combined. The focus solely on 'error' misdirects attention from creating safer systems—the systems needed to reduce the opportunity for errors to combine" (R. I. Cook, 2001).

As you read through the following summary of the research on medical accidents, remember that suppression of error will not create a safer system. What will create a safer system is to make error, hazardous conditions, and deviations visible or transparent. Learning from these inform actions to create a robust and resilient system to prevent hazards from creating harm. For progress on patient safety to occur, the focus must be on the system and on understanding the nature of technical work, not on individuals. The epidemiology of medical accident merely lays a basic foundation for understanding the scope and nature of failure and harm in health care.

Epidemiology of Health Care Accidents

How frequently do accidents happen? What types of medical accidents are the most common? How much do medical accidents cost health care organizations and the public?

These are the questions that draw a picture of medical accident for health care leaders and the public. Their answers provide a beginning place to learn about the inner workings of the organizations. This information can help leaders understand what accidents are likely to occur where, and reduce the risks that patients face when they come through the doors. External influences also create a motivation for leaders to understand the research surrounding medical accident: increasingly, purchasers of health care are balking at paying the high health care costs associated with death and injury and are demanding action to reduce adverse events to patients.

Three major themes have emerged from the epidemiologic patient safety research: the frequency of adverse events, the types of medical accidents, and the cost of adverse events. As health services research continues to reveal when and under what conditions adverse events occur, leaders will have access to better information and tools to improve their organization. They will also be better prepared to address the powerful external influences, such as the reaction of purchasers to the cost of medical accidents, that will increasingly affect the contracting and financing of health care services.

Frequency of Medical Accident

Decades ago, research documented that as many as 36 percent of admissions to a general medical unit and 13 percent of admissions to intensive care units followed adverse events, most often due to medications (Caranasos, Stewart, and Cluff, 1974).

The research that followed explained medical accidents as the unfortunate and unavoidable consequence of powerful, modern therapies (Sharpe and Faden, 1998; Moser, 1956), or the suspected causes were not addressed at all (Trunet and others, 1980). In the mid-1980s, a single study implicated human error, suggesting that up to half of all admissions related to adverse events were due to "lack of attention on the part of physicians or patients" (Lakshmanan, Hershey, and Breslau, 1986).

The Harvard Medical Practice Study. In 1991, the subject of medical accident received formal academic study with the publication of the **Harvard Medical Practice Study (HMPS)**. Analyzing medical records from fifty-one hospitals in New York State, the HMPS reported that 3.75 percent of all patients suffered adverse events as a result of their medical care. An adverse event was defined in this study as an extended hospitalization, disability at the time of discharge, or death that resulted from medical care rather than from the natural course of disease. Negligent care accounted for 28 percent of these adverse events, and of these, in 25 percent of cases the affected patients died and in 6 percent the patients were permanently injured (Brennan and others, 1991). A study of discharges from acute care hospitals in Colorado and Utah confirmed the HMPS findings (Thomas and others, 2000). These results have been extrapolated to more than 300,000 patients injured each year (Becher and Chassin, 2001). Another replication of the HMPS, conducted in Australia in 1995, reported that half the adverse events were predictable and therefore highly preventable (Wilson and others, 1995). Table 2.1 summarizes major studies of adverse events.

Understanding the Consumer's View. In 1997, the National Patient Safety Foundation commissioned a survey of how the public perceives risk when interacting with the health care system. Of those who responded, 42 percent reported that either they or someone they knew had experienced an injury when visiting a physician's office (Louis Harris and Associates, 1997). Studies by the Kaiser Family Foundation and the Commonwealth Fund support these results. A 2002 Kaiser Family Foundation survey found that one-third of U.S. physicians reported that they or a family member had been harmed by medical error (Blendon and others, 2002). The Commonwealth Fund found that one in ten consumers reported

TABLE 2.1. A SUMMARY OF MAJOR STUDIES OF ADVERSE EVENTS

Study	Adverse Events (AEs)	Patient Outcomes
Leape, Brennan, and Laird, 1991	3.7% AE rate from 30,121 randomly selected records of hospital admissions	70.5% of the AEs resulted in nonpermanent disability, 2.6% caused permanent disability, and 13.6% caused death
Studdert, Brennan, and Thomas, 2000	2.9% AE rate from 15,000 medical records randomly drawn in 1992 from acute care hospitals	2% of AEs were considered serious; death occurred 0.3% of the time, and permanent disability occurred in 1.3% of injuries
Wilson and others, 1995	16.6% AE rate from 15,000 medical records	2% of AEs were considered serious; death occurred 1.7% of the time, and disability was the result 8.4% of the time

that they or a family member had become sicker as a result of an event in the doctor's office or hospital (Davis and others, 2002). About half of these problems were reported to be very serious. Another 16 percent reported that they or a family member had experienced a medication error, and this was the largest category of adverse events. In more than 20 percent of the cases, the medication event had caused a serious problem. Physicians and consumers alike believe that the current national efforts are not the most effective way to reduce medical error (Blendon and others, 2002). For example, just 40 percent of physicians and 45 percent of the public believe that limiting certain high-risk procedures to high-volume centers would be an effective solution, and just one-third of physicians agree that using only physicians trained in intensive care medicine in hospital ICUs would be very effective (see the material later in this chapter about the **Leapfrog Group**, under the subhead "The Business Community," in the section titled "Background of the Patient Safety Movement"). Table 2.2 shows the findings of studies surveying health care consumers.

Types of Medical Accident

The data are inconclusive about the incidence and prevalence of medical accident by care setting, but we do have information about where unanticipated events occur (see Table 2.3).

TABLE 2.2. CONSUMER STUDIES

Survey	Study Size	Percentage Affected
Louis Harris and Associates (National Patient Safety Foundation, 1997)	Telephone survey of 1,513 adults	42 percent of Americans reported they or a family member had experienced a medical error of some kind.
Commonwealth Fund (Davis and others, 2002)	Telephone survey of 6,722 adults	22 percent of Americans reported they or a family member had experienced a medical error of some kind; 33 percent of those reporting an error said it happened in the hospital
Harvard School of Public Health/ Kaiser Family Foundation (Blendon and others, 2002)	1,207 adults, 831 physicians	42 percent of the public said that either they or a family member had experienced medical error in the course of receiving medical care; despite this reality, only 6% of the public felt that medical error was a top problem facing health care.

Acute Care. Prescribing drugs is one of the most common clinical activities in hospitals, so it is not surprising that **adverse drug events** produce the most common type of medical accident. Research indicates that 2 percent of hospitalized patients experience preventable adverse drug events, and that 20 percent of these events are life-threatening (Bates and others, 1995). Approximately 7,000 people die of preventable adverse drug events in hospitals each year, more than the total number who die from workplace injuries (Kohn, Corrigan, and Donaldson, 1999). It is notable that each prescription contains the opportunity for six to eight errors.

Other common types of adverse events in hospitals are preventable infections, surgical and diagnostic mistakes, and events involving equipment use. Two million patients are estimated to acquire infections in the hospital each year, and 25–70 percent of these infections are preventable; 90,000 of the affected individuals die (Centers for Disease Control and Prevention, 1996; Weinstein, 1998; Haley and others, 1985). Between 87,500 and 350,000 patients are exposed to life-threatening infections every year because of hospital-acquired bloodstream infections alone (Wenzel and Edmond, 2001).

TABLE 2.3. AVAILABLE RESEARCH ON TYPES AND FREQUENCY OF MEDICAL ERROR

Type of Event	Frequency
Acute care: Adverse drug events (ADEs)	1.8% of hospitalized patients suffer preventable ADEs; of the 20% that are life-threatening, 42% are preventable (Bates and others, 1995); 7,000 deaths per year (Kohn, 1999)
Ambulatory: Adverse drug events (ADEs)	218,000 patient deaths in 2000 (Ernst and Grizzle, 2001); 18% reported a drug complication, with 3% of those being ADEs, and 5% of that number requiring hospitalization (Gandhi and others, 2000); 350,000 ADEs per year in nursing homes, involving 1.55 million residents, with 20,000 of these being fatal or life-threatening and 80% of that number preventable (Gurwitz, 2000)
After discharge	19% had AEs; of those, 6% had preventable AEs and 6% had AEs whose impact could have been reduced (Forster and others, 2003)
Inpatient: Preventable infections	2 million cases per year (MBGH, 2002); 90,000 deaths every year, 25–70% of them preventable (Haley and others, 1985)
Surgical events: Inappropriate surgeries, wrong-site surgery, etc.	1,858 AEs found in 1,047 cases reviewed; 44% of cases had at least 1 event; a total of 4 events per patient; 14% of the events were considered to have caused serious injury (Andrews, 1993)
Diagnostic adverse events: Misdiagnosis, failure to perform a test, improper performance of a test, delays in diagnosis, etc.	20% of reviewed deaths contained a misdiagnosis; 44% of these cases would have been treated differently with correct diagnosis (Tai and others, 2001)
Medical equipment misuse	No systematic research on frequency or type

Surgical adverse events, including inappropriate surgery, wrong-site surgery, and mistakes during a surgical procedure, were observed in a study of 1,047 surgical cases. The study identified 1,858 events of all types, with 14 percent resulting in serious injury, defined as disability or death. In almost one-third of the serious injury cases, the surgery itself was inappropriate (Andrews, 1993). The findings from this study suggest that a single patient can suffer more than one event. As already mentioned in Chapter One, orthopedic surgeons are estimated to have a 1 in 4 chance of performing wrong-site surgery sometime during a thirty-five-year career, a finding that has prompted the American Academy of Orthopedic Surgeons to promote a "sign your site" program, requiring surgeons to initial the site of surgery with a permanent-ink pen, in the presence of an alert and informed patient and another member of the surgical team, before starting a procedure (Canale and others, 1998).

Diagnostic mistakes include misdiagnosis of an existing condition, failure to perform or improper performance of a diagnostic test, recommendation of tests or therapies that are inappropriate for the diagnosis, and delays in diagnosing. Some diagnostic mistakes are unavoidable (as when the cause of illness or death can be identified only through some sort of retrospective review, such as an autopsy or a pathology report), but a study in an intensive care unit found a misdiagnosis in 20 percent of deaths (that is, the presumed cause of death was different from the cause as determined through an autopsy). A correct diagnosis would have resulted in altered treatment in 44 percent of these cases (Tai and others, 2001).

The Food and Drug Administration categorizes events related to the use of medical equipment, or equipment malfunctions, as "use errors." To date, no systematic research exists on the frequency or type of these events, but many would be preventable with the application of human factors principles in equipment design that recognizes human abilities and limitations, training and clear instructions for users, an environment that is conducive to proper use (lighting appropriate to tasks, a low level of distractions, and sufficient space), or other ergonomic strategies (see the 1996 Center for Devices and Radiological Health article "Human Factors and Medical Devices" at www.fda.gov/cdrh/humfac/hufacgen.html).

Who Is at Risk? No patient is immune from harm, but research tells us that the most vulnerable patients are the elderly, those who are most critically ill, and those who are subjected to the most heroic interventions (Weingart, 2001). The youngest of patients, such as fragile neonates, are likely in the most vulnerable group, but there is a paucity of research on medical accident in the pediatric environment. Not surprisingly, surgery results in a greater proportion of adverse events; negligent injury, however, is no more common among patients undergoing high-risk surgery than among medical patients. Patients undergoing high-risk surgical interventions, such as neurosurgery, vascular surgery, and cardiothoracic surgery, are the most vulnerable to experiencing preventable injury, but patients requiring this type of care are also the most complex and are more vulnerable to harm because they often are quite ill and in need of urgent care that relies on potentially lifesaving but high-risk interventions (Thomas and others, 2000).

Ambulatory Settings. Although the majority of health care is provided in ambulatory settings, research on harm in outpatient settings is still in its infancy. Medical patients, not outpatient surgical patients, are more likely to experience preventable adverse events, a finding that reflects the type of care provided. One study found that drug-related events in the ambulatory setting resulted in 218,000 patient deaths in 2000 (Ernst and Grizzle, 2001). A chart review of medication-related complications in primary care sites identified adverse drug events in 3 percent of patients. The most frequent complications were allergic reactions, of which 13 percent were preventable (Gandhi and others, 2000). Another study estimates that 350,000 adverse drug events occur in nursing homes each year, approximately half of which are preventable (Gurwitz and others, 2000).

Other common adverse events that occur in ambulatory settings are failures in diagnostic **judgment** (the formal terms in patient safety language are **active failures**, or incorrect acts) and failure to implement preventive care (failures to act, or **errors of omission**) (Midwest Business Group on Health, 2002). An analysis of 344 reported errors in family practice settings identified 4 percent that had resulted in adverse outcomes, and it documented that 84 percent were related to systems and processes. These errors included administrative mistakes, such as failing to take a message, failure to include contact information in a medical record, losing laboratory reports, and miscommunicating. Clinical mistakes, such as a misdiagnosis or a wrong treatment decision, accounted for 13 percent of the errors (Dovey and others, 2002).

The Cost of Medical Accident

Preventable medical accidents are estimated to cost the nation $17–$29 billion a year, a total that includes litigation costs and direct health care costs, the latter accounting for more than half the total (Kohn, Corrigan, and Donaldson, 1999). The total economic impact, including lost income and disability, is estimated to be $38–$50 billion a year. Using the estimate (reported in *To Err Is Human: Building a Safer Health System*) of 98,000 inpatient deaths and 300,000 inpatient injuries each year, two automotive companies calculated that at least one of their employees or dependents died each day because of inpatient medical accidents—a total of 500 deaths a year, as reported by the Midwest Business Group on Health (2002), a nonprofit coalition of leading employers who are committed to improving both the quality and cost-effectiveness of health care services. This coalition also estimates that each of its member corporations loses three employees or dependents each day.

Costs have been calculated for two types of adverse events: infections and drug events. If the direct cost of each infection is estimated to be $12,500, preventable infections add $6.2–$18.6 billion each year to the burden of direct health care costs (Midwest Business Group on Health, 2002).

Inpatient costs related to preventable adverse drug events that occur in hospitals are estimated at $2 billion per year. In the ambulatory setting, drug events may equal more than 12 percent of the nation's total health costs, in excess of $175 billion (Ernst and Grizzle, 2001).

Costs associated with drug events can be reduced. For example, researchers from Brigham and Women's Hospital found that 6.5 percent of the hospital's inpatients experienced adverse drug events each year, and that 28 percent of these events were preventable. They estimated that each preventable adverse drug event cost $4,500, for an annual total of $2.8 million each year for the 700-bed hospital. Installing a computerized physician order entry system helped reduce adverse drug events by almost 80 percent, from 140 to 30 adverse drug events per 1,000 inpatient days. The order system reduced costs by $5–$10 million per year through reduction of adverse drug events and through increased efficiency in the use of drugs and tests (Bates and others, 1997).

Purchasers of health care are following the research on the cost of medical accidents. Employers, learning that most events are preventable, and realizing that they are paying for them, have taken action. (Beginning initiatives are described later in this chapter, under the head "The Business Community," in the section titled "Background of the Patient Safety Movement.")

Debates about Numbers

Like all other research, patient safety research involves some methodological issues. There are important factors that may cause both under- and overestimation of the number of medical accidents in the U.S. health care system. Some methodological concerns focus on the reliability of clinicians' judgments about the events themselves (Brennan, 2000) and their failure to account for the morbidity of hospitalized patients before calculating adverse event rates (Leape, 2000). When studies have not been able to address these issues, they may have overestimated the extent of medical accidents.

Most patient safety research relies on review of medical records. This approach represents a concern in research because medical records are often incomplete, and events are likely not to be recorded. Experts agree that the number of events undocumented in medical records is substantial (Weingart, Wilson, Gibberd, and Harrison, 2000). This concern is validated by observational studies that demonstrate higher adverse event rates. For example, observational studies document that 17.7 percent of patients on an intensive care unit experience a medical event (Flynn, Pearson, and Barker, 1997; Andrews and others, 1997; Donchin and others, 1995). By comparison, studies using medical records found injury in only 3.7 percent of patients in New York in 1991 (Brennan and others, 1991), 2.9 percent of patients in Colorado and Utah in 1999 (Thomas and others, 2000), 13 percent of patients in Australia in 1995 (Runciman and others, 2000).

More studies of medical accident are needed. These should include research on events in different types of health care settings, with different medical conditions, and in different population groups. The purpose of such research should not be to create an accounting of events but rather to create an entry to identifying **system vulnerabilities**. According to Leape (2001), "Studies are windows that allow us to see faults in the complex system of care. There is no precise metric." Academics may debate the precise number of deaths and injuries, but even the low end of the reported figures represents an unacceptable number of deaths from preventable medical adverse events. In fact, many experts believe that the research findings represent the tip of the iceberg (Ernst and Grizzle, 2001).

Irrespective of the exact numbers, whether 50,000 or 100,000 deaths per year, preventable medical injury is a serious problem. For health care leaders, the message is clear: allowing system vulnerabilities to cause harm to patients is unacceptable. Academicians may continue to debate methodology, but the leader's job is to focus on the design and implementation of safe care delivery systems.

In this section, we have summarized the medical literature on safety for instructive reasons. You are cautioned that the literature can be misleading, and we do not want this overview to create a deceptive sense that the patient safety movement is orderly, evolving in a logical sequence. Rather, we have provided an overview best characterized as a string of explorations and disagreements about substance and form, not the recounting of a single coherent story. The epidemiological studies have been driven by diverse experiences with health care accidents and by similarly diverse attempts to measure the nature and scale of the "error" problem in health care, without an understanding of the basic principles of safety science. The underlying, and largely unstated, assumption has been that these two topics—accident and "error"—are related, and that the problems health care is having with accidents arise from the presence of error. As we shall see in Chapter Three, however, this association is incorrect.

For leaders, the issue is this: responsible management is not about suppression of risk. Leaders do well to heed Leape's words (2001): "Do what you want with the studies. The issue is not error; the issue is injury." Harm-free care is our goal. Our response is a matter of attitude, belief, and will. The question is, will we surrender to the hazards that exist, taking an attitude of inevitability, or will we take action to understand and eliminate harm through building systems that do no harm? Patient safety problems will not be solved through the study of points in time before and after an intervention, because there is too much bias. Safety is a dynamic, emerging, and adaptive process. What will move patient safety forward is continual dialogue and sharing about the technical work (Cook, 2001).

Background of the Patient Safety Movement

The history of organized patient safety activities is conflicted, driven in the context of widely published deaths and injuries, and influenced by managed care and the threat of government intervention, associated with the ill-fated initiative of the Clinton administration.

The first seeds of the patient safety movement were planted more than twenty years ago in the work of individual practitioners who applied specific approaches to improving care in their respective domains. In the 1970s, anesthesiologists amid media and malpractice pressures, desired to minimize adverse outcomes. They launched an effort to improve their practice through systematic research initiatives and advanced technology (Pierce, 1996). Reporting efforts and discussions of problems with medications began to appear in the pharmacy world at the same time (Cohen, 1975).

Patient safety efforts broadened in the mid-1990s when a small group of researchers, educators, and clinicians joined forces to respond to a series of highly publicized accidents. A seven-year-old Florida boy died before minor surgery when the wrong anesthetic was given. A Massachusetts health care columnist died from a chemotherapy overdose. A Florida man had the wrong leg amputated. An infant from Texas died after a drug overdose. Media coverage of these events coming one right after another challenged the idyllic views held by the public and shed light on the dark side of U.S. health care, increasing awareness: accidents do happen (Belkin, 1997).

The health care community was jolted. The hospitals where these events occurred enjoyed solid reputations and received commendations from the Joint Commission on Accreditation of Health Care Organizations during their triennial surveys. Published research from the Harvard Medical Malpractice Study (Brennan and others, 1991) lent credibility to the severity of the problem (despite strident academic debates about the study's methodology), and the patient safety movement was born. At this early stage, a compelling statistical analogy, now well known in health care circles, was repeated to convey the severity of the problem: the 180,000 deaths that occur each year partly as a result of iatrogenic injury are the equivalent of three jumbo-jet crashes every two days; an estimated two-thirds of these deaths are preventable, a calculation that equates to one jumbo-jet crash per day (Leape and others, 1994). This analogy created a horrific image for the audiences who heard it. Exposure of the scope of medical accidents was a sentinel event for the health care industry, and the term "silent epidemic" was coined.

National Patient Safety Foundation

The movement spread incrementally for the first few years, then escaped the confines of the academic community and gathered increasing numbers of concerned, committed clinicians through the seminal conference titled "Examining Errors in Health Care: Developing a Prevention, Education, and Research Agenda," which took place at the Annenberg Center for Health Sciences at Rancho Mirage, California, in October 1996. After this meeting, an unprecedented partnership was formed, one that transformed patient safety from an issue into an organized effort. Through the generosity of the American Medical Association, CNA Health-Pro, the 3M Corporation, and the Schering-Plough Corporation, key stakeholders in the health care industry were able to work together toward safety through the formation of the National Patient Safety Foundation (NPSF). NPSF, an independent, nonprofit research and education organization, thus became the first national, multidisciplinary organization formally dedicated to the improvement of patient safety in the delivery of health care. Working collaboratively with a broad base of constituents to accomplish its mission, NPSF seeks to guide the transition from a culture of blame to a health care culture of safety by raising awareness, building a knowledge base, creating forums for sharing knowledge, and facilitating the implementation of practices that improve patient safety.

National Center for Patient Safety

Also at this early stage, health care organizations administered by the U.S. Department of Veterans Affairs (the Veterans Administration, or VA) became the first to demonstrate a consistent commitment to reducing and preventing adverse medical events. Under the umbrella of the National Center for Patient Safety (NCPS), all 172 VA hospitals participate in a unified and cohesive patient safety program supported by dedicated patient safety managers. Research on human factors and high-reliability organizations, with a focus on prevention rather than punishment, is applied to identifying and eliminating system vulnerabilities in health care.

The Harvard Executive Sessions on Medical Error and Patient Safety

The number of **early adopters** (Rogers, 1995) of patient safety tenets expanded when a select group of nationally recognized leaders of health care organizations participated in the invitation-only Executive Session on Medical Error and Patient

Safety sponsored by the John F. Kennedy School of Government at Harvard University. The executive session is a leadership model developed by the Kennedy School to instigate "sea change" for seemingly intractable social problems. In the late 1990s, patient safety was chosen as a target. The participants, CEOs of leading health care organizations, were hand-picked for their potential to influence the health care industry. The goal of the executive session was to change conventional wisdom among the participants about the nature of medical accident and stimulate them to action within their organizations. Participants went on to create learning labs in their own organizations, producing some of the **best practices** for improving patient safety that exist today.

The Business Community

The Business Roundtable, a coalition of prominent business leaders who purchase health insurance for 25 million Americans, mobilized in 2000 to confront the problem of medical accident. The coalition named itself the Leapfrog Group and established a voluntary program to reward the health care industry for breakthrough improvements ("big leaps") in patient safety. The Leapfrog Group members steer their employees toward facilities that have implemented the group's recommendations. The Leapfrog Group also provides consumers with information to help them make more informed choices about hospitals. The group has endorsed three practices to improve patient safety:

1. Implementation of computerized order entry systems in hospitals
2. Preferential referrals to identified hospitals for certain procedures in which there is evidence that outcomes are positively affected by volume of procedures performed
3. Staffing of intensive care units with physicians certified in critical care medicine (intensivists)

The Leapfrog Group, in collaboration with the Foundation for Accountability (FACCT), a not-for-profit organization dedicated to helping Americans make better health care decisions, offers information for consumers on its Web site.

The work of the Leapfrog Group has caused other purchasers to insist that providers implement these three safety "leaps" as a condition of contracting. As more purchasers begin to question their costs related to medical events (health benefits, time lost from work, employee death and disability), additional actions will be implemented. Patient safety language will be required in contracts for health plans. Enrollment will be frozen in health plans that fail to comply. Pay for performance is on the horizon. Payment systems will be revised from a simple per-transaction model to one that rewards improved outcomes and withholds payment when a patient is the victim of a preventable medical accident, complication, or infection (Midwest Business Group on Health, 2002).

The Midwest Business Group on Health offers purchasers the following list of suggestions for future contract language:

- Establish patient safety as a priority in the organization's mission statement.
- Create an accountability system (such as reports to the board) for patient safety.
- Designate a **patient safety officer** and create an internal reporting system.
- Provide practitioners with feedback as a reward for reporting hazardous conditions.
- Maintain the **confidentiality** of all individuals (both staff and patients) involved in events.
- Declare that involvement in events and reporting will not result in disciplinary action.
- Promote proactive quality improvement initiatives designed to enhance systems for addressing accidents, near misses, and hazardous conditions.
- Establish safe workloads and ensure proper breaks.
- Using national data as benchmarks, require hospitals to develop and share a plan for incorporating appropriate technology for efficiency and safety.
- Use periodic safety self-assessment guides to help with implementation of needed enhancements.
- Develop or participate in national or regional initiatives related to medical accident reduction, including reporting and agreed-upon approaches for collecting, sharing, and following up on data.

The Institute of Medicine

The Institute of Medicine's report *To Err Is Human: Building a Safer Health System* (Kohn, Corrigan, and Donaldson, 1999) appeared later in the patient safety movement. Its effect was to break open the secrecy that had surrounded medical accident by recounting research from two separate studies, one reporting 44,000 deaths per year from preventable medical accidents and the other reporting 98,000 such deaths per year. Even at the low end, these figures placed preventable medical accident as the eighth leading cause of death in the United States, ahead of car accidents (43,000 deaths per year), breast cancer (42,300), and AIDS (16,516).

Its substance was based on a few studies that have been widely debated. The report captured the attention of both the lay public and professionals worldwide and dramatically changed the landscape of patient safety. Almost overnight, patient safety was established as a top priority on this country's national agenda.

The report introduced three powerful new concepts that have the potential to transform health care (Leape, 2001):

1. Harm to patients occurs largely because of flaws in the system and not because of individual performance.
2. Harm will be reduced only as safer systems of care are designed.
3. To design safer systems of care, the culture of health care must change.

The Institute of Medicine published a second report, *Crossing the Quality Chasm: A New Health System for the 21st Century* (Institute of Medicine, 2001), that mandates fundamental change in the organization and delivery of health care in America. It criticizes the health care system's failure to translate knowledge into practice, to apply new technology in a safe and effective manner, to make the best use of its resources, and to restructure clinical services to meet the needs of patients.

Crossing the Quality Chasm provides a beginning road map to a safer health care system. Noting that outmoded systems of work must be redesigned to protect both the patient and the caregiver, the report points out such realities of clinical work as "information overload." Using current scientific evidence, the report describes and quantifies the severity of the problem: practitioners are inundated with information from knowledge bases that have become vast and that continue to expand with no end in sight, as the number of drugs, medical devices, diagnostic techniques, and other technological supports continues to grow. The report also notes that the need for leadership in health care has never been greater, and it calls for leaders to commit themselves to a shared agenda of improvement. *Crossing the Quality Chasm* asserts that a quality health care system must meet six aims: it is safe, effective, patient-centered, timely, efficient, and equitable. The report places responsibility for creating a culture of safety, one that can protect patients from harm, squarely on the shoulders of health care's administrative and clinical leaders. Almost immediately after this report appeared, the nature of patient safety activity changed. Having lived with the burden of medical accident while bound by the fear and secrecy of the health care culture, leaders were now given permission to acknowledge the problem and ask for help.

U.S. Government Initiatives

The investment in the notion of "error," reflected in the medical literature, set up the framework for government action. When *To Err Is Human* was released, there were four major federal initiatives to reduce medical harm. These intensified immediately after the report's publication. The federal government's largest single investment to address medical injury is the more than $50 million appropriated for research and administered through the Agency for Healthcare Research and Quality (AHRQ). In the year after the report, this appropriation funded ninety-four new research grants, contracts, and projects. The activities that were funded are now being conducted in state agencies, major universities, hospitals, outpatient clinics, nursing homes, physicians' offices, professional societies, and other organizations across the country. As this book was going to press, the agency had funded several special categories of patient safety–related research, including research on the topics listed here:

- The use of information technology in accident prevention
- The impact of working conditions on innovative approaches to improving patient safety
- Effective ways to disseminate research findings

A 1998 presidential directive established the Quality Interagency Coordination (QuIC) Task Force to ensure that all federal agencies involved in purchasing, providing, studying, or regulating health care services in the United States worked in a coordinated manner. The common goal is to improve the quality of care and especially to improve patient safety. In 2000, a patient safety task force was established in the U.S. Department of Health and Human Services to coordinate a joint effort among several departmental agencies aimed at improving the existing systems for collecting data on patient safety. With the goal of identifying the data that health care providers, states, and others must collect in order to improve patient safety, the federal agencies leading this effort are the AHRQ, the Centers for Disease Control and Prevention (CDC), the Food and Drug Administration (FDA), and the Centers for Medicare and Medicaid Services (CMS).

To Err Is Human spawned legislation at the state level that requires the development of voluntary and mandatory reporting systems, with legal protections (Prager, 2000). To date, twenty states have legislated the implementation of mandatory reporting systems; the National Academy of State Health Policy writes informative reports on patient safety initiatives that are under way at the state level.

The National Quality Forum

In 1998, the President's Advisory Commission on Consumer Protection and Quality in the Health Care Industry proposed the creation of the National Quality Forum (NQF) as part of an integrated national agenda for quality improvement, and NQF was incorporated as a not-for-profit membership organization in 1999. Members include leaders from consumer organizations, purchaser organizations, provider organizations, health plans, and health service research organizations. Their mission is to implement a national strategy for measuring and reporting on health care quality.

Broken System, System Solution

All the efforts just described provide a strong foundation for the patient safety movement and have pushed it forward. And although the report *To Err Is Human* created an intense and lengthy surge of patient safety activity, bringing patient safety to the forefront of the nation's consciousness, health care's culture of blame and denial remains largely unchanged.

Harmful outcomes occur in the finest hospitals, despite the best intentions of competent, hardworking, caring professionals. Why?

One answer lies in the myriad work processes that make up today's complex health care system. The health care culture and its inadequate infrastructure can no longer accommodate the massive medical and technological advances that are continuously introduced into today's health care delivery system. As Charles Denham put it at the 2003 NPSF congress, health care today is operating with a Concorde engine in a Wright Brothers chassis. The following case illustrates the risk of introducing new technology into a delivery system not up to the task:

A twenty-year-old woman experienced kidney failure after the birth of her baby. She was placed on continuous venovenous hemodialysis, at the time a new and expensive type of dialysis used for critically ill patients from which complications can develop.

The patient died twelve hours after her admission to the hospital. The attending physician (a pulmonologist) and a nurse were blamed for failing to monitor the new equipment adequately. Root cause analysis revealed that the technology was extremely difficult to monitor. Moreover, no oversight for implementing the new procedure had been assigned, nor was it clear whether accountability for this new type of dialysis belonged to pulmonologists or nephrologists.

As this case demonstrates, danger is introduced into the health care delivery system when organizational structures and procedures fail to accommodate new technology. In this case, the medical specialty responsible for the new technology was unclear. Departments, specialties, and clinical services have evolved into "silos" around specific organ systems (such as the renal, respiratory, and cardiac systems) that function autonomously. The result is that the whole picture—that is, the whole patient—is lost. Moreover, work processes belonging to an earlier time, when care was simpler and more predictable, have become a danger to the patients for whom they were created. Organizations have become crippled by the unremitting innovation that characterizes modern medicine. The conflict between medicine's scientific achievement and health care's limited organizational capacity has produced a deadly paradox: success, in the form of treatments and cures unthinkable mere decades ago, has introduced unforeseen types of failure because the system of care has not been redesigned to accommodate innovation.

The expense of new technologies creates huge economic pressure to increase production and thereby offset their costs. In an industry already stressed by inadequate financial resources, production pressures ("seeing more patients") are accompanied by reengineering ("cutting staff") in an attempt to accommodate the cost of innovations. Health care becomes more vulnerable as it becomes more successful (Cook, 2002).

Health care has evolved into a high-risk industry as advanced technology has been overlaid on unaltered, archaic work processes. The health care culture, inflexible and secretive, was and is the major obstacle to the crucial redesign of organizational structures and work processes.

Accident Rates in Health Care

Accident rates in the health care industry far exceed those in other high risk industries. Few health care organizations are using the safety practices common to other high-risk industries, such as aviation and nuclear power. These practices include incorporating safety goals into mission statements, reviewing safety performance indicators at board meetings, and holding CEOs accountable for creating a culture of safety. Not surprisingly, other industries are far ahead of health care in reducing accident rates. Today's health care executives do pay close attention to two proxies of vulnerability in their care delivery systems: patient complaints and litigation. These two indicators, monitored regularly and closely, cause great concern. The executive worries about what the board will think of the high cost of malpractice suits and about how the organization's image will be tarnished in the community if the media expose an injury or death due to a preventable accident. Physicians worry about malpractice suits and about their own reputations. They face increasing pressure from patients who know about and fear medical mishaps. Nurses and pharmacists worry about losing their licenses. Despite these anxieties, leaders tend to accept these organizational vulnerabilities as inevitable, without reflecting on their underlying causes.

Leadership in Health Care

Managing a complex, high-risk business is the work of the leader in health care today. But health care leaders have not received training in safety science during their schooling or their careers, and so they have little foundation on which to build the vision of a safe culture in health care. Strategies exist to mitigate risk beyond using indicators of patient satisfaction and tracking instances of litigation. Many of these strategies have proved successful in industries outside health care. After setting out, in Chapter Three, an overview of basic concepts in patient safety science, we will discuss, in subsequent chapters, the various strategies that can help health care organizations harness hazard as a teaching tool to reach the ultimate goal of eliminating harm to patients.

Summary Points

Three major research topics have emerged from the work on patient safety to date: topics involving the frequency of medical accidents (98,000 inpatient deaths every year, and more than 300,000 patient injuries), the types of medical accidents (involving medication, diagnoses, wrong-site surgery, infections, and other largely predictable and therefore preventable events), and the cost of medical accidents (estimated at $17–$29 billion per year for such direct costs as litigation and health care, and $38–$50 billion per year for expenses that include lost income and disability).

1. Medical accident is a serious problem—the reported figures represent an unacceptable number of deaths and injuries from preventable events—and many experts believe that these findings represent only the tip of the iceberg. Even at the low end, the reported figures place preventable medical accident as the eighth leading cause of death in the United States, ahead of car accidents, breast cancer, and AIDS. Accidents in health care far exceed those in other high-risk industries.
2. Health care does not make safety its top priority, but the message to leaders is clear: it is unacceptable to let system vulnerabilities cause harm to patients. The health care leader's job is to focus on the design and implementation of safe care delivery systems.
3. Most accidents do not happen because of a single mistake or one faulty work process. Instead, they are due to multiple small causes, each insufficient to create an accident, but potentially deadly when combined with others. Progress in patient safety requires a focus on the system and on understanding the nature of technical work, not on individuals. Continual dialogue and sharing about technical work is what moves the aims of patient safety forward. Weaknesses must be made visible and transparent in order for a safer health care system to be created.

4. The Institute of Medicine report *To Err Is Human* introduced new concepts that have the potential to transform health care:

- Accidents occur because of flaws in the system and not because of individual performance.
- Harm will be reduced only as safer systems of care are designed.
- For safer systems of care to be designed, the culture of health care must change.

CHAPTER THREE

UNDERSTANDING THE BASICS OF PATIENT SAFETY

This chapter introduces the fundamental concepts of patient safety. Research underlying the basic concepts of patient safety comes from outside health care, primarily from engineering, aviation, psychology, and sociology. These areas of inquiry replace the impoverished conceptualization of error reduction with the more robust concept of complex adaptive systems. The framing principles are:

Medical accidents are symptoms of a disease of the health care system.

Medical accident must be studied, without judgments, as if it were a physiological state.

Identified system vulnerabilities are useful as initial data sources to prevent failure from reaching a patient.

Health care's fear-based culture has thwarted exploration of weaknesses in the system's work processes, causing the industry to lose rich information about how individuals, technical work, and organizational processes interact. When accidents and near misses are thought of as the symptoms of an underlying problem, they become sources of information and valuable tools to understand how a system functions. Accidents and near misses are useful tools that help define the margins of risk and safety and help us to learn about how harm can be prevented (Amalberti, 2001).

The Systems Approach

The Institute of Medicine publications *To Err Is Human* (Kohn, Corrigan, and Donaldson, 1999) and *Crossing the Quality Chasm* (Institute of Medicine, 2001) endorse a systems framework for patient safety in health care organizations. If a system is defined as "an interdependent group of items, people, or processes with a common purpose" (Kohn, Corrigan, and Donaldson, 1999, p. 211) then "systems thinking" emphasizes the interdependence of people, technology, and organizations as opposed to considering these in isolation. Systems thinking requires consideration of connections both within and outside the organization. These entities must be considered as a whole, even though they are separated by distance and time, management infrastructure, and culture. For example, people in an organization who want to disclose near misses to patients and families may feel unable to do so because of the threat of litigation. Litigation brings in an external entity, the culture of the legal system with values and goals that are different from, if not opposed to, those in health care.

Within a systems framework, harm to patients is viewed as a consequence of flaws, usually hidden in the system, that need to be identified and corrected (Reason, 2000). The **systems approach** makes the fundamental assumption that harm in health care, with rare exceptions, is not caused by incompetent or uncaring physicians, nurses, or pharmacists. It accepts the proposition that accidents and near misses are symptoms of an underlying problem, just as fever is the symptom of a disease or disequilibrium. The symptom, the accident or near miss, is used to understand the underlying disease process, composed of multicausal variables that interact to create the conditions in which harm can reach a patient.

The systems framework does identify individual human action or inaction as part of a complex system but places greater emphasis on systemic vulnerabilities. These include the design, construction, and maintenance of work processes; allocation of resources; technology; expectations; training; and development of operational procedures (Leape, 1994).

When the systems approach is applied to medical accident, the multiple interactions among the various components that make up the care delivery system are evaluated as being more or less susceptible or resistant to failure. To prevent vulnerability (hidden flaws) from causing harm to a patient, the same interactions are designed so that they facilitate detection and correction of vulnerability (Reason, 2000; Leape and others, 1995). Efforts to reduce harm must target the work processes within the system of care delivery to be effective. For example, designing checks and balances ("fail-safes") can catch and correct or mitigate flaws in the system to intercept harm from reaching a patient. Successes are also examined for lessons of resilience that prevent injury.

The traditional knowledge bases that undergird the work of health care cannot provide the guidance needed to understand failure in the complexity of the health care system. To build applications that will effectively mitigate harm to patients, a distinct science of patient safety that builds on bodies of knowledge outside health care, primarily human factors and organizational analysis, is needed.

Human Factors

The term *human factors* originated in World War II as military aviation grappled with "people problems," such as fatigue and responses to stress (Reason, 2001). In the ensuing decades, human factors concepts spread beyond aviation and were applied to a broad range of hazardous technologies. Concerns expanded to include such topics as psychomotor performance, cognitive factors, social factors, and organizational factors. Today the field of human factors is concerned with understanding and enhancing human performance in the workplace, especially in complex systems.

Among the significant contributions from human factors research to the field of patient safety is the notion that fallibility is part of the human condition. Therefore creating safety requires changing the conditions in which human beings work. Although individual failures and system vulnerabilities are inevitable, adverse events and harm resulting from them need not be.

Organizational Analysis

System-oriented studies of the normal **cognition** and behavior of individuals and the work environment are replacing studies that count error as the target for patient safety research. Researcher Jens Rasmussen, noting problems with the concept of human error (for example, the notion is hard to define and is a function of the biases of the observer), believes that error is only "an indication of experts exploring the boundaries of acceptable performance in an unkind environment" (Rasmussen, 1998, p. 4), and believes (p. 3) that safety "depends on the control of work processes to avoid accidental side effects causing harm to people, environment, or investment."

Expert performance depends on the individual practitioner's effective adaptation to the characteristics of the work tasks at hand and to the overall surrounding work environment. Characteristics of the work environment (such as financial pressure, often characterized as "doing more with less"), coupled with antiquated management and regulatory structures that cannot support ever-advancing technology at the practice level, are likely to push practitioners to exceed the boundaries of safe practice (Rasmussen, 1998; Amalberti, 2001). Rasmussen states that human error neither can nor should be removed from the design of safe work systems; humans are basically boundary-seeking beings, and errors often reflect efforts to adapt effectively to work requirements (Rasmussen, 1998). These boundaries or margins of safety, defined by understanding error, are called **boundaries of excediency** (Amalberti, 2001), a term that refers to times when practice moves into zones of intolerable risk. Errors, when made transparent, become early warning signals to reassess, slow down, pull back, and ask for help in the clinical environment to reestablish safety. To design a safe work system is to design an **error-tolerant system**, that is, a system in which errors do not cause irreversible effects because system interfaces support the immediate detection of errors and allow practitioners to take corrective action to recover from errors.

The study of patient safety is the study of complexity. The study of complexity invites us to understand key concepts that can be applied to patient safety. Basic concepts from the field of patient safety are: sharp and blunt end; active and latent failure; the Swiss Cheese Model of Accident Causation; **slips**, **lapses**, and mistakes; and hindsight bias and the **fundamental attribution error**. Key concepts from organizational analysis, such as normalization of deviance, **diffusion of responsibility**, **tightly coupled work processes**, and sensemaking, introduce practical lessons from high-reliability organizations. Application of specific lessons to health care are explored in Chapter Five.

Basic Concepts

The Sharp End

In the language of patient safety, health care workers who provide direct patient care work at what is known as the "sharp end" (Reason, 1990). This term refers to those points of vulnerability in the care delivery system where expertise is applied, where failure is visible, and accidents are experienced. Work at the sharp end is characterized by management of competing demands for production and for failure-free performance. Professionals at the sharp end are always weighing the probability of various outcomes of their actions: successful operations are the rule and failure is rare.

At the sharp end, decisions, actions, and inaction contributing to accidents are called "active failures," a term that connotes the immediacy of adverse effects (Reason, 1997). Active failures are direct operational errors (Reason, 1997; Weick, 2000). Weick has identified four processes, familiar ways of doing things, that can emerge under stress and become sources of vulnerability for sharp-end providers in complex systems: interruption of important routines, regression during a crisis, fragmentation, and miscommunication. These are summarized in Table 3.1, adding examples of common sources of stress and external pressure. The sources of vulnerability are not meant to match up with specific sources of stress or external pressure, as these are dynamic and interacting forces, not categories. Vulnerabilities emerge from sources of stress that have been shaped in turn by external pressures.

The Blunt End

In contrast to the delivery level (the sharp end), the work of management is referred to as the "blunt end." In addition to management, the blunt end includes governance, regulators, suppliers, payers, and purchasers. The world of technical sharp-end work is fashioned by the blunt end, and it is the blunt end that produces the latent failures that are hidden in work processes. Individuals at the blunt end generate predicaments and force trade-offs among competing goals for those at the sharp end (Cook and Woods, 1994). Blunt-end decisions and actions (policies, procedures, resource allocation) and expectations for productivity contribute to adverse events by producing hidden but powerful **latent conditions** for failure. That is, they create an environment that increases the probability of a sharp-end failure to be transformed to harm at some point in time. Latent conditions, rooted in the work processes of the organization, can provoke operational vulnerability in certain circumstances or may present hazards on their own. Examples of latent conditions

TABLE 3.1. SOURCES OF VULNERABILITY UNDER STRESS

Vulnerability	Sources of Stress	External Pressures
Interruption of important routines	High workloads	Insufficient resources
Regression to more habituated ways of responding to crisis	Fatigue	Unworkable regulations
Breakdown of coordinated action (fragmentation)	Repetitive crises	Lack of planned processes
Miscommunication	Time pressures, over-tasking, lack of teamwork and sensemaking, understaffing	Faulty education and training

Source: Adapted from K. Weick, "The Vulnerable System: An Analysis of the Tenerife Air Disaster," *Journal of Management,* 1990, *16*(3), 571–596.

for failure include inadequate training, unworkable procedures, denigration of preventative maintenance and quality standards, poor or inadequate technology, information overload, unrealistic time pressures, understaffing, and fatigue (Reason, 1997). Latent conditions for failure frequently arise from high-level decisions and actions and they are reflective of organizational culture. Conditions for latent failure in clinical environments typically become visible only after they provoke unsafe acts or adverse outcomes. Rasmussen (1993, 1994) notes that accidents are most likely to be caused by systematic migration toward conditions favoring accidents when organizations operate in an aggressive, competitive environment, or when organizations are working under pressures of time and funding.

In the health care culture, the sharp and blunt ends tend to function as separate entities, despite the fact that clinical, operational, and financial processes are interdependent. Figure 3.1 illustrates this interdependence.

Cook and Woods (1994) lay out a model that depicts how success (defined here as harm-free care) for individual practitioners and their teams requires three overlapping cognitive functions to work in sync: *knowledge factors,* which can be drawn on to solve problems in context; *attention factors,* which govern the control of attention and the mental workload as situations change and evolve over time; and *strategic factors,* or goals, which are in conflict and require trade-offs to be made, especially in conditions of uncertainty, risk, and limited resources (Cook and Woods, 1994). These cognitive factors are influenced in turn by the demands presented by the problem at hand, which may be simple or challenging, and by the available resources, such as sufficient personnel and adequate training, time, and supplies. Each of these factors interact to determine whether practitioners and teams are vigilant and flexible in their thinking so that relevant knowledge is activated when needed.

There are always two different stories or realities about accidents in health care (Woods, Johannesen, Cook, and Sarter, 1994). The first story, attention-grabbing and sensationalistic, is the one told in the media about accidental deaths and wrong-site surgeries. Because it focuses solely on the sharp end, this story is superficial and incomplete. The second story is quieter and less dramatic, but it gives a truer picture of the reality of the situation. This story explains how changes in technology are imposed on existing organizational procedures and how these changes combine with economic pressures to create management policies that produce new forms of failure at the sharp end.

Active and Latent Failure

Work processes in the health care environment are so complicated that series of minor failures that by themselves would do no harm inevitably combine with latent or hidden flaws. Unexpected interactions produce chains of events that lead

FIGURE 3.1. SHARP END/BLUNT END

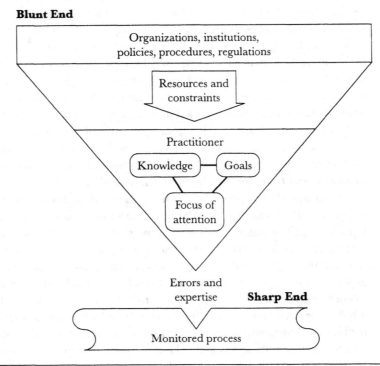

Source: Adapted from R. I. Cook, D. D. Woods, and C. A. Miller, *Tale of Two Stories: Contrasting Views of Patient Safety* (Chicago: National Patient Safety Foundation, 1998), p. 14.

to disastrous outcomes. Figure 3.2 illustrates how this can happen by laying out the failure sequence in complex organizations.

The triangle in the figure shows that there is no single cause that produces an accident. Rather, it takes three layers of "causes" to produce an accidental injury or death. The first layer is visible: failure at the delivery level. This is where active failures occur. Here, failures are obvious in the actions of an individual, and they have a direct impact on safety in the system and on the safety of the patient. This is where most investigations of health care begin and end; hidden are the conditions that produced this failure. As Reason (1997, p. 10) explains, "Latent conditions are to technological organizations what resident pathogens are to the human body. Like pathogens, latent conditions—such as poor design, gaps in supervision, undetected manufacturing defects or maintenance failures, unworkable procedures, clumsy automation, shortfalls in training, less than ade-

FIGURE 3.2. HARM TRAJECTORY IN HIGH-RISK SYSTEMS

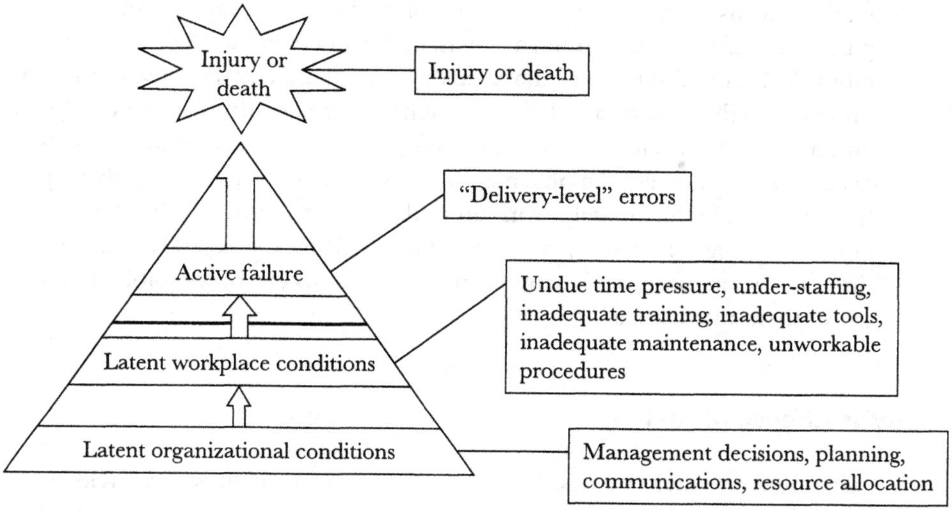

Source: Adapted from J. Reason, *Managing the Risks of Organizational Accidents* (Brookfield, N.Y.: Ashgate Publishing Company, 1997), p. 12.

quate tools and equipment—may be present for many years before they combine with local circumstances and active failures to penetrate the system's many layers of defenses."

Latent conditions nurture an environment that becomes vulnerable to failure and harm. Latent conditions are linked to conditions in the work environment, not to the active failures of individual actors. In contrast to the active failure, latent failure is hidden, an invisible hole in the work process, and stems from management decisions. Policies that determine the working conditions and affect communication, resource allocation, and planning are examples of blunt-end work that can contribute to failures at the sharp end. Human factors experts identify four different management dimensions that apply directly to improving patient safety: the design of equipment or tools, the design of tasks, the environmental conditions of work, and the selection and training of staff (Wickens, Gordon, and Liu, 1998).

Latent conditions can lie dormant for a long while before hazardous conditions emerge. One example of a latent condition at play in today's health care environment is deferred preventive maintenance on equipment to reduce costs. As equipment continues to be used, risk increases for glitches and problems.

The "work-around" is an example of a sharp end–blunt end interaction that facilitates failure. Health care professionals are masters at work-arounds, those work patterns an individual or a group of individuals create in order to accomplish a crucial work goal within a system of dysfunctional work processes that prohibits the accomplishment of that goal or makes it difficult. Because so many work processes in the health care delivery system are broken, practitioners at the sharp end must find ways to work around them and figure out ways to complete their tasks. Doctors, nurses, and pharmacists view work-arounds as the only way to get the job done. Unfortunately, work-arounds create an environment that is ripe for failure, although the participants do not realize it. As Cook (2001) has said, "Fish don't see water, because they live in it. All accidents are preventable if you know about them in advance."

The Swiss Cheese Model

James Reason's Swiss Cheese Model is well known in patient safety circles as a useful tool for describing how a combination of multiple small failures, each individually insufficient to cause an accident, combine to create failure in a complex system (Reason, 1990). Figure 3.3 depicts the trajectory on which active failures combine to form an accident by slipping through holes (latent failures). These holes occur at different levels of the care delivery system—institutional, organizational, professional, team, individual, and technical. More often than not, the vulnerabilities are deflected from the path toward an accident, either because the failure results in no harm or because normal defenses—organizational, human, or technological—successfully defend against the failure reaching a patient. For example, a physician may miscalculate a drug dosage, but a pharmacist may catch the mistake and call the physician to correct it. It is when patterns shift, because of any of a number of factors (for example, the pharmacist is distracted by an influx of orders and forgets to call the physician, or staffing is insufficient for pharmacy review of all orders), that the holes—the latent failures—can line up, and the active failure can slip through the defenses, allowing an accident to occur.

An important component of the Swiss Cheese Model depicted in Figure 3.3 is the "individual plane." This plane represents the protective defenses put up by workers at the sharp end to deflect failure and vulnerability from becoming transformed into harm. Individual workers create safety at the sharp end all the time as they encounter hazards and opportunities for failure and continually stop them before they reach patients. It is when workplace stresses erode the coping resources

FIGURE 3.3. THE SWISS CHEESE MODEL

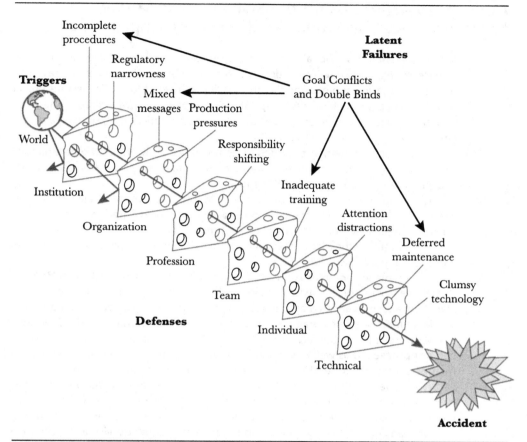

Source: Modified from J. Reason, *Human Error* (Cambridge, England: Cambridge University Press, 1990).

of those at the sharp end, through overwork, inadequate resources, and fatigue, that the defensive mechanisms for deflecting failure are weakened by what can be understood as rescue fatigue. Individuals and teams defend against working in unmitigated risk by losing situational awareness and normalizing deviance. In other words, they become resigned to their environment and increase the probability of risk. Progress on patient safety depends on understanding front-line technical work and the ways in which practitioners overcome hazards (Cook, 2001). Protecting and understanding sources of success and resilience at the sharp end is a critical factor in creating safety.

Concept to Action: Using the Swiss Cheese Model to Deconstruct Risk-Prone Conditions and Improve Safety

As a participant in his hospital's patient safety initiative, pediatric emergency physician Tom Hellmich attended several educational sessions where he learned about basic concepts in safety, such as hindsight bias and the Swiss Cheese Model. The lessons proved useful during a particularly busy week at work. In one day, two children, one in the hospital's emergency department and the other in an inpatient unit, suffered a cardiac arrest, requiring a code to be called.

"The code in the emergency department was probably one of the best-handled codes ever," Hellmich remembers. "The child's heart rate and pulse came back quickly, and she walked out of the hospital the next day."

The code in the inpatient unit was less smooth. It prompted Hellmich to think about how, in the same hospital, a code could proceed so differently. After a short break, Hellmich assembled the involved staff members.

"I could see on their faces, they were thinking, 'Now, here it comes.' And, instead, it became a great discussion."

On a table in the break room, staff members gathered around while Hellmich sketched a version of the Swiss Cheese Model on a piece of paper. He began to explain how a team is affected by the systems that surround it. The discussion grew into a series of meetings where staff members conducted a multicausal analysis of the code.

With Hellmich as the facilitator, staff members discussed reasons why the code had not proceeded as well as it could have. They identified a variety of factors: staff members' difficulty in reaching the unit in a remote location, unfamiliarity with the cart (the code team's nurse was from a different unit, and the carts were not standardized), confusion about who should participate in the code (it had occurred during a shift change), the rarity of the code's occurrence (the specific inpatient unit experienced codes infrequently and did not perform frequent drills), and equipment difficulties (there had been mechanical problems with the bedside equipment).

Staff members identified ways to improve performance during future codes. The improvement ideas included training, equipment and cart standardization, and regular **simulations** of emergency response.

"They were impressed that it wasn't a blaming session," Hellmich recalls. "Today, Swiss Cheese is our brand for patient safety in our hospital."

Whereas other businesses commonly distribute promotional "stress balls"—squeezable foam balls imprinted with the business's logo and used by employees to vent stress—Hellmich's organization elected to produce a squeezable foam wedge of Swiss cheese in place of the popular stress ball. The small yellow giveaway sits on many desks and at many nurses' stations and helps remind staff members to focus on risk identification, learning, and systems thinking. It serves as a conversation starter, allowing employees who are enthusiastic about safety to educate new employees.

"I was in the emergency room the other day, when I overheard one nurse say to another nurse, 'What's this about?'" Hellmich says. "The other nurse started to explain the little piece of Swiss cheese, saying, 'It's part of the patient safety initiative here,' and then explained its significance. It's become a rallying point for education and for identifying risk."

Concept to Action: Using Human Factors Science and the VA Triage Cards to Analyze Medical Accidents and Near Misses

The Swiss Cheese Model, based on knowledge from human factors, guided the Veterans Administration's National Center for Patient Safety in developing a tool to help organizations analyze and learn from medical accidents and near misses. The tool, a pocket-size, laminated cognitive aid designed to enrich and guide analysis of medical accidents and near misses, is called the NCPS Triage Cards for Root Cause Analysis (see Figure 3.4). The Triage Cards help teams avoid hindsight bias and focus on learning and systems improvement (National Center for Patient Safety, 2001).

To get a sense of how the Triage Cards can be used, suppose that a fifty-five-year-old man undergoes an outpatient lung biopsy and is recovering in a short-stay unit (SSU). After a delayed assessment, a nurse discovers the patient in acute discomfort: the pulse oximeter alarm has been turned off, and the patient's lung has partially collapsed. An emergency chest tube is inserted, and the patient recovers. But how is it possible to discover what happened?

To resist the natural human tendency toward hindsight bias and thoroughly explore an adverse event like this one requires disciplined commitment and a methodical analysis. Through a **process flow diagram** (also known as a "sequence of events diagram") and questions gleaned from knowledge of human factors science, it is possible to develop a list of factors, action statements, and outcome measures to reduce the probability of an accident or near miss from recurring.

Creating a Process Flow Diagram

A team might begin by creating a process flow diagram of the activities surrounding the event. The team could begin with an overview that starts from the first contact with the patient, when an X ray reveals a spot on his lung. A radiology visit is scheduled and a biopsy is performed. Then the patient is transferred to the SSU. The transfer is delayed by fifteen minutes, however, and there is minimal reporting between the patient's escort and the SSU staff. Patient assessment is delayed by another thirty minutes after the patient arrives. While the patient is waiting, he is acutely uncomfortable. He becomes annoyed with the pulse oximeter alarm and silences it.

FIGURE 3.4. NCPS TRIAGE CARDS FOR ROOT CAUSE ANALYSIS

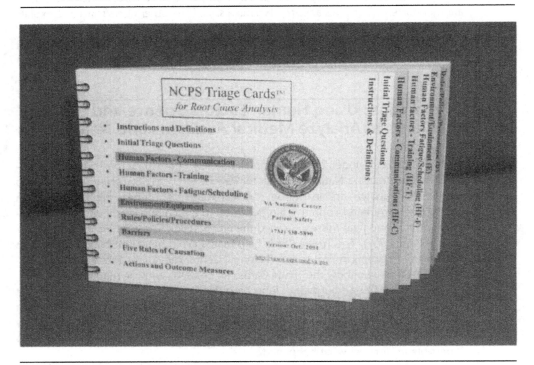

Source: National Center for Patient Safety, 2001.

Using the Questions from the Triage Cards

After the process flow diagram is completed, the team can select a step from the process flow and work through the sections of questions on the Triage Cards chart, including the areas of communications, training, fatigue/scheduling, environment/equipment, and barriers (the controls in place that should have stopped a medical accident or, in the case of a near miss, that did successfully stop the sequence of events from reaching the patient). Every question is re-asked for each step identified in the process flow diagram. For example, the team can work through each question to explore the time the patient spent undergoing the surgical procedure, the time that elapsed while he was being transferred from radiology to the escort, the time involved in the delayed transfer from the escort and the SSU, and the time involved in the delayed assessment in the SSU. Then, if the delayed assessment in the SSU is chosen as an example, the team can begin by answering the fourteen questions in the communications section of the flipchart:

1. Was the patient correctly identified? *Yes.*
2. Was information from various patient assessments shared and used by members of the treatment team on a timely basis? *Don't know.*
3. Did existing documentation (assessments, consultations, orders, program notes, medication administration record, X ray, labs) provide a clear picture of the workup, the treatment plan, and the patient's response to treatment? *Don't know.*
4. Was communication between management/supervisors and front-line staff adequate? *Doesn't immediately seem to be applicable.*
5. Was communication between front-line team members adequate? *Don't know.*
6. Were policies and procedures communicated adequately? *Don't know.*
7. Was the correct technical information adequately communicated twenty-four hours a day to the people who needed it? *Doesn't immediately seem to be applicable.*
8. Were there methods for monitoring the adequacy of staff communication? *Don't know.*
9. Was the communication of potential risk factors free from obstacles? *Don't know.*
10. Was there a manufacturer's recall/alert/bulletin on file for equipment-, medication-, or transfusion-related elements at the time of the event or close call? Were relevant staff members aware of the recall/alert/bulletin? *Nothing was on file; not applicable.*
11. If relevant, were the patient and his family/significant others actively included in the assessment and treatment planning? *No.*
12. Did management establish adequate methods of providing information to employees who needed it in such a way that it was timely and easy to access/use? *Doesn't immediately seem to be applicable.*
13. Did the overall culture of the facility encourage or welcome observations, suggestions, or "early warnings" from staff about risky situations and risk reduction? *Doesn't immediately seem to be applicable.*
14. Did adequate communication across organizational boundaries occur? *Don't know.*

Other portions of the Triage Cards can also be explored:

- *Training.* Questions might include the following: Was the training adequate? Had procedures and equipment been reviewed to ensure that there was a good match between people and the tasks they did, or between people and the equipment they used (human factors engineering)?
- *Fatigue/Scheduling.* Questions might include the following: Did scheduling allow personnel adequate sleep? Was there sufficient staff on hand for the workload at the time? (Was the workload too high or too low, or was there the wrong mix of staff? Was the level of automation appropriate?)
- *Environment/Equipment.* Questions might include the following: Were the work environment's stress levels (physical or psychological) appropriate? Was the equipment designed in such a way that mistakes in using it would be unlikely?
- *Rules, Policies, and Procedures.* Questions might include the following: Was there an overall management plan for addressing risk and assigning responsibility for risk?

Had a previous audit been done for a similar event, were the causes identified, and were effective interventions developed and implemented on a timely basis? Would this problem have gone unidentified after an audit/review? Was the care that the patient required within the scope of the facility's mission, its staff expertise, the staff's availability, technical resources, and resources for and support service?

- *Barriers.* Questions might include the following: What barriers or controls were involved in this adverse event or close call? Had these barriers been evaluated for reliability? Did the audits/reviews related to barriers include evaluation of plans, designs, installation, maintenance, and process changes?

After working through all sections, the team can pinpoint several areas for further information gathering and analysis. The process can then be repeated for each step in the process flow diagram.

Constructing a Causation Summary

Next, the team can construct a causation summary for root cause analysis. The Triage Cards can guide participants in constructing statements about root causes if the following guidelines are observed:

1. Root cause statements must clearly show the cause-and effect relationship. For example, instead of saying, "A resident was fatigued," the statement would say, "The resident was so tired that she probably misread the instructions and inserted the tube incorrectly."
2. Negative descriptions should not be used in root cause statements. A negative description is often a placeholder for a clearer, more accurate description. Words like *carelessness* and *complacency* are poor choices because they are broad, negative judgments that do little to describe the actual conditions or behaviors that led to the mishap. For example, instead of referring to a "poorly trained nurse," a helpful root cause statement might say, "The nurse probably didn't have enough training to understand the IV pump controls, and that's probably why he missed steps in the programming sequence of dose and rate."
3. Each human error must have a preceding cause. A statement like "The lighting level was low" should be further explored and explained to produce a more complete statement: "The lighting in the patient's room was too low for the tripping hazard to be seen."
4. The violation of a procedure is not itself a root cause. It must have a preceding cause. The goal is to identify the positive and negative incentives that create informal norms or accepted ways of doing things.
5. Failure to act is causal only when there is a pre-existing duty to act. For example, a doctor's failure to prescribe cardiac medication after a myocardial infarction can be causal only if he was required to prescribe the medication in the first place.

In the incident involving the pneumothorax in the SSU, the team will likely find that the "off" or "silencing" mechanism on the pulse oximeter alarm is easy to identify, and that it is a simple matter for even a bedridden patient to reach it and disable it. The sentence the team might construct for the contributing factor would show cause and effect without placing blame: "The patient's access to the pulse oximeter, and his ability to silence the alarm, increased the likelihood that his deteriorating condition would not be observed." Contributing factors can be paired with actions and outcome measures. For example, personnel in biomedical engineering can be instructed to deactivate the "off" or "silencing" mechanism on all pulse oximeter alarms in the SSU. Random, unannounced checks of all pulse oximeter alarms in the SSU can also be conducted quarterly, to ensure continued compliance.

The overall goal of the Triage Cards is to steer participants away from hindsight bias and blame and toward an iterative exploration of what has happened. The tool continually prompts users on what questions to ask and where to ask them, to fuel a productive process of inquiry. The set of cards was originally constructed for use during medical accidents and near misses, but the cards can also be used "upstream" to explore risk-prone conditions before they turn into near misses or accidents (see Chapter Nine for a case study on "thinking dirty"). The Triage Cards, available through the American Hospital Association (see Resources), are sent with kits of case studies and other support materials intended to help teach organizations how to use them.

Cognitive Concepts

New students of patient safety quickly discover that the Swiss Cheese Model can alter perceptions.

There are other basic concepts that drive home the point that the key to improving safety lies not in punishing human beings for their part in accidents but rather in changing the conditions in which they work. Accidents are more likely to occur under predictable environmental circumstances that mark the work life of the health care clinician: dealing with complex events, high levels of uncertainty, ill-defined problems, competing goals, time pressures, and fatigue (Reason, 1990).

Slips, Lapses, and Mistakes

The pursuit of human error does not aid but rather impedes our understanding of how complex systems fail and the ways in which human clinicians contribute to or detract from safety. The path to safety lies in understanding the normal cognition and behavior of interacting individuals and the environments in which they work; such understanding points to modifications that will reduce the likelihood of accidents (Cook and Woods, 1994).

Slips, lapses, and mistakes are three basic concepts that have been used to describe types of active failure in health care. Although they characterize all human activity, they can produce deadly results in the health care environment. A slip, lapse, or mistake occurs at one of three levels of cognitive control that experts use in interacting with their work environments (Rasmussen, 1998): the level of skill-based control, the level of rule-based control, and the level of knowledge-based control. The skill-based level encompasses work routines that run without conscious control. The rule-based level entails tasks that rely on a plan, a guideline, or a protocol; these organize a sequence of steps that prior experience has shown to be effective. When no such plan is available, cognitive control is at the knowledge-based level. Here, a plan must be built de novo on understanding the problem at hand, and of the work environment, that is sufficient to make predictions about outcomes.

Slips. Slips tend to occur in automatic, skill-based activities. Common examples include slips of the tongue, slips of the pen, and slips of action (Reason, 1990) as in brushing one's teeth (grabbing a lookalike tube of ointment rather than toothpaste), driving a car (taking the wrong exit off a freeway), or answering the telephone (going to answer the door when the telephone rings). Distractions create fertile environmental conditions for slips. A distraction may be an external stimulus in the environment (such as noise or interruptions) or an internal stimulus (a nagging worry; focused concentration on an upcoming task or event; a physiological state such as fatigue).

Lapses. Lapses differ from slips in that they are not visible. An example would be a memory failure. Lapses occur in such **rule-based activities** as following a treatment protocol or a regimen for entering an order or typing blood. The person who commits a lapse knows what he or she should be doing but for some reason does not follow the expected protocol. For example, if the protocol is too difficult or unwieldy, the person who is following it under time constraints may be tempted to leave out a step or two in service of production or may simply forget a step.

Mistakes. Reason (1990) defines a mistake as a deficit or failure in the judgment involved either in selecting an objective (such as picking a treatment goal) or in specifying the means to achieve it (such as formulating a treatment plan). Mistakes are most common in **knowledge-based activities** where workers have to deal with new and unfamiliar situations. Mistakes turn up in complex processes, such as diagnostic judgments, and they tend to be more subtle and complex than slips. They can pass unnoticed for a long time. When they are detected, mistakes sometimes remain a matter of debate: witness the discussion in traditional morbidity and mortality conferences. Similarly, the quality of the treatment plan is open to a diversity of opinions (for example, there may be different opinions about which drug regimen should be selected).

Mistakes take us into the realm of individual intention: has an individual worker knowingly relied on what is accepted as a best practice? As Marx writes (2001, p. 7), "Most rules, procedures, and duties will require or prohibit a specific behavior. The intentional rule violation occurs when an individual chooses to knowingly violate a rule while he is performing a task. This concept is not necessarily related to risk-taking, but merely shows that an individual knew of or intended to violate a rule, procedure, or duty in the course of performing a task." Marx provides a clinical example of a mistake made consciously but not maliciously:

A new transfusion service phlebotomist is on the early morning shift drawing samples on the hospital floor. She checks Ms. Jones's requisition and armband before she draws her samples.

Ms. Jones is really annoyed about the bright lights the phlebotomist has turned on, and the phlebotomist is trying to placate Ms. Jones by turning them off quickly. She knows that there is a strict procedure to label tubes at the bedside, but as she has already positively identified the patient, and this is the only set of tubes she has, she decides to label the tubes at the nurses' station (*intentional rule violation; mistake in selecting means to achieve objective*).

She lays the tubes down at the nurses' station and begins labeling. However, a nurse comes to the nurses' station with an unlabeled tube of blood and lays it down nearby. Not noticing this, the phlebotomist mistakenly thinks one of her tubes has rolled away. She picks up the nurse's tube and also labels it with Ms. Jones's information.

Ms. Jones is a new patient and her blood type is unknown. The mislabeled tube is used to type and cross units for her. Ms Jones has a moderately severe transfusion reaction when the first unit is being transfused [Marx, 2001, p. 9].

The phlebotomist knowingly violated procedure because she experienced an internal conflict: trying to meet the need of the patient versus following the blood handling protocol.

Compensating for Slips, Lapses, and Mistakes. Slips, lapses, and mistakes, common in any work setting, can be disastrous in health care. There are many strategies for compensating for them. Here are a few strategies derived from engineering:

- *Forcing functions.* In health care's recent past, one common slip was the deadly infusion by an overworked nurse of concentrated potassium chloride instead of its lookalike, benign saline solution. To compensate for this problem, potassium chloride has been removed from nursing units in hospitals. This is a **forcing**

function. Nurses now have to order the solution specially when needed (a condition was purposefully created that makes it impossible to mistakenly use potassium chloride instead of saline solution).

- *Constraining functions.* If bags of potassium chloride were placed in a spot not readily accessible, for the purpose of causing a worker to think before using them, then that would be a **constraining function**. In this circumstance, automatic action is interrupted by a need to pause and take deliberate action. For example, sometimes solutions are placed in a "bread box" container, requiring workers to perform an extra step to retrieve them from the shelf, thus interrupting automatic behavior by creating a pause. Another strategy would be to change the packaging of drugs to make them dissimilar.
- *Redundancy functions.* A **redundancy function** is basically a checking function that builds double checks into a work process. Requiring countersignatures on a procedure is a simple form of redundancy.

Consider the application of these terms in the following example from Marx's primer on a "just culture":

A medical technologist receives a sample for type and cross-match. As she brings up the patient record on the computer, the computer flashes a warning that the patient has autologous units on hold (*constraining function*). She goes to the refrigerator to retrieve the autologous units. Before she can get the units, someone asks her a question about an antibody identification problem (*distraction*). She takes a few minutes to help the other technologist (*interruption*). When finished, she remembers she was going to the refrigerator for two A Pos units, but gets two homologous units rather than the two autologous units. The two homologous units are crossmatched and labeled for the patient (*lapse*).

The issuing technologist looks at the pickup slip and goes to get the two units off the shelf. During the computer crossmatch, a computer warning indicates that the patient has autologous units available (*constraining function*). The issuing technologist notices that she has two homologous units. The issue is delayed until the autologous units are made available [Marx, 2001, pp. 7–8].

Marx notes that this event involves a simple memory failure: the technologist did not remember the exact blood specification she was to pull. The system is robust; its defenses caught the failure before the blood made it to the patient. Marx goes on to point out that the design of any high-risk system should attempt to prevent solitary human missteps (**single-point failures**) from leading to a catastrophic result. From the perspective of learning about system safety, the technologist should participate in the process of learning how the system can be improved. For example, the system could be further enhanced by the following measures:

- Analyzing the typical kinds of distractions that can arise during the procedure
- Training employees on how to react to inevitable interruptions
- Altering the system to reconfirm computer orders before continuing after any interruption

Hindsight Bias and Fundamental Attribution Error

Two critical concepts are essential in understanding our reactions to medical accidents: hindsight bias (see Figure 3.5) and the fundamental attribution error. The phenomenon of hindsight bias is based on research that demonstrates that knowing the outcome of an event influences the way we view it (Fischhoff, 1975; Slovic, 1989). Hindsight bias is always present and cannot be avoided. It is a judgment of human performance that tends to be applied only when accidents or near misses that could have produced a bad outcome occur (Cook and Woods, 1994). There are two parts to hindsight bias (Reason, 1990):

- Observers of past events exaggerate what other people should have been able to anticipate in **foresight**.

FIGURE 3.5. HINDSIGHT BIAS

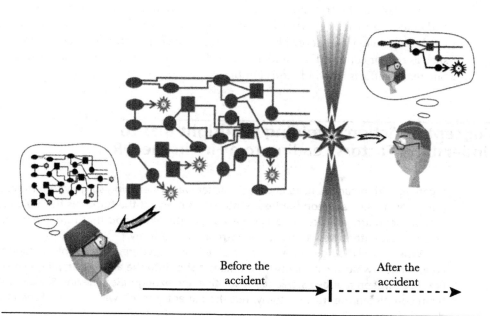

Before the accident ⟶ After the accident ⤏

Source: Cooke, 2002. Copyright © by Richard I. Cook, Cognitive technologies Laboratory, University of Chicago. Used by permission.

- Observers of past events are unaware of the great influence that knowing the outcome has had on their perceptions.

The need for second stories comes in large part from the presence of hindsight bias in all accidents, and especially in the local types of investigation common in health care. This is because the interests and knowledge limitations of the stakeholders create biases that are likely to obscure real issues and limit the explanations of the accident, and this tendency is amplified by the severity of the consequences. As Reason puts it:

> There is one obvious but psychologically significant difference between ourselves, the retrospective judges, and the people whose decisions, actions, or inactions led to a disaster: we know how things were going to turn out, they did not. Outcome knowledge dominates our perceptions of the past, yet we remain largely unaware of its influence. Before judging too harshly the human failings that concatenate to cause a disaster, we need to make a clear distinction between the way the precursors appear now, given knowledge of the unhappy outcome, and the way they seemed at the time [Reason, 1990, p. 215].

Fundamental attribution error is the pervasive human tendency to attribute bad outcomes to an actor's personal inadequacies (dispositional causes) rather than attributing them to situational factors beyond his or her control (situational causes), such as role or context (Fiske and Taylor, 1984). The following case study describes one team's efforts to avoid hindsight bias.

Concept to Action: Avoiding Hindsight Bias to Understand Factors Leading to a Fire in the OR

A patient with recurrent head and neck cancer was undergoing surgery to remove a tumor. As the first surgeon finished removing as much of the tumor as he could, an ENT surgeon arrived (prescheduled because of the likelihood that tumor removal would cause extensive swelling) to perform a tracheostomy.

When the ENT surgeon was ready to begin the procedure, he brought the cautery equipment toward the neck. Just then, flames shot into the air. The draping was on fire. The surgeon grabbed sterile saline solution and extinguished the fire. Shaken, the team completed the tracheostomy, but the patient was left with first- and second-degree burns on his neck.

What happened?

"At first people were shaking their heads, saying, 'This was an act of God. Spontaneous combustion.' There was a sense of disbelief," remembers an executive working with surgical services. "Then people started blaming each other."

First, talk rippled through the staff that the surgeon may have been rushing through the surgery and hadn't allowed the prep solution to dry before using the cauterizing equipment. Then the questioning focused on the nurse. She may have used excessive draping, the theory went, which allowed the prep solution to pool in the material. Finally, the prep solution itself became suspect. Was it too flammable for use with cautery equipment? Did the label have the warnings and cautions it should have had to prevent such a situation?

The medical director and director of surgical services met with the family and explained what had happened and what they knew about the event. They assured the family that a detailed analysis of the event was taking place, that the family would be informed as the analysis proceeded, and that all medical costs related to the burns would be absorbed by the hospital. They apologized for the event's occurrence and for the injury to their family member.

Next they began an extensive review of the case.

"We knew a simple assignment of one cause, especially the cause of 'human error,' was shortsighted and lacked an understanding of the process that would prevent something like that from happening in the future. But the team was stuck—the high emotions and unbelievability not only of what had happened but also of what could have happened were overwhelming," said the executive.

The executive and the lead physician for medical accident investigation decided to ask a researcher from the field of human factors to help them uncover the conditions and factors that had created the fire. The prep solution, they discovered, was the solution of choice for the majority of the hospital's surgeons. No other problems with it, including problems encountered during procedures involving cautery, had been reported. The ENT surgeon had painted the solution onto the neck as directed by the label and had waited the instructed length of time to allow the solution to dry before beginning a cauterization procedure. The nurse had draped the patient according to the procedures of the hospital.

With the facilitation of the human factors researcher, team members began to disclose their roles in the procedure and began an analysis and reconstruction of the sequence of events.

"Each participant, from case cart technicians to scrub and circulating nurses to the surgeons and anesthesiologists, knew their part of the procedure, but there was a lack of shared understanding of the sequencing, procedures, and risks that eventually had led to the fire," explained the executive.

As the analysis continued, other variables began to emerge. Because there were two procedures, the patient, as was the routine, had been draped twice. Although the solution typically spread out and dried fast, the double draping had created an absorbent reservoir for the liquid. The patient's previous head and neck surgeries also contributed to the fire. They had left him with significant skin deformities that created small crevices in his neck, where the solution pooled. A plume of gas from the prep solution, it was theorized, may have been trapped between the two layers of draping, igniting and causing the flames to shoot into the air. The 100 percent oxygen being administered to the patient contributed to the fire starting.

Moreover, the team discovered, fires in the OR weren't uncommon. Fifty to one hundred fires occur during surgery each year in the U.S. (Emergency Care Research Institute, 2000).

The group generated a list of changes that would help prevent similar conditions from realigning to create another fire. In addition to creating educational sessions around the event, staff members called each hospital surgeon individually, reported what had happened, and, if requested, changed the surgeon's "preference card"—the card that tracks the prep solutions, equipment, and procedures each surgeon prefers when performing surgery at the hospital—to reflect a different prep solution of choice. Few surgeons elected to change their preferences, and the prep solution is still in use today. The manufacturer has added additional alerts in labeling, and additional drying time is used when the patient's anatomy or procedure adds risk. Surgery team members started holding team meetings before all complex procedures to mentally simulate the upcoming sequence of events, identify possible risk scenarios, and create plans for reducing risk and recovering in the face of risk.

"According to the field of human factors, seeking a person to blame is a typical and understandable human reaction," said the executive. "Everyone was looking for an individual actor to blame because we wanted to put such a frightening scenario to rest. If we had identified a scapegoat, we wouldn't have learned anything from the incident. We would have lost our ability to predict and reduce the probability of a similar event in the future. Using a defined process and facilitator based on human factors research, we've reduced the possibility that a future patient and surgical team will become victims to the conditions that could have eventually reassembled to cause another fire."

Normalization of Deviance

Normalization of deviance is the acceptance of, or failure to recognize, faulty and risk-prone processes because they are so familiar, pervasive, and entrenched in the work environment. This results in failure to attend to problematic conditions. Diane Vaughan describes the role of normalization of deviance in her book about the 1986 *Challenger* accident, noting that normalization of deviance is common in organizations and often results in failure and frequently in disastrous consequences (Vaughan, 1996). This is more fully examined in Chapter Ten.

Work-arounds and interceptions of failure have become commonplace in the highly complex environment of health care, normalized as "how we do things here."

A prime example of normalization of deviance in health care is the excessive work hours for residents, a tradition described by Leape as "the hazing period that must be endured because those before have done so." Another example is the **er-**

gonomics nightmare that is the modern operating room, with its hodgepodge of equipment, cables, hoses, tubing, and activity. Normalization of deviance is all around us in health care. Structure process auditing is required to detect and make it visible. Cook and Woods (1994) relate the following story about a busy weekend operating room schedule:

> On a weekend in a large tertiary care hospital, the anesthesiology team (consisting of four physicians of whom three are residents in training) was called on to perform anesthetics for an in vitro fertilization, a perforated viscus, reconstruction of an artery of the leg, and an appendectomy, in one building, and one exploratory laparotomy in another building. Each of these cases was an emergency, that is, a case that cannot be delayed for the regular daily operating room schedule. The exact sequence in which the cases were done depended on multiple factors. The situation was complicated by a demanding nurse who insisted that the exploratory laparotomy be done ahead of other cases. The nurse was only responsible for that single case; the operating room nurses and technicians for that case could not leave the hospital until the case had been completed. The surgeons complained that they were being delayed and their cases were increasing in urgency because of the passage of time. There were also some delays in preoperative preparation of some of the patients for surgery. In the primary operating room suites, the staff of nurses and technicians were only able to run two operating rooms simultaneously. The anesthesiologist in charge was under pressure to attempt to overlap portions of procedures by starting one case as another was finishing so as to use the available resources maximally. The hospital also served as a major trauma center, which means that the team needed to be able to start a large emergency case with minimal (less than 10 minutes') notice. In committing all of the residents to doing the waiting cases, the anesthesiologist in charge produced a situation in which there were no anesthetists available to start a major trauma case. There were no trauma cases, and all the surgeries were accomplished. Remarkably, the situation was so common that it was regarded by many as typical rather than exceptional [Cook and Woods, 1994, pp. 277–278].

Diffusion of Responsibility

"If everybody is in charge, nobody is in charge." In a widely publicized case in the 1960s, thirty-eight people watched as Kitty Genovese was raped and murdered in front of an apartment building in New York City (Rosenthal, 1999). Social psychologists studied the situation and found that no one called for help because every bystander thought somebody else was contacting the police. The phenomenon was labeled "diffusion of responsibility" (Darley and Latane, 1968). Applied to health care, diffusion of responsibility means the assumption that someone else will do a specific task, such as checking on the correct dosage of a drug. In health care's busy working environment, it is easy for failures to quickly turn to accidents because someone who gets busy is more likely to assume that someone else will finish the task.

Tightly Coupled Work Processes

Organizational accidents are an expected risk in complex industries that employ high-risk technologies. Health care shares characteristics with other high-risk organizations, such as myriad of interrelated, tightly coupled work processes. Visually represented by interlocking the fingers of two hands, tightly coupled work processes mean that one person's actions are directly tied to another's, and this second person's actions are tied to yet another's, and so on. The more tightly coupled the work processes, the greater the likelihood of accident (Perrow, 1999). For instance, a physician writes an order with the intention of benefiting a patient. The probability that this intervention will be successful goes far beyond the intentions of the physician. Other factors also influence success. They include the physician's skill in diagnosing the condition and selecting the appropriate treatment, the physician's skill in calculating the correct dosage, the legibility of the physician's handwriting, and his or her use of appropriate notations. All these are separate, complex, interrelated processes in and of themselves. The successful administration of the drug relies on still other people and work processes. The pharmacist must select and label the right drug. The nurse must administer the right dose of the right drug to the right patient at the right time. In larger medical centers, these three different groups of professionals may never interact directly with each other, nor may these practitioners know the scope of the others' practices and the intersections of the process.

Mindfulness and Sensemaking

Two concepts—sensemaking and **mindfulness** (Weick, 1995; Weick and Sutcliffe, 2001)—characterize high-reliability organizations and refer to the ways in which workers in HROs remain individually and collectively alert and prepared to deal with unforeseen events. These concepts tie together the domains of human cognition and organizational functioning. Mindfulness describes a culture that cultivates alertness and vigilance and enables people to notice and, if necessary, halt unexpected developments. According to Weick and Sutcliffe (2001), mindfulness is a "struggle for alertness" in which HROs continually share and update information as events unfold. Organizational mindfulness has five key features: preoccupation with failure, reluctance to simplify interpretations, keen attention to operations, commitment to resilience, and deference to expertise.

HROs know that mundane problems can escalate to crisis situations, so they are keen to detect and organize to take action to early and weak signs of peril. Workers are encouraged to conduct simulations and mental rehearsals to increase their repertoires and gain confidence in alternative ways of responding to risk. By staying open to new information, workers better adapt to changing conditions and innovate when confronted with new challenges.

Sensemaking is the process that transforms raw experience into intelligible collective worldviews by taking the time to make sense out of new and changing circumstances. The process represents the collective, cognitive work of the team to make meaning of events and the environment. HROs develop a fascination with failure in their cultures and refuse to take shortcuts or simplify reality. When an organization faces a crisis or is in transition, multiple conflicting interpretations, all plausible, are considered. The process creates a greater repertoire of responses so that the team has flexibility in the face of crisis. Alternative possible courses of action and their consequences are considered so that the list of interpretations is narrowed to a manageable size. The meaning the team derives from the events converts interpretations into action. Trust is a product of sensemaking.

Summary Points

1. The systems framework views harm to patients as a consequence of flaws that are hidden in the system, particularly in the design, construction, and maintenance of work processes; these flaws need to be identified and the systems redesigned to eliminate conditions that create harm.

2. Among the significant contributions that the field of human factors makes to understanding accidents in health care is the notion that the conditions in which human beings work must be altered.

3. Different branches of knowledge outside health care come together to inform our understanding of patient safety:
   - Human factors science
   - Organizational analysis
   - Safety science

4. Among the concepts outlined in this chapter, some that are particularly useful as leaders begin their journey toward high reliability in health care are the following:

- The "sharp end" and the "blunt end" describe how expertise is applied, and how error or accident is experienced, at different levels in the organization. The sharp end is where providers and patients interact, and it is the place where system failures will appear. The blunt end is where the table is set for encounters at the sharp end. Here, governance and management make decisions involving policy, production expectations, and resource allocation. Leaders need to close the distance between "front office" and "front line" by understanding the complexity of technical work in health care and anticipating the effects of their decisions on the technical work and on those who perform it.
- The Swiss Cheese Model represents the nature of emerging risks in complex systems, with their defenses and vulnerabilities. Undetected vulnerabilities or denigration in defenses create conditions for errors to concatenate to produce medical accidents.
- Hindsight bias is a phenomenon of human nature whereby people simplify and reduce conditions in retrospect and underestimate the complexity with which the people involved in an accident were dealing at the time of the event. The most common effect of hindsight bias is attributing the cause of a medical accident to "human error." All learning stops, and hazardous conditions that have been present are allowed to lie in wait and realign to produce another accident in the future.
- Fundamental attribution error is the pervasive tendency to attribute bad outcomes to an actor's personal inadequacies (dispositional causes) rather than attributing them to situational factors beyond his or her control. In contrast, the actor tends to attribute bad outcomes to environmental factors rather than to individual action.
- Normalization of deviance is the phenomenon of accepting aberrations as a natural course of doing business and is a symptom or defense of people working in a hazardous environment of unmitigated risk.

CHAPTER FOUR

ASSUME EXECUTIVE RESPONSIBILITY

Chapter Four returns to the patient safety manifesto and continues with the committment: "Assume executive responsibility." This chapter focuses on what it looks like to accept responsibility on a personal and organizational level, whether in a clinical discipline, a department, a clinic, a single hospital, a large system of care, in the academic health sciences, or on a governing board.

For leaders to assume responsibility, it is essential that they be grounded in the basic principles of safety science and have the courage to challenge the conventional wisdom that pervades the health care industry. These safety principles are as follows:

- Risk of failure is inherent in complex systems.
- Risk is always emerging.
- Not all risk is foreseeable.
- People are fallible, no matter how hard they try not to be.
- Systems are fallible.
- Alert, well-trained clinicians create safety every day through recognizing and compensating for risks in the workplace.

These principles stand in sharp contrast to the beliefs that permeate health care today:

- Clinicians are supposed to be infallible.
- Bad things happen only when people make mistakes.
- People who fail are bad.
- Blame and punishment sufficiently motivate people to be more careful, thereby avoiding future mistakes.

These beliefs are myths. In his commencement address at Yale University in 1962 John F. Kennedy said, "the great enemy of the truth is very often not the lie—deliberate, contrived, and dishonest—but the myth, which is persistent, and persuasive—and unrealistic." Creating a culture of patient safety requires dispelling myths and anchoring the culture in the principles of safety science. This requires a leader to rethink the beliefs that you have held and perhaps even perpetuated in the health care environment. Accepting responsibility means that you own your part for the current state. No longer is it a matter of trusting that careful people with good intentions will provide safe care at the sharp end; now you will examine each decision you make and every action you take through the lens of safety. Your decisions influence whether safety is compromised or facilitated, whether in the design and operations of a **microsystem** of care or across an entire health care enterprise.

Leaders Become Personally Involved

Jim Conway, chief operating officer at Dana-Farber Cancer Institute, Boston, has created guidelines for executive leaders who are launching and sustaining patient safety agendas in their organizations. This leadership resource has been distributed through the American Hospital Association and is being linked with executive and management compensation levels in some organizations. It contains the following checklist for leaders:

- Read *To Err Is Human: Building a Safer Health System.*
- Read other primers on patient safety.
- Participate in external safety education programs, continuing medical education, conferences, etc.
- Hold detailed conversations with in-house experts on our realities of practice.
- Walk my hospital with a human factors expert.
- Walk my hospital as a patient.
- Familiarize myself with enhanced JCAHO Patient Safety Standards.

- View Bridge Medical video "Beyond Blame" and Partnership for Patient Safety video "First Do No Harm."
- Speak publicly to various audiences on the unacceptability of the current state of and my commitment to patient safety as a personal and corporate priority.
- Include safety focus in hospital publications, strategic plan, etc.
  - Board and hospital leaders
  - Medical and hospital staff
  - Patients/consumers
  - Media
- Implement a proactive effort on patient safety design, measurement, assessment, and improvement. Include direct care, administrative, and clerical staff and patients and family members in all aspects.
- Set the goal of establishing an environment of trust with a non-blaming, responsibility-based approach to the causation of incidents and errors; establish policy in this area.
- Set the expectation for timely and interdisciplinary error and near miss investigations with an emphasis on: patient/family impacted by the error; the broader institutional implications of and learning from the error; and the support of staff at the sharp end (closest to care).
- Build quality improvement and patient safety policies into staff orientation and continuing education offerings.
- Set the expectation for executive involvement in significant incident investigations.
- Establish a policy to ensure patients/families are notified ASAP when an error reaches a patient.
- Establish effective grievance systems for patients/families who see themselves as "victims of error."
- Establish mechanisms to train leadership and other experts in patient safety.
- Openly engage with medical staff, nursing, and other leaders in patient safety planning.
- Continuously articulate the business case for safety improvement.
- Personally participate in a significant incident investigation/root cause analysis.
- Tell "my story" around incidents/errors that I have been involved with and the systems improvements that could have prevented them.
- Routinely involve myself, all levels of our staff, and our patients and family members in direct and ongoing communications around the patient safety work of our institution and areas for improvement.
- Routinely bring patient safety matters, trending data, and specific cases to the board and other hospital leadership committees.

- Routinely probe staff perceptions of risk areas from existing or proposed systems and take immediate actions wherever possible.
- Openly support staff involved in incidents and their root cause analysis.
- Ensure that there is ongoing prioritization and achievement of safety improvement objectives.
- Ensure that articles on patient safety matters regularly appear in my organization's communications vehicles.
- As part of annual budget preparation, ensure resources are funded for priority safety areas.
- Request and routinely receive reports on facility utilization of and comparison with best-practice information from the AHA, NPSF, and ISMP.
- Ensure self-assessments from the AHA and others are completed and used internally for quality improvement activities.
- Cultivate media understanding of patient safety and my organization's efforts to improve safety.
- Ensure effective systems are in place to assess individual accountability and competence [Conway, 2001].

The checklist further identifies ways for leaders to help advance the field of patient safety:

- Share my personal and the institution's patient safety learning outside the organization.
- Participate in local, regional, and national conferences, coalitions, and other efforts to improve patient safety.
- Engage in initiatives to drive enhancements in regulatory, facility/professional licensing, and accreditation agencies that support safety improvement and cultural change in consort with the specific goals of the agency.
- Advocate for my professional association to make/keep patient safety a high priority.

Expertise is applied and error is experienced directly at the sharp end, where care is delivered and received. However, leaders shape the context for sharp-end care delivery at the blunt end of health care through management and governance expectations and decisions. This checklist can help leaders establish a patient safety culture through personal responsibility and commitment.

The following sections explore what a safety culture looks like, the leaders' role in nurturing such a culture, embracing failure and successes, and changing language, policy, and personal reactions to failure in order to influence the development of a safety culture.

Leaders Create a Generative or Learning Culture

A safety culture is a culture that constantly seeks and learns from failure and also from anticipating failure, using mental simulations of possible failure scenarios. Figure 4.1 adapts the work of Westrum (1992) and outlines three different organizational cultures. These cultures are differentiated by how they use information: **pathological culture**, a **bureaucratic culture**, and a **generative culture**. A culture of safety is generative relative to its pursuit of information and its use of information.

FIGURE 4.1. PATHOLOGICAL/GENERATIVE CULTURE

How Different Organizational Cultures Handle Safety Information

Pathological Culture	Bureaucratic Culture	Generative Culture
• Don't want to know	• May not find out	• Actively seek it
• Messengers (whistle blowers) are "shot"	• Messengers are listened to if they arrive	• Messengers are trained and rewarded
• Failure is punished or concealed	• Failure leads to local repairs	• Failures lead to far-reaching reforms
• New ideas are actively discouraged	• New ideas often present problems	• New ideas are welcomed

Safety culture is generative, constantly "uneasy," seeking, learning, changing.

Source: Adapted from Westrum, R. "Cultures with Requisite Imagination" in J. A. Wise, V. D. Hopkin, and P. Stager (eds.), *Verification and Validation of Complex Systems: Human Factors Issues* (Berlin: Springer-Verlag, 1992), p. 402.

Pursuit of Information

Generative organizations encourage workers to bring observations about safety and risk to the attention of management. In contrast, pathological organizations do not want to know about safety problems. They punish reporters and cover up failures. Most health care organizations fall into a third category: bureaucratic. Bureaucratic cultures compartmentalize safety management (for example, appointing a patient safety officer instead of holding senior leaders accountable for safety), deal with error on an isolated, local basis, and do not integrate lessons from failure throughout the organization. Reporters are not penalized, but neither does the organization know what to do with new ideas. In a culture of safety, workers are not only trained to report but also encouraged and rewarded for reporting. Leaders publicly thank and celebrate reporting and hazard identification. The following is an example of celebrating hazard identification (Berwick, 1999):

Jerry Gonsalves was one of thousands of front-line workers at NASA who had been involved in preparing a Titan rocket for launch. The day before the launch, a problem was diagnosed in the tank of liquid oxygen fuel. Metal baffles bolted onto the bottom of the tank were interfering with the way the tank was draining. To fix the problem, the NASA team came up with a solution that was effective but expensive: the tank had to be completely drained so that a worker could enter it and reduce the size of the metal baffles bolted to the bottom of the tank. The task would involve removing pieces of metal and four of the bolts that secured the metal to the tank.

With his supervisors looking on, Gonsalves donned a diving suit and harness and lowered himself into the emptied tank. Using metal shears, he pared down the baffles and placed the extra metal and bolts he had removed into a small cloth bag. Finished with his task, he exited.

When Gonsalves emptied his cloth bag, out came metal fragments and three bolts—not four. He looked to his supervisors. "There must have been only three," he said. Just in case, the team decided to unbolt the hatch and look for the missing bolt.

Each leaned far into the tank, systematically sweeping the bottom in search of the loose bolt. One official passed out from the toxic fumes. All agreed that there must have been only three.

That night, NASA's director of quality, safety, and reliability, the senior official for quality in the organization, whose boss reported directly to the president of the United States, was sleeping at home when his phone rang. Jerry Gonsalves was calling. Gonsalves, unable to sleep, knowing that a loose bolt or fragment could cause an engine explosion during launch, had left his house at midnight, driven an hour to a storage facility where another Titan liquid oxygen tank was stored, and entered the tank. Over and over again, he had placed a bolt in different spots in the tank, then walked to the hatch and shined his flashlight down. In his search, he found two places where a bolt could escape illumination.

The director of quality, safety, and reliability called the flight director. At 5:00 A.M. they gathered near the rocket, observing as the fuel tank was emptied yet again, at extremely high cost, so another worker could don the diving suit and be lowered into the tank. While Gonsalves and the administrators looked on, the worker emerged with the bolt in hand.

A few days later, the rocket was ready to launch, and administrators and front-line workers looked on. The administrators pulled Gonsalves aside—they had something for him. They had saved the bolt, gold-plated it, and mounted it on a plaque. They dedicated the launch to him for his persistence and vigilance.

Use of Information

The second dimension of a generative safety culture is the productive use of information after risk is identified. A culture of safety faces reality, acknowledges that risk is present and always emerging, and confronts risk with informed and effective action. This begins with the leader facilitating a continual pursuit of information—persistently asking "Why?" until all potential contributing factors have been explored—and assigning accountability for the changes that must occur to close gaps in safety. In the case of the missing bolt, NASA officials, although grateful the bolt had been retrieved, did not stop there. They continued their quest for fail-safe procedures that would prevent another loose bolt from ever again falling undetected into the engine of a spacecraft.

Architecture of Safety: Generative Learning Culture

A generative culture is in a state of perpetual learning and deepening of knowledge. It is a **learning organization.** Learning takes many forms. The following case study profiles an organization that used minicourses with national patient safety experts, dialogues to invite informal exploration of safety, self-learning packets, orientation and training modules, and ongoing internal publications to teach, reinforce, and stimulate learning among all members of the health care community.

Concept to Action: Changing Culture through Educating Health Care Professionals about Patient Safety

The evolving science of patient safety is a required knowledge base for organizations that seeks to prepare to meet new and increasing expectations to deliver harm-free care. One hospital system launched its safety agenda and nurtured the ongoing development of patient safety champions, designing an ongoing system of safety education.

Education of executives, managers, physicians, and all staff who provided or supported bedside care began with a series of educational minicourses, offering continuing education credits on a set of fundamental concepts. Each course created the theory to ground the actions for the organization's safety initiative. The first session, an all-day course, was titled "Beyond Blame." Eric Knox, a physician and expert in medical risk and safety, used videos and personal stories from his own practice to explore how normalization of deviance occurs in the workplace and how the culture of shame and blame blunts the ability to learn from near misses and accidents. As in all the other minicourses that followed, the participants formed multidisciplinary groups and engaged in discussions about how to apply what they had learned.

The speaker told carefully crafted stories and then asked the course attendees to define where normalization of deviance could be discovered in their own practice. The organizer of the minicourses reported, "It was eye-opening for participants to understand how this behavior [normalization of deviance] occurs in a practice setting, that it isn't unique but is evidenced in everyday life and is a danger in health care." The content of the discussions was bold and rich in detail as new knowledge was applied and routines of everyday practice were reframed.

The second minicourse described the concept of high-reliability organizations and how health care can learn from them to improve safety performance. John Nance, aviation expert and author, was the invited faculty member.

"Nance provided a base of knowledge surrounding crew resource management and team communication," said the organizer. (See Chapter Five for more about this training process.) "He related his own experience of being the captain of the cockpit and how he personally became more open and responsive to team communication, and how he had learned that team communication is a requirement for creating safety. He told compelling stories of how failures in team communication had directly contributed to near misses and aviation disasters."

The third minicourse introduced Richard Cook, a physician and the director of the cognitive technology laboratory at the University of Chicago, who explored human factors research and its applications to creating safety in high-risk environments. Then Henri Manasse Jr., chief executive of the American Society of Health-System Pharmacists, discussed evidence-based specifics of safe prescribing practices and the aim of a zero-defect medication administration system. Next the course participants learned from a panel composed of a physician, a nurse, a pharmacist, and parents who had been involved in an actual near miss during the hospitalization of their child. Dr. Cook moderated the panel to extract lessons learned, pull forward principles from human factors research, and highlight the complexity inherent in responses to medical accidents.

A fourth minicourse focused on creating a culture for blameless reporting, featuring three faculty members: Paul Barach, a physician in the department of anesthesia and critical care at the University of Chicago, presented a study of communication, culture, and simulations; Caryl Lee, a nurse and program manager at the U.S. Veterans Administration's National Center for Patient Safety; and James Bagian, physician, astronaut, and leader of the National Center for Patient Safety, via videotape. The session captured stories from practitioners about risk-prone conditions, near misses, and medical accidents, and it harnessed the power of storytelling as a method of understanding how systems work and how they can be improved.

"We started with broad key principles, and each course built on a theory construction to application," said the minicourse organizer. "We carefully invited faculty with expert knowledge, presence, and ability to create interactive learning experiences." Several other strategies also guided the minicourses:

- *Promotion.* Articles appeared in all hospital system publications. Advance notices were sent to key leaders of the medical-professional staff, the executive team, union leaders, patient care managers and directors, and direct-care clinical staff. A respected staff physician was selected as the sponsor of each minicourse, and a quote from this sponsor set the tone for the course and was prominently displayed in the publicity brochure. The promotion differentiated the minicourses from other educational offerings. The first course attracted one hundred multidisciplinary participants. These early adopters' enthusiasm about the courses generated additional interest. The process of attraction led to progressively higher attendance in subsequent courses.
- *Investment in attendance for registered nurses.* "The decision was made to compensate registered nurses for their attendance," explained the organizer, and this decision helped increase attendance by nurses. "Paid time for attendance was seen as a pledge of support by management." Whenever possible, minicourses and other patient safety educational events were repeated at different times of the day, to improve access for staff who were assigned to evening and night shifts.
- *Patient and family participation.* Through the hospital system's family advisory council, families were invited to each minicourse. One early minicourse included family as faculty. "It was an illustration that the families are viewed as equal partners in creating safety," said the organizer.
- *Distributed learning strategies.* The *Patient Safety Learning Packet* (Morath, Malone, and Anderson, 1999a), a binder of reference materials, articles, and presentations, was made available in each department and distributed to each medical-professional staff member. Continuing education credits were offered for completion of a posttest that was based on patient safety scenarios included in the guides. The *Patient Safety Resource Guide* (Morath, Malone, and Anderson, 1999b) is a manager's toolkit, with "talking tips," videos, and articles to help managers engage in ongoing dialogues with staff. Case studies, constructed from incidents that had taken place inside and outside the organization, and using deidentified information, were circulated to staff members via an e-mail list.
- *Leveraged exposure.* The course organizers linked their efforts to prescheduled quarterly professional medical staff meetings, bringing the message to as many people as possible. The minicourses were conducted during the day and then excerpted by attendees for sharing at in-house professional staff meetings.
- *New learners as teachers.* Other educational formats have developed to provide ongoing education. As new areas of emphasis are added to the agenda, they are

launched with a relevant minicourse to teach the theory base underneath the strategy. Members of a systemwide patient safety steering committee engage in a learning-teaching model by bringing new ideas and knowledge into the meetings and safety-related projects in which they participate. The steering committee operates as a learning lab, and sets direction and policy for the safety agenda. The members receive e-mails and monthly distributions of new research and journal publications to learn from and examine for applications of new ideas and findings." One-hour patient safety dialogues, held monthly by steering committee leaders, facilitate discussions among staff members. The dialogues have titles like "Family-Centered Care: A Strategy for Patient Safety" and "Lessons Learned: A Near Miss Can Become a Medical Accident if Not Addressed."

The leaders of the organization periodically try new formats to deliver education and encourage dialogue. Over time, the nature of the dialogues has changed as a new patient safety culture has emerged. The minicourse organizer reports having begun by learning from external experts, but now can showcase sources of success within the organization and learning takes place by sharing new ideas among its members.

Leaders Accept Responsibility for Mitigating Risk and Building Resilience

The Swiss Cheese Model of Accident Causation is a prerequisite for understanding the dynamics of the emerging risk and organizational defenses that are necessary to improve safety. Figure 4.2 illustrates the model, using its **metaphor**, a wedge of Swiss cheese. The model was described in detail in Chapter Three; here, a metaphorical exploration of the model amplifies its implications for accepting leadership responsibility.

Note the slab of cheese without holes added in Figure 4.2b. This can be thought of as a slice of cheddar, and it tells the rest of the story. The slice in Figure 4.2b represents the final line of defense for deflecting errors traveling through the holes, or vulnerabilities, before they reach a patient and cause harm. This important concept represents the ability of the individual or the team to recover a situation. In a culture of safety, leaders recognize, reward, and learn from stories of recovery, or "sources of success," in addition to reporting stories of failure. In health care, we depend on people to continually create safety through their vigilance and their ability to intercept error and recover from failure. Safety is a story of both risk and recovery. As we reduce risk, we also seek to build resilience and a capacity for anticipating and recovering from harm.

If organizations expect people to continually intercept error, without improving the conditions and systems in which they work, the phenomenon of rescue fatigue

FIGURE 4.2. SWISS CHEESE: ANIMATED MODEL

**The Swiss Cheese model
of accident causation**

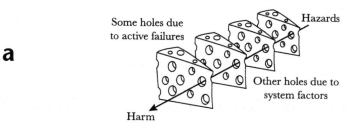

a

Successive layers of defenses, barriers, and safeguards

**But that is not the
end of the story**

b

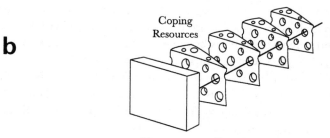

The team can still recover the situation

**Limited coping resources
can get nibbled away**

c

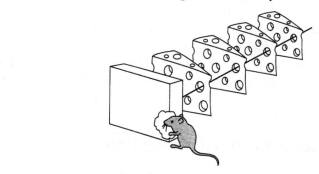

Accumulation of minor events weakens defenses

Source: J. T. Reason, "The Basics of Human Factors," paper presented at the Salzburg Seminar on Medical Safety and Human Error, Apr. 25–May 2, 2001.

FIGURE 4.3. SIMPLE RULES

Rules for Accelerating Change

- Fix what you can

- Tell what you fixed

- Find someone who can fix
  what you cannot

Source: E. Knox and J. Morath, *Simple Rules* (Minneapolis: Children's Hospitals and Clinics, 1999).

sets in. Imagine now, as depicted in Figure 4.2c, a mouse nibbling away at the cheese, eroding the coping and rescue mechanisms at the final line of defense.

If the management system fails to respond to risks and near misses pointed out by the front line, a sense of resignation will grow among staff members over time. Thus people who work in conditions of unmitigated risk lose situational awareness and defend themselves by normalizing deviance. They accept vulnerabilities and risk as the way it is. The mouse in Figure 4.2c is the metaphor for deterioration of situational awareness, increased normalization of deviance, and erosion of the front line's capacity to recover over time. This kind of deterioration undermines the organization's final defenses of harm prevention, and leads to erosion of trust and denigration of quality standards.

The antidote is vigilance. Like the cat that stands guard against a mouse, an organization maintains a constant, catlike vigilance through continually paying attention and taking action. Vigilance and simple rules help build the mutual trust and reciprocal responsibility that are required for reducing risk and building robust defenses. Simple rules that empower front line staff to take action were developed by Dr. Eric Knox while working with front line staff (see Figure 4.3): "Fix what you can. Tell what you fixed. Find someone to fix what you cannot."

Leaders who accept responsibility for safety take into account what is reported and provide resources to the front line to reduce risk. This is known as "reciprocal accountability." It is not passive acknowledgment but active, visible leadership.

Leaders Embrace Error to Eliminate Harm

The idea of eliminating harm rather than stamping out error is a relatively new concept in health care. Not long ago, when error was attributed to the carelessness of individuals or to human mistakes, and blame and punishment were thought to be sufficient to create safety, leaders were divorced from direct responsibility. Once the sharp end target, the individual, was identified, blamed, and removed, the leader could proceed under the illusion that safety was restored. But now we know better. Harm to patients is recurring; it has systemic causes, and the front-line operator is only one variable in a complex system of causation. Efforts toward harm-free care must continue past the individual if lessons are to be extracted from the system.

The concept that medical accident is the result of faulty systems—not faulty people—is transforming health care. The issue is not error; the issue is injury or harm. Errors are not intrinsically bad. What is important is to make them transparent and learn from them about the system's performance. A danger in working to create safety is the tendency to focus exclusively on eliminating error. Here is a paradox. Trying to manage error has the unintended effect of suppressing error. Instead, error must be made transparent and harnessed as a rich source of information to help prevent future harm (Amalberti, 2001). Removing fear of blame and punishment, and learning to talk about and learn from error, are significant parts of creating a culture of patient safety. As Blumenthal says (1994, p. 1868), "The paradox of modern quality improvement is that only by admitting and forgiving error can its rate be minimized. . . . Every defect is a treasure."

Leaders Use Language to Shape a Patient Safety Culture

Language shapes culture, and a safety culture requires thoughtful and deliberate use of a new vocabulary. Leadership responsibility includes redefining how we talk about safety. Consider how the following terms and phrases, and the ideas they represent, frame safety differently and how terminology can be used deliberately to build a new vocabulary for leadership and management (Minnesota Hospital and Healthcare Partnership and Minnesota Medical Association, 2000):

- *What happened* versus *whose fault it is.* The question "What happened?" invites analysis of the conditions surrounding and contributing to an error or accident. Asking, "Whose fault is it?" immediately seeks to place blame and attributes the cause to human error.
- *System* versus *isolated event.* An accident does not just happen. An accident evolves from latent failures or weaknesses in a system. These failures or weaknesses are cumulative and interactive. Nearly always, a single error is insufficient to create an accident, but the same error combined with others will be cumulatively successful in creating an accident. Research has revealed that at least four errors must align to produce an accident. A recent analysis of a catastrophic medical accident revealed over fifty latent system failures contributing to the

event (Smetzer and Cohen, 1998). Isolated single-cause accidents, such as those attributed to simple "human error," are rare.

- *Analysis or study* versus *investigation.* A process of analysis or study is used to learn how systems work and how the pieces fit together to create the whole. The knowledge gained through rigorous analysis can be applied to predict accidents and create interventions to prevent or reduce the probability of future failures. An investigation carries the connotation of a process for assigning blame, as in the phrase "criminal investigation." An investigation is typically a linear search to determine a single cause or "bad apple."

- *Accountability* versus *blame.* Health care professionals are accountable for their work. They have a responsibility to possess current knowledge and competence in the work they perform; they also have a responsibility to acknowledge the interdependence they have in their performance. In addition, they must appreciate how systems work and understand that people are the human components of systems, both contributing to failure and creating safety. Blame focuses on a scapegoat rather than on the pursuit of deeper understanding about failure. The traditional "blame, shame, and punish" methods have not worked to improve safety.

- *Blameless* versus *punitive* or *retaliatory.* A **blameless environment** is one where the front line is comfortable reporting failures and near misses so they can be studied; in this kind of environment, the front line even feels compelled to report failures. A **punitive or retaliatory environment** creates an atmosphere where sharp end staff members are afraid to disclose failures and near misses, and in this way opportunities to learn from mistakes are eliminated.

- *Just* versus *arbitrary* or *avoidant.* Although they are rare, there are **blameworthy actions** that present barriers to patient safety. These include impairment, felony, malfeasance, reckless behavior, and failure to learn over time. Such actions need to be addressed with administrative processes that are timely and fair.

- *Heedful procedure* versus *routine procedure.* **Heedful procedures** are designed to be performed with attention. They include steps that require situational awareness and verification before action is taken. **Routine procedures** are those that are performed so many times that they can become automatic; as such, they introduce greater risk.

- *Functional Hierarchy* versus *bureaucracy.* A functional hierarchy is not the hierarchy that exists as a barrier in health care today, such as the hierarchy of power differentials between physicans and nurses, physicians and patients. Rather, a functional hierarchy is a system of **formal rules**, structures, procedures, training, and decision making in the service of organizational mission and values. In a safety culture, there is a clear chain of command so that people at the sharp end know where to go for help, but hierarchies are flexible and can be modified when organizational conditions so warrant. Senior managers see the big picture and therefore do not micromanage; instead, they attend to patterns and systems. Decisions are made by the person with the most expertise. A **bureaucracy** is a system of administration marked by adherence to fixed rules, red tape, authority by position rather than expertise, specialized and isolated "silos," and political decision making designed to obscure and protect the status quo.

- *Accident* or *failure* versus *human error.* The term *accident* describes a breakdown in a system that is complex and needs analysis. The term *error* suggests that only one factor, usually noted as the mistake of a human being, is the cause. If human error is assigned as the cause of harm, learning stops because a scapegoat has been identified.

- *Multicausal* versus *root cause.* The Swiss Cheese Model illustrates the multicausal concept, hypothesizing that multiple failures or errors must align to produce the conditions for an accident. An understanding of this concept, and the pursuit of the deeper story of an accident, will disclose the contributing conditions and latent vulnerabilities where accidents can occur. Analysis of the deeper story also allows for systemic actions to reduce the probability that a similar accident will occur in the future. Although the term *root cause analysis* is used in describing a retrospective exploratory process aimed at understanding what has happened when an event has occurred, a single root cause is seldom the product of such an exploration.

- *Learning* versus *judgment.* To build safer systems, an organization must be committed to learning from mistakes. Such a mind-set directs a passionate curiosity to dig deeply into the sources of failure and also into the sources of success, where harm was averted. Judgment presupposes a conclusion, introduces bias, and closes down inquiry.

Leaders Anchor a Safety Culture with Culture Carriers

Culture carriers ensure that change is enduring. They are interventions that define and shape the culture of an organization. Policies are strong culture carriers because they codify expectations and give guidance to behavior. Broad policies such as those that support blameless reporting are building blocks for creating safety.

Introducing a policy can create unintended effects. A new policy should be introduced judiciously. It should focus on broad organizational versus technical domains. Setting organizational policy is the responsibility of leaders. The following broad policies are suggested as anchors for the safety culture:

- *"Nothing about me without me"* (Delbanco and others, 2001). Recognizing patients and families as an active part of the system of care and not passive recipients brings an abundance of expertise and safety nets to the sharp end of care. This policy embraces practices and tools that involve the patient and family in decision making and participation in the care process. It includes providing information to patient and family through multiple vehicles, such as printed materials, the Internet, videos, educational courses, counseling, and conferencing, in a timely manner and in a way that can be understood. This includes ensuring not only that translators and translated materials are available for multicultural communities but also that cultural understanding and mediation are available to support effective care. Informational content focused on what patients and families want and need to know, on what they wish and need to ask, and on how they can engage to create safety with their providers is empowering and an essential part of care.

- *"If it looks wrong, it is wrong."* This policy gives anyone who perceives a risk to safety legitimate authority to stop a care process. This includes a patient and family. All participants have the responsibility to stop care processes until the question of risk has been thoroughly examined and safety has been established. This policy, fashioned after the **andon cord** policy in industry, empowers all participants in the health care system to act to establish safety without regard to hierarchy, and without risk of retaliation (Flinchbaugh, 2001).

- *Disclosure and truth telling.* This policy provides guidance for working with patients and families in the face of adverse events, near misses, or medical accidents. It establishes and guides expectations for communication. Elements of disclosure include a prompt and compassionate explanation of what is understood about what happened; information about the probable effects; information about what is being done to ensure safety; assurances that a full analysis will take place and that the findings of the analysis, as they are known, will be communicated; information about changes that are being made on the basis of the analytical findings, to reduce the likelihood of a similar event happening to another patient; and an acknowledgment of accountability including an apology. Professionals need to develop skills in this critical type of communication. The CEO has responsibility for ensuring that the necessary resources for this training are made available. Additional information on partnering with patients and families through disclosure is provided in Chapter Seven.

Leaders Define and Shape the Culture When Things Go Wrong

The leader's responses in the face of a medical accident are crucial to determining whether an organization advances or retreats from a culture of safety. Understanding how a leader should respond to a medical accident requires a detailed discussion about the leader's accountability to the patient and family, to staff members, and to external agencies. The leader's role in managing the inevitable tensions between accountability and blamelessness in an organization, and the leader's use of that tension as energy for change, is also a subject needing detailed discussion. Those subjects are the topic of Chapter Seven.

Failure and accidents contain critical information about how an organization is performing. Reactions to these failures are painful, powerful, and potent. How a leader chooses to react to failure will shape how an organization responds to the events of failure and perceptions of risk. Organizational cultures tend to defend and wall off information, thereby limiting ability to learn from and thus anticipate failure. Organizations that are successful in creating safety have discovered ways to change their reactions to failure. Changing expectations, and thus changing reactions, allows learning about performance.

Changing the reaction to failure begins with the leader. The question "What happened?" (versus "Who did it?") is an essential first step. A leader who personally reviews medical accidents and sentinel events demonstrates responsibility and commitment to learning.

Understanding a Family's Response to Medical Accident

The literature regarding psychological trauma is useful in understanding the experience of the patient and family who are victims of a medical accident (Vincent, Young, and Phillips, 1994), but the trauma associated with medical accident is unique. Betrayal is a prominent feature. The patient has been harmed in a situation in which they placed great trust. There is also fear of further harm when patients continue to be cared for in the same organization. This is very different from being harmed in a car accident and then taken to a hospital or another place of safety (Vincent, Young, and Phillips, 1994). Failure to recognize these features leaves family members feeling that their experience has been trivialized.

Accepting responsibility for safety includes continuing the duty of care to a family with ongoing communication, truth telling, and offers of support from an outside expert. Communication is a core competency of the health care professional and a core duty in a safety culture. The duty for leaders is to try to maintain a healing relationship with patients even in the face of tragedy.

A statement of responsibility and accountability and a sincere apology—"I am so sorry this happened" or "I apologize for the terrible event that has occurred to you"—are important elements of interaction with families and can be codified in a disclosure policy.

Responding to the Second Victim

The concerns of providers in circumstances of harm mirror those of families. Both need to be addressed. Leaders who accept responsibility for patient safety are cognizant of the impact that medical accidents have on "the second victim," the involved staff. Harm to patients affects the staff's confidence and sense of self-worth

(Hickson and others, 2002). The degree of blame in these situations has long-term consequences for staff members' personal adaptation after an event (Tennen and Affleck, 1990). The leader's initial responses to providers involved in a medical accident can deeply affect the providers' short- and long-term recovery. Skilled resource personnel outside the situation must be made available to take hold of and guide the situation. The management system must be meticulous in ensuring that verbal and nonverbal communication is compassionate and free of blame.

Concept to Action: Closing the Gap between a Patient's Family and a CEO

A teenaged patient was diagnosed incorrectly. After initial improvement, he failed to respond to treatment, and his family and the managing physician began seeking new answers. They arranged for further diagnostic testing, evaluation, and an outside opinion. When the correct diagnosis was established, months of treatment had been lost. The young man died of an elusive cancer.

Family members worked hard to learn from the organization how a misdiagnosis could have happened but were provided with little information. In a regulatory environment where error is punished severely, and where courts can award settlements that have the potential to cripple an organization, the organization feared retribution and refused to respond to the family.

When family members threatened to tell their story to the media, the CEO agreed to meet with them, asking the hospital's risk manager and attorney to join him. The family members—the young man's parents and his siblings—arrived at the CEO's office and laid out a framed photo of their son and brother. They demanded to know who was at fault and what was being done to make sure this type of event would not happen again.

This was the first meeting the CEO had ever had with a family regarding a failure in care. The CEO, following the counsel of the hospital's attorney and risk manager, avoided disclosing any significant information. After the meeting, the attorney and the risk manager congratulated the CEO for his ability to demonstrate sympathy without disclosing any information.

"It was the worst meeting of my career," the CEO said later. "We stonewalled this family."

The hospital was in the process of creating a policy of disclosure to families in cases of medical accident, but progress was advancing slowly with extreme caution. After the CEO's meeting with the family, leadership team members sat down to explore other ways the meeting could have unfolded. They asked each other, "How would we want to be responded to if we were the family faced with this situation?"

A second meeting was scheduled with the family. This time the chair of the board, the chair of the board quality committee, and a member of the executive leadership staff were present. Again the family members brought pictures of their lost son and brother. There were no attorneys or risk managers present. It was agreed that the meeting would be held with full disclosure. The family was told the sequence of events in the young man's care and what was understood about the incorrect diagnosis. They were told what the organization had learned from the experience and the changes that had been made to prevent such an occurrence from happening again. In an emotional and tearful exchange, the officers of the organization apologized to the family and accepted responsibility for failures in the system of care.

The family asked that specific persons involved in the event be named and singled out for sanction. Hospital leaders remained firm that the misdiagnosis had occurred because the system had failed and not because of careless or incompetent individuals.

The sorrow of failing a family inspired the organization to accelerate action around improving patient safety. Staff members and leaders discussed how an organization devoted to families could act this way in the face of a family's loss. They discussed the lessons learned from this family, including how to respond to tragedy and how to build a foundation of disclosure in the organization. A new commitment was forged to create a comprehensive culture of disclosure, truth telling, and responsibility, built on full partnership with families.

The staff caring for the patient and his family throughout the ordeal also required healing. Early reactions of blame, defensiveness, and criticism had damaged their trust in each other and in the organization. They felt isolated, guilty, and angry. Relationships had fractured, and staff members needed to find closure and move forward through their grief. Leaders met with the staff and providers who had been involved in the patient's care, apologizing for the organization's failure to respond to them as well as to the patient's family. Outside expert resources were offered and healing began.

Finally, the leaders fully accepted executive responsibility for patient safety. They made a commitment to design and operate safe systems. They promised patients' families and health professionals that the organization, as its first priority, would do no harm.

The Business Case for Safety

In addition to providing safe high-quality care, an overarching role of leaders is to operate their organizations cost-effectively. Such financial stewardship provides affordable care and services, ensures the ability to reinvest in growth and capability expansion, and ensures long-term viability of the organization. Leaders face questions about how pursuing a safety culture will affect the bottom line or produce a return on investment (ROI). Little information exists on the costs of a comprehensive safety initiative, but the costs of not having one are immense:

- Organizations invest substantial resources to address each preventable accident, each increase in the cost of care for reversal and recovery from the effects of error, and each investigation to ferret out wrongdoing. In the end, the "shame and blame" culture of medicine drives away experienced, talented employees who are assets to an organization.

- Organizations risk regulatory sanction and possible litigation after medical accidents.
- Organizations whose accidents are made public risk the loss of public confidence and a tarnished reputation.
- Indirect costs are borne by society and business interests. These costs include lost income, increased disability rates, and increased burden on caregivers when patients are injured as a result of error (Weeks and Bagian, 2003).

Overarching this discussion are the incalculable costs in lives and human suffering. The practice of medicine is grounded in the Hippocratic oath to do no harm. Beyond all financial and business arguments stands the moral imperative to deliver safe care, or do no harm, for the good of patients, health professionals, and the public.

Calculating the Costs of Adverse Events

The original Harvard Practice Study concluded that 4.7 percent of people admitted to a hospital experienced an adverse event, and of these events two-thirds were estimated as preventable (Leape, 1993). Applying these early findings, leaders can estimate the predicted number of patients to experience an adverse event. The studies have further shown that each preventable medication adverse event adds $4,685 to costs of care (Bates and others, 1997). An economic estimate can be made for increased costs due to preventable adverse events. Analyzing actual adverse events in an organization to determine their cost is a worthwhile initiative. Engaging the chief financial officer in this exercise is an important strategy for developing awareness and appreciation of the issue.

It is important to note that an accurate economic model of this problem is impossible to construct. Adverse events are not caused by unusual or rare circumstances (Johnson and Bootman, 1997). Rather, these events make up a familiar list, including wound infections, drug overdoses, administration of the wrong drugs, bleeding from anticoagulation, insulin reactions, missed diagnoses, and falls. Because these risks and events are known and predictable, they are also preventable. It is estimated that these preventable events represent 69.6 percent of medical accidents (Leape and others, 1993).

Studies have also found that preventable adverse events occur across sites and locations and are not concentrated in what are often perceived as higher-risk settings (such as surgeries or intensive care units). Therefore, attention can be focused on the system as a whole: the hospital, the clinic, the emergency department, free-standing ambulatory care units, and diagnostic settings (Leape, Lawthers, Brennan, and Johnson, 1993). The work of patient safety is not limited to the highest-risk clinical inpatient environments; it is the work of the entire system of care, with particular attention to hand-offs and transitions between areas and functions, which create gaps in which risk is amplified and the probability of medical accident is increased.

Improving Quality and Patient Safety

Improving safety improves care and eliminates the costs of poor quality. Safety serves as a more compelling rallying point for efficiency and productivity than the cost-cutting messages that often have caused morale to plummet in the health care industry and may have caused increased risk.

The business case for patient safety rests on reducing the costs of poor quality. The development of aligned and effective systems of care delivery at every point along the continuum, from supply of products to the care encounter will eliminate waste, reduce cost, and mitigate risk. When patient safety becomes an explicit business strategy, near misses and accidents must be examined in detail. The organization must be examined from the perspective of process flow. As Jerry Massman, a chief financial officer, stated, "Efficient and effective systems are safe systems" (Shapiro, 2000).

In most health care organizations, people have learned to work around unnecessary complexity, **process failures**, and other system issues. When people adapt their practices to faulty systems, waste is usually produced. Waste in processes adds additional cost burdens and frustration to the work of patient care. Chronic process failure becomes normalized deviance that is not only costly; it also adds risk of accidents in the care system.

An engaged and stable workforce contributes to safety and reduces the costs of turnover and declining productivity. A safe organization builds confidence and enhances its reputation in a way that can be translated into loyalty and market share. However, there is an investment required. Designating an operating budget to support patient safety and funding applied research are leadership roles.

Making Decisions about Investments in Patient Safety

Patient safety is not a domain over which to preside. It requires active involvement and investment. Investment in patient safety requires investment in budgeting and staffing for the number of competent, well-trained personnel it takes to do the job. Planning for this investment involves several dimensions:

- *Leaders assume failure will occur.* This assumption leads to planning for recovery and automatic course corrections, such as radiology film "over-reads" and call-backs. The goal is to prevent harm from reaching patients and to harness the failure that occurs, learn from it, and use it to create a more robust system.
- *Leaders ensure that staffing levels and staffing plans are aligned with the findings of human factors research about human limitations.* Staffing levels can detract from or contribute to safety. Levels should match workloads well enough to provide for periodic breaks and to minimize extended work hours. This planning prevents fatigue and decreases the probability of slips, lapses, and mistakes. Safety demands a skill level that comes from training. This training, including simulations, drills, and debriefings, requires financial resources in order to be successful. Appropriately staffed teams also allow for work simplification and reduced hand-offs, which will reduce the probability of error. Fatigue, sleeplessness, illness, boredom, frustration, fear, and stressful working conditions are physiological and psychological contributors to error. Creating systems designed to remove or reduce them will help increase safety.
- *Leaders plan work environments and technology to ensure and improve safety.* Charts, protocols, preprinted orders, calculators, decision supports, checklists, checks, and alerts can all be used to reduce reliance on memory and manual calculations. The ergonomics of the environment, involving distractions, noise, lighting, levels of activity, clutter, temperature, and faulty workflow, also affect safety. The layout and design of work environments can contribute to safety or produce barriers for staff to work around or overcome.
- *Leaders plan for the introduction of changes to minimize the potential of increased risk.* The modern evolution of health care services has introduced complexity into the workplace, and this is a major factor in the rate of medical accidents. The manner in which new technologies are introduced to the workplace can add risk and lead to unanticipated consequences. Leaders are responsible for ensuring that increased risk does not accompany the increased capabilities that come with progress. The following case study illustrates how one organization used incremental steps to reduce the risks of new technologies.

Concept to Action: Planning for Changes to Improve Safety through Information Technology

In the near future, Dr. Jim Levin, medical director of informatics, will be able to walk into one of the patient rooms in his multihospital system and see the patient's bedside dramatically changed by technology: a nurse will be able to call up the patient's medical record on the computer by the patient's bedside. A physician will use a mobile wireless computer to order new prescriptions. Online knowledge bases, such as those for medication references and clinical standards, will help physicians make decisions about medications. Bar codes will be used to ensure that the right medication is given to the right patient at the right time. Prompts built into software will help verify the kind of medication and the dose ordered. Specialists will be able to use the computer to call up the latest lab results to show the patient, and, with a few clicks, be able to show in graphic format how the new results compare with previous tests. When a patient leaves the hospital and continues treatment in an outpatient clinic, the patient's medical information will automatically follow the patient.

These changes enabled by the hospital system's information technology investments are immense, but they are being phased in slowly over several years.

"The implementation of each element needs to be successful," says Levin. "So as each module of the technology matures, we bring it live. Benefits are achieved earlier and, at each step, we leverage the available functionality to advance patient safety and to increase efficiency."

Busy staff members have a chance to get used to the changes gradually and understand any potential unintended consequences and recovery mechanisms.

"It emphasizes the reality of implementation to the organization with gradual introduction of change—and it minimizes the training needs," says Levin.

The organization plans regular quarterly "releases" of modules of the technology. The releases are usually rolled out on one hospital campus at a time. "Clinical decision support," or the use of technology to inform clinical judgments, is seen as a theme, not as the outcome of one specific project.

"Clinical decision support is part of every project, not the last project," says Levin. "It's an approach that brings knowledge resources directly to care providers."

Along the way, information technology leaders have learned valuable lessons about implementing large-scale technology changes:

- *Expect change and plan for change.* "Contingencies and slippages will happen," says Glenn Galloway, chief information officer at Children's Hospitals and Clinics, Minneapolis/St. Paul, Minnesota, "and 'course correction' is a core competency for this work. It helps to attune management to think about flexibility in their planning."
- *Planning requires detailed and ongoing assessment of your vendor.* "Our project leaders meet quarterly with our vendor for ongoing reality checks of product timelines. The meetings help us identify the changes we need to make on our end to ensure that project implementation is successful."

An implementation task force that oversees all project teams was needed for an effective rollout of new modules. While project teams are immersed in the details of their individual efforts, the overall task force takes a broader perspective on the effort, looking across departments to plan training, identify barriers, and communicate about the implementation to the departments involved. The task force takes a broader perspective, looking at the project from the point of view of the departments that will use the technology, and determining the impact of multiple projects on the end user.

The leader's role in accepting responsibility for patient safety is pivotal in defining, inspiring, and developing an organization's responses to failure and designing and operating safer systems. Dedicating the resources to educate and advance patient safety underlies the leader's role and organizational commitment. The willingness and enthusiasm to engage in the work of patient safety, and the courage to stay the course and model the way, are the leader's responsibility.

The more you know and do as a leader in patient safety, the more you will see what has to be done. As our industry effectively tackles the known risks of today's environment, new and emerging risks will be continually introduced by new knowledge, technology, and pharmaceutical agents, changing workforce demographics, patient vulnerabilities, and availability of resources. Aggressively learning the lessons of today will create greater intelligence and capacity to address the challenges of the future. It is a worthy pursuit for the leader, one that adds value to health care delivery.

Summary Points

1. The leader sets the stage for the safety culture by embracing error and learning from failure. Hazards and vulnerabilities and perceived unsafe conditions are identified, examined, made visible, and mitigated. Leaders in a culture of safety face reality, acknowledge that risk is present and always emerging, and confront risk by taking informed, effective action.

2. Leaders facilitate a continual pursuit of information—persistently asking "Why?" until all known potential contributing factors have been exhausted—and accountability is assigned for the necessary changes that must occur to close gaps in safety.

3. Accepting responsibility to create a culture of patient safety requires leaders to accept their part in the current state and rethink the beliefs that they have held. Leaders' decisions and actions influence whether safety is compromised or facilitated.
   - Leaders redefine how the organization talks about patient safety by using a new language comprising a thoughtful, deliberate vocabulary.

- Leaders anchor the safety culture through such culture carriers as policies that include patients as partners and that guide communication with families when an accident occurs.
- When the system has failed, how a leader chooses to respond to patients, families, and staff members shapes how the organization will respond to future failures and perceptions of risk.

4. Leadership accountability is at the heart of culture change to create patient safety.

CHAPTER FIVE

IMPORT NEW KNOWLEDGE AND SKILLS

The knowledge base required to instill safety throughout operations and perform as a high reliability organization is lacking in health care. New knowledge and skills need to be learned and adapted to health care. A high-reliability organization is one in which failure is not an option, because lives are at stake. Although the performance of hazardous activities is the norm in such organizations, accident or harm rates are low. Poole (1997, p. 40) asks readers to envision the following scenario:

> Imagine that it's a busy day, and you shrink San Francisco Airport to only one short runway and one ramp and gate. Make planes take off and land at the same time, at half the present time interval, rock the runway from side to side, and require that everyone who leaves in the morning returns that same day. Then turn off the radar to avoid detection, impose strict controls on radios, fuel the aircraft in place with their engines running. Now wet the whole thing down with salt water and oil, and man it with 20-year-olds, half of whom have never seen an airplane close up.

These are the conditions of *Nimitz*-style aircraft carriers. Danger and risk are clear and present in their operations, and yet they have a remarkable safety record. Other HROs, such as those in the fields of aviation, aerospace, nuclear energy, and smoke-jumper organizations, face similar dangers. They also have a signifi-cant history of safety from which health care can learn.

Health care has much in common with other high-risk industries. High-reliability applications from nonmedical high-risk domains (such as aviation, aero-space, and nuclear power) can be adapted to advance safety in health care.

Characteristics and Structure of High-Reliability Organizations

Health care and its high-risk counterparts are **large-scale complex systems** in which decisions are made with less than perfect information, in stressful con-ditions that are full of uncertainty. To add to these challenges, large-scale complex systems have specific organizational characteristics that challenge the pursuit of safety (Grabowski and Roberts, 1997):

- *Simultaneous autonomy and interdependence.* Tightly coupled work processes frequently create situations in which individuals, although socialized to be independent op-erators, must rely on each other if they are to execute tasks successfully.
- *Multiple cultures.* Many distinct cultures operate simultaneously in large-scale complex systems. Doctors, nurses, and pharmacists are all socialized and trained in distinct ways, even though successful outcomes in their fields require highly aligned teamwork.
- *Intended and unintended consequences.* In a large-scale complex system, every action has intended consequences, but may have unplanned outcomes as well. For ex-ample, given the complexity of the human body, one person may suffer an al-lergic reaction to a drug, whereas another tolerates the drug well.
- *Long incubation periods during which risk can arise.* A risk can be planted in a large-scale system and lie dormant long before an effect, benign or adverse, appears. For ex-ample, deferred maintenance on a bedside ventilator or fire extinguisher may eventually lead to equipment failure and a catastrophic outcome.
- *Risk migration.* Risk that is mitigated in one part of a large-scale complex system can move to another part. For example, an intensive care unit may discharge a patient at 11:00 A.M. in order to maximize its own efficiency and function-ing, but that hour may also be the time that is most chaotic and risk-prone in the unit to which the patient is being transferred.

Although health care shares characteristics with other large-scale complex sys-tems, there are differences that challenge high-reliability performance. Roberts (1999) has studied HROs and found several characteristics that define high reliability.

Foremost is the explicit aim that *the lives and safety of everyone is the number one goal.* The structure of the organization flows from this goal. HROs may appear solely hierarchical on the surface, but they are actually quite dynamic, with three layers of organizational structure that emerge for different situations. The workforce organizes itself into different patterns to meet the demands of particular situations:

1. *In day-to-day operations, a structure of functional hierarchy, not bureaucracy, makes everyone accountable to the goal of safety.* The organization has a functional **command and control** for routine operations. There are **formal rules and procedures** that purposefully create an environment of thoughtful and intelligent adherence (what in HROs is called "heedful attention") versus automatic or routine (versus heedful) compliance. Training is a priority, and investments in training particular to the work situation are made for the workforce. Training includes mental rehearsals and simulations to anticipate and respond to contingencies, as well as discipline and guidance around communication and teamwork. Required competencies are clearly designated, and there is ongoing verification of competencies. Expertise is developed by training to cope with expected problems. A **structure of hierarchy** promotes clear decision-making authority and accountability. Senior managers see the big picture, identify patterns and potential risks, and make regular course corrections as needed. This practice is exemplified by the senior officer standing on the bridge of an aircraft carrier, overseeing the on-deck activity of a well-trained and well-rehearsed team.

2. *A structure of collaboration takes over in situations of increased risk.* When risk is emerging, for example when planes are landing and taking off, the hierarchical structure gives way to a highly interactive and **collaborative structure**. Positional authority gives way to expertise. There is constant communication and eye contact among members of the team. They watch each other, listening for what is unusual so that problems can be rectified before intolerable risk emerges. The capacity to be constantly alert leads to situational awareness and is aided by **ambient listening**, or listening to detect anything unusual in the noise or nature of communications in the work area. Anyone can ask a question, and the team member with the most expertise provides the answer. Any member of the team may stop an action if they perceive that conditions of risk may overwhelm the team's ability to manage and recover. When this stop-the-line policy is invoked to restore safety, it is respected and adhered to. If the call is incorrect, the mistake is viewed as an opportunity for further learning. If the call is correct and has prevented an accident, the team member is publicly recognized and rewarded.

3. *A predetermined structure with clear roles and responsibilities is rehearsed and emerges in situations of clear and present danger.* This third organizational structure mobilizes in circumstances such as a fire on the flight deck of an aircraft carrier. In this situation, team members move into predetermined roles that have been carefully rehearsed and that everyone understands. Decisive, coordinated, competent action is required in these circumstances because there is no time for delegation or role negotiation.

These examples of high-reliability performance can be extended to the health care environment, as in an emergency department, an intensive care unit, an operating suite, an acute medical or surgical unit, or a clinic. Patients arrive and depart, much as airplanes land and take off, as assessments, treatments, procedures, medications, and care are being provided. Risks are continually emerging: life-threatening emergencies such as a cardiac arrest, trauma stabilization, hemorrhage, suicide attempt. The team of providers, caregivers, and support staff can be organized to function in a way that reflects the resilience found in high-reliability organizations, or team members can function in a more fragmented, "siloed" manner.

Despite hierarchies and regulations, HROs are constantly changing; questioning is an accepted practice, and team members who continually search for ways to improve are valued. Front-line workers strive to avoid errors of omission and commission that may have unexpected consequences. Employees are vigilant, constantly thinking about actions to avoid harm. HROs are both centralized and decentralized, hierarchical and collegial, rule-bound and learning-centered. Leaders in HROs continually anticipate the future and question what adaptations are being made at the front line and why they are occurring. This type of leadership focus keeps the culture nimble and underscores the idea that safety is a dynamic, emerging, adaptive process.

Barriers to High Reliability in Health Care

There are numerous examples of how health care organizations have begun to successfully adapt concepts from high-reliability organizations, but there are considerable forces that present barriers to achieving high reliability performance. As health care leaders begin to apply the lessons from HROs, they need to anticipate these barriers and plan to address them.

Health care professionals are, by and large, caring and conscientious people and are devastated when an accident occurs. The typical response—to blame, criticize, and punish the individual who happens to be closest to the failure or accident—compounds personal feelings of failure, isolation, and shame. These effects also damage the organization. Fear causes professionals to push errors, near misses, and accidents underground, masking hazards in the workplace. If blame is assigned to failure, all learning stops. Any opportunity to correct the underlying vulnerabilities in the system is lost. The conditions, seen and unseen, that produced the accident persist unchanged, and it is just a matter of time until they reassemble to produce an accident involving different people.

Health care can benefit from the work of James Reason and colleagues, who have identified a group of core pathological elements: blame, denial, and the pursuit of the wrong kind of excellence, that, when present, cause organizations to be more susceptible to adverse events. This group of core elements creates what they have termed the "Vulnerable System Syndrome (VSS)" (Reason, Carthey, and de Leval, 2001). Blame and denial have been addressed earlier in this volume. Single-minded pursuit of the wrong kind of excellence has to do with such management goals as efficiency, cost savings, and patient satisfaction with such ancillary services as a hospital's décor or its menu at the expense of patient safety. Each of the three core pathologies identified by Reason and his colleagues interacts with and increases the strength of the other two, and together they create a self-sustaining cycle that is a malignant, undermining influence on efforts to change culture, rendering the organization vulnerable rather than resilient to patient harm. Reason and his colleagues have developed a checklist for assessing institutional resilience, which is included in Appendix One.

There are three different kinds of domains of work: simple, complicated, and complex. Simple problems can be managed by a recipe or protocol. Complicated problems require multiple steps of analysis and multiple perspectives for system design and control. Complex problems require more individual freedom, with reminders and alerts, and with sharing and understanding of deviations from protocol. Creating patient safety and developing a culture of high reliability is a complex problem, and it cannot be solved through study of points in time or use of the complicated problem solving well known to medicine and to health care.

Agreement and certainty are high in simple problems. The question of how to bake a cake is a simple problem, and following a recipe is a clear map. A complicated problem introduces more variables, less certainty, and a broader zone within which agreement must be negotiated. Examples of complicated problems include the question of how to conduct open-heart surgery or a quality improvement project. A complex problem is characterized by ambiguity, and dynamic and changing interactions of parts that combine and propagate in unpredictable ways, with nonlinear effects. Disagreement is high; continual trade-offs and negotiations are required. McCandless and Zimmerman (2002) illustrate this domain by the example of raising a child. Creating a culture of patient safety is complex work. Complexity-inspired approaches are likely to have the highest probability of success, whereas simple and complicated approaches may use numerous resources and require great effort and yet have little impact or sustainability. In a complex system, small changes can have big effects and big changes can have little or no effect because of the complex system's attribute of nonlinearity.

Tables 5.1 and 5.2 depict a developmental trajectory for health care's journey to greater safety. Table 5.1, from left to right, shows three types of organizations that evolve from simple to complicated to complex. In a complex system, there is no single strategy; rather, there are multiple sources of information from people, events, and relationships that continually provide input into decision making. In a **complex adaptive system**, one single event can have a big result, whereas big initiatives can bring about very little change.

Table 5.2 integrates the terminology of Roberts (1999), Reason (2001), and Westrum (1992). It depicts an evolution, again from left to right, in terms of maturing development toward a safety culture.

As explored in previous chapters, organizations committed to safety make errors and near misses transparent for learning. Strategically, errors and near misses are valued as learning opportunities that will make the delivery system safer. Ascribing error solely to individual failure is not part of the thinking; rather, it is recognized that such an approach only serves to drive errors underground.

Unfortunately, regulatory and legal systems often reinforce the pathological health care culture by emphasizing individual culpability and punishment for error (see Chapter Eight). Vulnerabilities hidden in system and process failures are not well addressed, either by the legal system or by licensing bodies. Licensing boards in medicine, nursing, and pharmacy often focus on individual responsibility for error and seek to limit or remove professional licenses. An environment of fear permeates the working lives of professionals, and errors are driven underground.

TABLE 5.1. DEVELOPMENTAL TRAJECTORY FROM SIMPLE TO COMPLEX

Simple	Complicated	Complex
Health care before the Information Age	Health care today	The health care system as a high-reliability organization

TABLE 5.2. DEVELOPMENT OF A SAFETY CULTURE

Vulnerable System	Large-Scale System	High-Reliability System
Pathological	Bureaucratic	Generative
Almost any health care system before the IOM	A health care system that is beginning the journey toward patient safety	A health care system that achieves a culture of safety

Another cultural barrier to using the lessons offered by HROs is the hierarchical nature of medical practice. The hierarchy that exists between patients and physicians places the doctor in the position of expert and the patient in the position of a passive, subordinate recipient of services. The hierarchy is replicated between the various health professions—doctor to nurse, nurse to nursing assistant, pharmacist to pharmacy technician. In a high-reliability organization, the knowledge and contributions of all members of the team are welcomed and respected, regardless of title or organizational status. When health care achieves a safety culture, the patient will be a partner in his or her own care, and collaborative teamwork will be the norm.

How to Adapt High Reliability to Health Care

High-reliability organizations share common factors that create safety (Roberts, 1999). The following factors are among the most relevant ones to be applied in health care:

- *Communication.* On a flight deck, everyone announces what is going on as it happens, to increase the likelihood that someone will notice and react if something starts to go wrong. Controllers constantly watch out for one another, listening and looking for signs of trouble, trading advice, and offering suggestions for the best way to route traffic.
- *Risk acknowledgment.* HROs acknowledge that practitioners face complexity in their work processes and appreciate that front-line workers must cope with ever-escalating change and information overload. Leaders of HROs respond to their workers' needs and design the work environment to accommodate these realities. In contrast, health care clinicians face increased expectations for perfect outcomes because of widely publicized technological advances and a decade-long emphasis on production and outcome, and because of increasing demands for service. Practitioners also grapple with new vulnerabilities in patients as peo-

ple live longer and trade death for difficult-to-manage chronic illnesses. With the modern technology that saves and prolongs lives, complexity increases. These conditions must be appreciated and acknowledged before they can be dealt with effectively.

- *Emphasis is on active learning.* In HROs, employees know why procedures are written as they are, but they can challenge them and look for ways to make them better and more relevant. Poole (1997, p. 44) gives some of the reasons for this provision: "Once people begin doing everything by the book, operations quickly go downhill. Workers lose interest and become bored: They forget or never learn why the organization does things certain ways; and they begin to feel more like cogs in a machine than integral parts of a vibrant organization. Effective organizations need to find ways to keep their members fresh and focused on the job at hand." As the organization ensures that employees do not become complacent, employees in turn will remain vigilant and ensure that the organization does not regress to an earlier unsafe state.

The following case study provides an example of how one hospital used lessons from HROs to modify and improve teamwork on a medical-surgical unit.

Concept to Action: Learning Team-Based Solutions from High-Reliability Organizations

Clinicians from a pediatric hospital visited an air traffic control tower to observe high reliability in action. They also engaged an expert from the airline industry to speak to staff members. Nurses from a medical-surgical unit became interested in the teamwork techniques used by the air traffic controllers.

Nurses' and air traffic controllers' jobs have many similarities. Both cope daily with "takeoffs" and "landings" (admissions, discharges, transfers) and other risks. Their jobs are inherently unpredictable. To be successful, team members must rely on each other, and yet the busy work environment makes it easy for an individual to slip into his or her own mental "to do" list.

Nurses began to identify the team work applications that they had learned from aviation. One application made was to develop a self-assignment system. When nurses arrived for their shifts, they selected their own patients on the basis of their individual expertise, their previous relationships with patients, and other factors.

Another application was the "huddle." In an air traffic control tower, team members engage in **ambient listening** to maintain constant situational awareness of the everyday activity around them and scan for irregularities or potentially emerging risk. When conditions are detected that are moving them into zones of intolerable risk, workers stand up from their cubicles to establish critical communication with each other, and reassess, reprioritize, and redistribute work to reduce risk and restore a zone of safety. The nurses developed a similar system that helped the team reassess and redistribute work each day in the face of changing circumstances that could add risk. Any nurse could call a huddle whenever conditions become especially busy or uncomfortable to reassess, redistribute work in the face of changing circumstances, and buddy-up as necessary to provide better care. Passing each other between patients' rooms, the nurses listened for signs of emerging risk. If a huddle was called, the team members asked each other, "Is anyone overwhelmed? Are there ways to change the patient assignments or workload to improve care and reduce risk?"

The techniques improved safety, patient flow, and morale on the unit, according to the patient care manager of the unit. "In the old system, sometimes a lone nurse would say, 'It's been a horrid day. I was behind all day, and I didn't get to take a break,' while other nurses had a very good day. We rarely hear that anymore. Staff members no longer express feeling left out or unassisted. When it gets harried, they can call the huddle to make sure everything happens that needs to happen for our kids and families."

Another Example of HRO Adaptation

The following case study describes how another organization used the lessons of HROs to design a strategy of identifying and mitigating risk in day-to-day operations.

Concept to Action: Acknowledging, Predicting, and Learning to Prevent Risk-Prone Conditions with the Zone Strategy

Every day, health care professionals at the sharp end create safety by compensating for risk-prone conditions. Predicting and preventing those risk-prone conditions is the goal of the zone strategy. Katharine Luther, director of performance improvement at Memorial Hermann Healthcare System, Houston, created the zone strategy to predict when conditions exist that have the potential to overwhelm a team's ability to protect patients.

The zone strategy, which categorizes risk at green, yellow, or red levels, is predicated on the concept of the **tipping point**, a single event that can propel a manageable situation out of control (Gladwell, 2000). The theory of the tipping point is that one occurrence, such as an unexpected admission, a code, or a clinician's calling in sick, can tip the balance in a situation from one of stability to one where conditions can spiral out of control. "Caregivers often fail to recognize destabilizing patterns that occur with great frequency in their work environments, attributing them to 'special cause' variation, the unpredictability of their work, or the unique needs of individual patients," says Luther (2001). Using human factors science, Luther developed a list of prompts to help caregivers identify these situations prospectively.

Clinicians are prompted to use the colors green, yellow, and red to identify current conditions in the workplace and to prevent conditions from escalating. Teams create their own definitions for the red, yellow, and green zones on their units, using the following steps:

1. *Risk categories are identified.* The team pinpoints the hazards of the unit and how normalization of deviance may have affected responses to risk-prone conditions. Team members discuss situations in which they have felt out of control and times when they have not thought that the resources available to them would allow them to recover.
2. Risks are quantified and categorized into one of three zones. The risks may include increases in census, increased patient acuity, and emergent activity. The green zone is described as comfortable, the yellow zone indicates risk-prone conditions and the need to be alert, and the red zone indicates conditions of moving into intolerable risk or what Amalberti (2001) calls "boundaries of excediency" (see Table 5.3).

TABLE 5.3. ZONE STRATEGY

Category	Green	Yellow	Red
Census	xxx–xxx	xxx–xxx	xxx–xxx
Agency/Float	1	2	4
Acuity	xxx–xxx	xxx–xxx	xxx–xxx
Emergent Activity: admissions, procedures, increasing acuity	2 procedures; 2 admissions	4 post-op admissions	1 code; 3 post-op admissions
Day/Shift	Monday–Thursday	Friday, Sunday	Saturday, Holidays
Initiate/consider:		No additional float; frequent rounds; screening of admissions	Direct on unit; close admissions; extra housekeeping; double the number of linen deliveries; "time out" for staff; delivery of sand-wiches; reliance on everybody for help
Identify for:	Hospital; units/areas (ED, ICUs, general floors); departments (radiology, dietary, housekeeping)		

Source: K. Luther, *Zone Strategy: Knowing Your Zone Keeps Patients Safe* (Chicago: National Patient Safety Foundation, 2001). Used by permission.

3. *Solutions are identified.* Proactive, individual, and team-based interventions are created, with an emphasis on ideas that are easy to implement.
4. *Zones are implemented and monitored.* At designated intervals, ranging from every shift to every hour, depending on the individual unit's preferences and daily circumstances, the zone status is revisited and revised if necessary (Luther, 2001).

In the end, staff members created lists of the unique tipping points for their units or teams.

"We worked with staff around the tendency to say, 'What a terrible day, and I hope it doesn't happen again tomorrow.' When they're not in the heat of the moment, we convene staff to talk about the variables that cause them to feel out of control," says Luther. "Staff can quickly finish the sentence, 'It's a good day when . . .' or 'It's a yellow day when. . . . '"

The risks and solutions vary widely by unit. In obstetrics, for example, the staff members identified that the time of day women in labor arrived affected their zone. If two or three patients arrived in labor before 10:00 A.M., the rest of the day was overwhelming, even when the 3:00 P.M. shift employees arrived to assist. As a solution, the unit chose 10:00 A.M. as a check-in time for identifying a zone. When two or more women were in labor by 10:00 A.M., the zone was elevated to yellow. Staff members devised a plan whereby a team member from the 3:00 P.M. shift was available by pager to come in early on yellow zone days. Often, reports Luther, the on-call employee was able to leave at the end of eight hours of work, but the knowledge of his or her availability during the busy time kept staff members from elevating into a red zone.

Some units created partnerships to address elevated zone conditions. The surgery and orthopedics unit found that their patient populations rarely kept both units busy at the same time. Therefore, the units arranged for unit clerks to be cross-trained in each unit and transferred as needed during the day coincident to workload fluctuations.

Memorial Hermann is experimenting with a team of two nurses, trained in critical care, who are available as short-term floats to any unit in a yellow zone.

"The idea is for them to arrive on the scene, size up the situation, move in, and help clear out the backlog," says Luther. "They are highly specialized and experienced, and are expected to move around all day." The nurses remain on a unit no longer than two hours, to prevent the units from relying on them as regular backup staff.

The solutions developed through the zone strategy have helped predict and prevent risk, have increased patient satisfaction and, along with other concurrent changes in process, have decreased serious adverse events. The positive results have compensated well for the investments in the zone strategy's implementation. Needs and solutions among the units have varied, but most units have found that small solutions can mitigate problems.

"It only took one of something to lower the zone of risk," says Luther. "One nurse for an hour, one patient discharging off the unit—one can get you out of trouble."

Leadership

The primary role for leaders is to design safe systems of care grounded in a culture of trust and shared values. This is accomplished through training in effective and varied communication that focuses on creating shared mental models and diverse decision making. (Using these methods to create accountability is discussed in further detail in Chapter Seven.) The following tools can assist leaders in meeting these accountability goals:

- *Risk/**process auditing.*** Ongoing checks and audits help spot unexpected safety issues. Analytical tools, such as **Failure Mode and Effects Analysis (FMEA)**, help leaders conduct prospective audits.
- *Process control.* This is a tool for developing meaningful rules, procedures, and training that emphasizes specific skills. It is also used for building strategic redundancies into areas of vulnerability.
- *Reward systems.* Recognition and reward systems drive the attention and behavior of the organization. People are thanked for reporting potential dangers and promoting safe practices and behaviors.
- *Risk Perception.* This involves training and reinforcing the members of an organization to recognize and report risk, and cultivating an alert "on-your-toes" attitude that pervades the organization.

The following case study explores how one organization used these tools, in addition to others discussed in this chapter, to improve safety after a medical accident.

Concept to Action: Using High-Reliability Tools to Reduce the Probability of Medical Accidents

"With ECMO, it's always an intense time, always a complex patient," states the medical director of an extracorporeal membrane oxygenation (ECMO) program in a busy neonatal intensive care unit.

A nurse in the program explains, "With ECMO, even with the best efforts, death may result, because ECMO is an extraordinary effort to save a child's life."

ECMO, a highly technical heart-lung bypass machine usually used on premature infants on the brink of death, is an example of the complexity of modern health care. The machine uses subsystems and parts from a variety of manufacturers. A team of forty highly trained people, covering twenty-four-hour shifts, is needed to care for one child requiring ECMO technology. Rapidly improved and changing technology has made the operating manuals obsolete for the pump systems in use.

The design of the system is predisposed to error; the complexity of the procedure has the potential to set a lethal sequence of events in motion. In one case, an error was identified, intercepted, and corrected before it reached the patient. An experienced and highly skilled team member had missed one of the seventy steps in the sequence of procedures necessary to place a child on ECMO. No report of the near miss was made.

Months later, the same error occurred, and again the trajectory was set in motion. This time, the error combined in a lethal combination with other variables, and the error reached the patient.

"It was devastating," said a senior leader at the time. "The conditions that had operated in the near miss had reassembled. We had the opportunity under much less painful conditions to reduce the probability of harm, and we missed it."

The accident propelled the organization to change the environment to reduce the potential for harm. The organization began an intensive case analysis of what had happened and began generating ideas for change.

After the initial training, most learning happened on the job and through verbal knowledge passed from team member to team member, and from shift to shift.

According to a nurse, the lack of a systematic, intentional method for transferring information created a tense environment.

"When I would come on and a child was going to be put on ECMO, I would be thinking, 'Will I remember everything? Would something on the machine break or happen?' These are the most skilled, knowledgeable, and experienced nurses on the unit. Yet ECMO is needed infrequently. We didn't have enough practice working together."

After the accident, safety became the explicit first priority in the ECMO program.

"We had talked about safety, certainly," says the doctor, "but we didn't look at every single thing we did and ask, 'Is this the safest way we can do it?' There was a mental shift after the accident, where we started to look at everything we do in order to minimize risk. And we realized we have to assume there will be human error—just priming the pump is a seventy-step process."

The team used many of the lessons from HROs in building a safer ECMO program.

Simulations

ECMO team members undergo simulations monthly, an increase from their previous annual review. An ECMO coordinator ensures that the simulations take place during each shift. The value of the simulations extends beyond testing individual performance, says the nurse.

"When we have to practice together as a whole team, if a team member makes a mistake in the simulation and I see it then I learn from it, too," she explains.

The simulations test basic skills and expected precision, as well as less common scenarios. For example, team members practice what they would do in the face of unexpected events, such as an equipment failure.

"We train the nurse who might be there at 2 A.M., when the tubing ruptures, to physically do it and think about what they need to do, until they can perform with confidence," explains the doctor.

The simulations also expose how the team members communicate and work together.

The simulations emphasize the team's collective responsibility to communicate assertively and to ask questions when something isn't clear.

"We train to empower people to question each other if something didn't seem right and train to raise the total educational level of everyone so they had a common knowledge base . . . so everyone understands why we do it the way we do," says the doctor. "The message was, it's everybody's job to get a baby on ECMO safely, so it's your job to watch others and question."

Protocols and Checklists

The simulations have helped create agreed-upon protocols for a range of potential events associated with ECMO.

"If a patient is dying, it's always an intense time, where people are on edge," says the physician. "The practice sessions help us sort out roles and the safety issues from the perspectives of all team members, so there is a shared understanding. We developed checklists for each team member so that roles and action sequences are validated: 'This is my job, and this is the order in which I will do it.'"

The group began with building the protocols and checklists for processes they thought were the most dangerous, like priming the pump. In the end, they built checklists for every process associated with ECMO.

Regular Competency Evaluations

Each year, ECMO team members are required to successfully complete a written and technical competency evaluation similar to the initial test required to qualify as a member of the ECMO team. Reaction to the evaluation has been positive.

"It was stimulating," says the nurse. "It felt good to confirm that our knowledge and skills were up to date."

Accelerated Communication

Every patient requiring ECMO presents a unique set of circumstances that creates new opportunity for learning. Communicating individual information to create team knowledge has been accomplished through several methods. Case journals, notebooks kept at the bedside, are used to record unique insights and ideas that are useful to the ECMO team to continually improve its performance.

The physician explains, "You might have a patient with some complex congenital heart condition, so the bedside journal is where a drawing of one cannula is located and where the other is in relation to it."

The bedside journal is read from shift to shift. E-mail has also played a role in speeding communication.

"Everyone needed to agree to communicate by e-mail," says the physician. "Everyone reads e-mail regularly, and if a safety issue or question about something arises, we can rapidly disseminate the information."

Training Manual

"There are lots of articles about individual patient management, but the technical manual was outdated," reports the physician. "So we had to write our own training manuals."

The team created a comprehensive ECMO resource book, with pages divided by tabs for easy retrieval of information. This reference has also been useful for experienced staff members.

"The information available is beyond what anyone with an I.Q. of 140 could memorize," quips the physician. "So if you're caring for the patient at 2:00 A.M., you have available decision support to help your practice, such as how to issue a specific drug."

Debriefings

The team conducts multidisciplinary reviews after treatment of every patient and uses the feedback from the debriefings to inform the content of simulations and educational sessions.

"We debrief very honestly about what could have been better," says the nurse. "Before, we would only debrief as part of mortality review. Now, we're analyzing how the system worked and how it could work better with every patient."

The new procedures have required a significant investment, but staff members report increased quality of care and increased satisfaction with their work.

"Staff are more comfortable with what they're doing and more satisfied that they're being properly trained and mentally equipped," says the physician.

The death that led to these changes also led to an extensive, blame-based, external review and negative press.

"To have the failure publicly displayed exacerbated the shame and doubt," the physician says, "but an external review doesn't have to be inconsistent with a safety initiative. It's important to remember that it's often your most experienced people, engaged in the most risky procedures, who are at most risk to be in the rubble of a medical accident. The risk is of losing those people who are your best."

Lessons from the Cockpit

Dr. Robert Helmreich directs the Human Factors Research Project at the University of Texas at Austin. With twenty years' experience conducting human factors research, he believes that aviation's approach to harm reduction can be cautiously adapted to health care (Helmreich, 2001).

Having placed expert observers in airline cockpits on more than four thousand flights, Helmreich's research team studied both the nature of errors and the strategies used to detect and mitigate them. Observed errors were classified into five types, listed in Table 5.4. We have added hypothetical analogies in health care.

Helmreich notes that an **error-tolerant culture** acknowledges errors but does not tolerate violations of formal rules, especially rules created and validated as strategies for avoiding or mitigating harm. The aviation industry responds to human failure by investigating and addressing systemic factors in accidents and incidents. Specific methods include developing confidential error-reporting systems (see Chapter Six) and initiating formal training in teamwork and decision making (known in aviation as **crew resource management**), which trains front-line workers in specific effective communication behaviors as countermeasures against error. Helmreich (2001) offers health care a six-step template for error management, taken from aviation:

1. Understand the organization's history and issues.
2. Diagnose the error-inducing conditions by obtaining accurate data on current practices (through confidential reporting systems, surveys of personnel, and observations of normal practices).
3. Change the organizational culture to a safety culture that recognizes the inevitability of error and actively seeks to identify and remove latent risks.
4. Train staff in effective teamwork, decision making, and error management as well as technical aspects of the job.
5. Provide feedback and reinforcement for effective teamwork and error management.
6. Recognize the continuing need for accurate data on threat and error management and ongoing training in threat management and error countermeasures.

Many health care organizations are adapting methods of high reliability to health care. Specific tools that leaders can use to promote accountability are covered in further detail in Chapter Seven; Chapter Six discusses HRO methods of auditing risk via a blameless reporting system, and Chapter Nine addresses acknowledging risk through HRO mechanisms of accelerating change. Here are

TABLE 5.4. AIRLINE COCKPIT OBSERVED ERRORS: FIVE TYPES

Type of Error	Definition	Example from Aviation	Example from Health Care	Examples of Remediation
Procedural error	Slip, lapse, mistake	Pilot inadvertently makes an incorrect navigational setting	Surgeon, working multiple cases, becomes distracted and leaves a sponge in a patient	Change in procedures
Proficiency error	Lack of skill or knowledge	Pilot lacks flight hours and experience to manage aircraft in changing weather conditions	Cancer patient is admitted to general floor unit; nurses, with no training in the administration of complex chemotherapeutic agents, administer a large pill, which causes the patient to choke	Training
Communication error	Faulty or inadequate communication	With ice on airplane wings, copilot fails to convey the gravity of the situation (authority gradient)	Nurse recognizes a lethal magnitude of digoxin but does not stop physician's order (authority gradient)	Training

TABLE 5.4. AIRLINE COCKPIT OBSERVED ERRORS: FIVE TYPES, *continued*

Type of Error	Definition	Example from Aviation	Example from Health Care	Examples of Remediation
Decision error	Chosen course of action unnecessarily increases risk	An air traffic controller, who knows that there is a mandatory distance between contiguous flights, decides to move air traffic more smoothly by relaxing the rules but misjudges the distance between two planes	Physician administering diagnostic contrast dye outside of scheduled work hours; patient has a severe allergic reaction and a stroke, and there are not enough support staff available	Modify organizational culture so that controller or physician asks for help
Intentional noncompliance error	Violation of procedure	Pilot deliberately chooses to ignore rules and does not complete preflight checklist.	Phlebotomist, to avoid bothering a patient, violates policy by not labeling blood at the patient's bedside	Education and/or discipline

presented additional innovations, adapted from HROs, that are being introduced into health care.

Teamwork, Rather Than Individual Heroes, Creates Safety

The same type of progress that has been realized in the aviation industry, in terms of managing threats to safety and minimizing the consequences of human error, is edging into health care, notably in areas (such as surgery, emergency medicine, delivery suites, and intensive care units) where frequent crises make teamwork essential.

Effective teamwork requires skill development and practice. Standardized teamwork training has been introduced into emergency departments, with staff being taught how to create work teams composed of tightly coordinated, mission-focused, technically skilled small groups (Risser and others, 1999). The objective is to reduce the risk that a team will make fatal errors or permit a fatal chain of errors to unfold because members failed to foster teamwork, solve problems, communicate, and manage workloads. Team members are encouraged to support and coordinate with each other in the course of executing their clinical tasks.

A consideration regarding teams is that teams generally are formed and have stable membership over a period of time. They have clear roles and responsibilities, shared goals and expectations. Teams use reliable communications with tools such as structured protocols and guidelines for assertive communication. They conduct training through rehearsals and simulation. Because teams work together over time, role substitutions and flexibility in responsibility and response repertoires can be developed. A management team, or a dedicated cardiovascular team, or an outpatient clinic are examples.

Contrast this to the daily operational realities of hospital care with 24/7/365 coverage requirements and increasing part-time employment. Instead of a team, a crew is working. A crew is assembled from a talent pool: unit staff, float team, physician practice, deployed staff from other disciplines and departments. Each member brings individual expertise and technical competence. They form together to complete work: by shift, by episode of care, or in brief encounters. After a time interval, they redistribute and may or may not reassemble again. This has serious implications for standardization and simplification of work processes, clearly defined roles and responsibilities such as attending physican and resident, and protocols for reports, communications, and physican notifications.

One organization, profiled in the following case study, has received national acclaim for its work in reconfiguring clinical teamwork to improve communication and safety.

Concept to Action: Using Human Factors Concepts and Aviation Techniques to Improve Communication among Providers and with Patients

Health care practitioners spend their days responding to ever-changing conditions, time pressures, risks, and uncertainties. Theoretically, the decisions they make are communicated to other practitioners on the health care team through notes in clinical records or through one-to-one hallway conversations. In fact, however, most clinicians spend a significant amount of time playing telephone tag, answering pages that interrupt their current work, and performing rework. Even when hallway conversations occur, they typically leave out a rich source of expertise, the patient and the patient's family.

Paul Uhlig, a surgeon at Concord Hospital, along with a team of Concord clinicians, has adapted the concept of the microsystem (the grouping of people and resources in response to specific patterns of customer need) to help reconfigure clinical teamwork for patient safety and communication effectiveness (Press Ganey Associates, 2002; Northern New England Cardiovascular Disease Study Group, 2001; Nelson and others, 2001). Together, Uhlig and his colleagues created and refined the Concord Collaborative Care Model, which modifies daily rounds to include a multidisciplinary team of providers, the patient, and the patient's family.

The Concord Collaborative Care Model emphasizes collaboration and teamwork and alters the way in which clinicians do their daily rounds. Uhlig and others (2002) describe the rounds this way: "Rather than coming one at a time throughout the day to see each patient, members of the extended cardiac team come together one time each day to make rounds at each patient's bedside. Family members are encouraged to be . . . active participant[s] in the rounds process. Every effort is made to speak in 'ordinary language' instead of medical terminology. Team members find it rewarding to see how much the process means to patients and families and feel that a complete picture leads to better decisions and fewer medication errors. Patients and families don't ask anymore, 'Don't you people ever talk to each other?' They know exactly what we planned."

An example of a clinical microsystem in an open-heart surgery unit would be a group that includes cardiologists, surgeons, nurses, pharmacists, therapists, nutritionists, social workers, and others who routinely interact to care for heart patients. The following steps, known as the Collaborative Communications Cycle, developed in consultation with a human factors expert, are repeated each day for each patient:

- The plan from the day before is reviewed.
- All team members (patient, family members, nurse, pharmacist, therapists, social worker, spiritual care provider, surgeon, and any specialists who are involved) discuss the patient's progress, medications, and concerns.
- The team members work together to develop a plan of care for the day.
- Roles and responsibilities are clarified.
- The plan is summarized for the patient's approval.

- All team members, including the patient and the patient's family, are asked about anything that has not gone as expected (events known as "system glitches").
- System glitches are discussed openly by the entire team and are recorded for further review and action.
- The team takes immediate action to rectify system glitches. If they cannot be rectified, they are recorded for review at a bimonthly team meeting (known as "system rounds").

Team members report that the Collaborative Communications Cycle is a significant cultural shift. It requires a physician champion and buy in from all disciplines. It also requires perseverance, in addition to trust among team members. Each patient takes an average of ten minutes (simpler cases take as little as five minutes, and more complex patients as much as twenty minutes), but the rounds save time throughout the day as rework is minimized.

"By the time the rounds begin, at 9:00 A.M.," says Valerie Cote, a nurse, "I've already done vitals, weights, morning assessments, etc., and I can bring up any issues that may come up. Everyone is there to answer, so I'm not telling the story five different times throughout the day. The issues are addressed right then."

The Concord Collaborative Care Model has produced measurable improvements in morbidity and mortality. Cardiac staff members who participated in a survey on quality of work life reported that the Collaborative Communications Cycle consistently helped them make better therapeutic decisions. According to staff members, a key motivator has been the reactions of patients and family members. Patient satisfaction has increased as family members have reported feeling comforted and empowered by the process.

Elise Kendall, a pharmacist, states that patients are "better informed, more reassured, and they have less anxiety." She believes that the Collaborative Communications Cycle "empowers a patient to become more participatory."

Teamwork Planning

Successful teamwork in aviation results from careful planning to establish and organize the team and from continual monitoring to maintain team structure and climate (Risser and others, 1999). On an effective team, members always know who the leader is, who the other members are, and what their respective roles are. Team members apply problem-solving strategies: conducting scenario planning, practicing decision-making methods, and engaging in error-recovery actions. They use structured communication, they prioritize tasks, and they manage resources and workloads. Continuous quality improvement is built into routine team functioning so that team skills are improved by specific follow-up actions. The following teamwork behaviors (Risser and others, 1999) have been identified as powerful tools for avoiding serious errors:

- Develop a plan or identify an established protocol that is clear to everyone on the team.
- Prioritize tasks for patient care and make sure that all caregivers understand them.
- Maintain situational awareness by cross-monitoring actions of team members so that caregivers watch each other's behaviors for errors and act to correct them.
- Confront the authority gradient, the tendency of human beings to "overtrust" the words and actions of a person in authority, by asserting a position or corrective action when any caregiver believes the patient is at risk.

The following case study profiles one organization that developed a simple, low-cost intervention to confront the authority gradient (see Figure 5.1).

Concept to Action: Challenging the Authority Gradient

In aviation, the authority gradient refers to people's tendency not to question the decisions of others who are perceived to have more authority; the greater another's authority, the stronger the tendency to accept his or her decisions. In any organization, rank or status, experience, and expertise all play a role in creating the authority gradient.

FIGURE 5.1. AUTHORITY GRADIENT

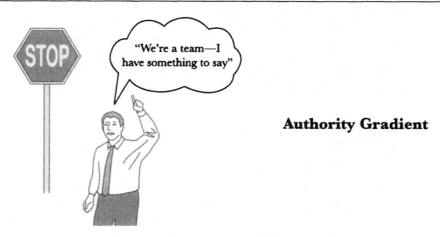

Source: K. Luther. Used with permission.

Katharine Luther, director of performance improvement at Memorial Hermann Healthcare System, has developed ways to encourage health professionals, from assistants to nurses to physicians to specialists, to resist the authority gradient in their environments. For example, she has identified a variety of reasons why a nurse may not want to question the authority of a physician.

"It may just be lack of knowledge, or the response that they're the doctor, so they must know," says Luther. "It may also be because of an attitude of being 'bulletproof'—the idea that we don't make mistakes here, so that person must be right. Lack of teamwork can contribute. If you have tried to speak up in the past and been reprimanded or embarrassed, you may have the attitude 'I'm not going to do that again.'"

Memorial Hermann instituted a broad-based educational program about the authority gradient, and about how to recognize when it is coming into play. Each year a brief presentation is given to staff members, who are then asked to describe situations in which the authority gradient may have come into play. The information is grounded in other, complementary topics involving patient safety, such as human factors research and the systems approach to safety.

At these annual sessions, Memorial Hermann distributes pocket cards that serve as guides to the authority gradient (see Figure 5.1). Employees are asked to carry these cards as reminders and to take multiple cards to share with colleagues. As they distribute the cards, employees teach and remind each other about the phenomenon of the authority gradient.

To encourage constant vigilance against the potential negative impact of the authority gradient, the subject is revisited throughout the year, in various venues (for example, in the daily safety briefing at the beginning of each shift on each patient unit). After discussing patient acuity, staffing levels, and other issues of the day, nurse managers periodically spend a minute or two reviewing a safety concept, such as the authority gradient, and its application to the unit.

Reinforcement of the concept keeps staff members from becoming desensitized to the effect of the authority gradient and reinforces assertive communication.

"The reminders help us avoid normalization of deviance," says Luther. "It's a reminder for people to speak up when they may not have spoken up before to protect patients from potential harm."

Summary Points

1. Health care organizations are large-scale complex systems. In large-scale complex systems decisions are made with less than perfect information, and in uncertain, stressful conditions. Other characteristics include simultaneous autonomy and interdependence, the existence of multiple cultures, intended and unintended consequences, long incubation periods during which risk can arise, and risk migration.

2. In a high-reliability organization, safety is the most important goal. Leaders of HROs continually anticipate the future, asking what adaptations are taking place and why. This kind of leadership focus keeps the culture nimble and underscores the concept of safety as a dynamic, energizing, adaptive process.

3. An HRO's organizational structure may appear hierarchical, but it is dynamic, with three different organizational structures that come into play, depending on the situation at hand:

   - A structure of functional hierarchy, not bureaucracy, for day-to-day operations makes everyone accountable for safety. It ensures training, procedures, and pattern detection.

   - A structure of collaboration takes over in situations of increased risk with deference to expertise.

   - A predetermined structure, with clear roles and responsibilities, is rehearsed and mobilizes immediately in situations of clear and present danger.

4. Culture is the barrier to high reliability in health care. Three core pathological elements, blame, denial, and the pursuit of the wrong kind of excellence, make health care a system that is vulnerable to accidents. The hierarchical nature of medical practice, based on power, is another barrier. In a high-reliability organization, the knowledge and contribution of all members of a team is encouraged and respected.

5. Strategies to move health care toward high reliability include communication, risk acknowledgment, an emphasis on active learning, teamwork, and crew resource management. Tools include risk and process auditing, process control, reward systems, and perception of risk.

CHAPTER SIX

INSTALL A BLAMELESS
REPORTING SYSTEM

Many medical accidents can be predicted and prevented if near misses and risk-prone conditions can be made transparent. High-risk industries employ systems of reporting to improve the safety of their environments and reduce harm. Health care can do likewise.

A safety culture develops a robust reporting system infrastructure. The management of the system is disciplined. The emphasis of this chapter is on developing a system to prospectively capture information about system performance, and uncover latent conditions and vulnerabilities. Practical lessons from high-reliability organizations are reviewed. The questions that preceed the design of a reporting system are posed. The principles that are crucial to the success of a blameless **voluntary reporting system** are laid out. There are two case studies. One case study profiles how an organization used key principles and lessons from high-reliability organizations to learn from stories of mistakes, hazards, and near misses. Another case study reports how an organization used a blameless voluntary reporting system to learn from adverse events. Both describe early efforts to make error transparent, identify risks, and build a system of learning and improvement.

Blame Prevents Learning

The concept of hindsight bias is important to the discussion of a health care reporting system. It is a major barrier. Hindsight bias is the human tendency to assign blame to a human being as the cause when things do not work out for the patient. It has a chilling effect on reporting. If analysis of medical accident starts and stops with a human being as the cause of the accident, a negative effect on reporting is created, and progress in patient safety is stalled.

Assigning human error as the cause of medical accident allows the health care culture to reinforce an illusion of restored safety when the individual in error is removed. This approach denies the existence of system failures, identifies a scapegoat, and prevents learning. It truncates the ability to predict and prevent future adverse events. Later, after the human "cause" of an accident is removed, another human being will step into place. The same conditions and factors can be reassembled, and the stage is set for the medical accident to recur.

A voluntary, nonpunitive reporting system helps create a culture that is resistant to the phenomenon of hindsight bias. It enables the collection of information, supports analysis of system vulnerabilities, and informs redesign of systems to prevent harm to patients. Rather than viewing individuals as the source of harm, a safety culture recognizes that sharp end professionals continuously create safety and prevent harm to patients by intercepting error and compensating for faulty and riskprone systems. The front line is the best source of information about how systems are operating and about the complexity of technical work. Focusing on systems, not people, a voluntary reporting system provides the vehicle for systematically collecting and learning from front-line wisdom.

Background of Safety Reporting in Health Care

The Institute of Medicine report *To Err Is Human* (Kohn, Corrigan, and Donaldson, 1999) calls for mandatory and voluntary reporting systems as part of a comprehensive strategy to improve patient safety. The IOM report concludes that systems for reporting adverse events are mechanisms for enhancing our understanding of failure and the underlying contributing factors. The report emphasizes that the purpose of a reporting system is to create an environment that encourages organizations to identify system vulnerabilities, evaluate the causes of those vulnerabilities, and take appropriate action to improve performance. While the report falls short in its attention to near misses, hazards, and systemic risk, it is a starting point in seeking to understand adverse events.

Why Create a Blameless Reporting System?

In December 2002, the *Washington Post* published an article with the headline "No End to Errors: Three Years After a Landmark Report Found Pervasive Mistakes in American Hospitals, Little Has Been Done to Reduce Death and Injury" (Boodman, 2002). How could a health care system known for saving millions of lives through the use of complex technology not be able to eradicate the problem of medical accident so thoroughly delineated in the IOM report? A primary reason is the continuing failure of health care to grasp the power of understanding the nature of error as a way of preventing medical accidents.

Although the health care industry has fulfilled minimal obligations of mandatory reporting, other efforts have been largely preoccupied with measurement. Berwick (2001a, 2001b) captures the limitations of this approach: "Reporting for measurement contains almost no information. Reporting that loses the 'story' is mostly a waste. We need to harvest the knowledge. We need firesides, not spreadsheets. The question 'How many?' isn't powerful. The question should be: What happened?"

The purpose of a blameless voluntary reporting system is to help people learn. It has the following clear and specific goals:

1. Designing fail-safe care delivery processes that deflect **system errors** and system vulnerabilities before they reach a patient to create harm
2. Facilitating more informed decision making for patients, providers, and clinicians
3. Feeding information back to the system to improve system design
4. Gathering information about the system that can be used for training staff

Reporting systems that serve these goals have the potential to fundamentally change the health care culture from one of blame, denial, and cover-up to one of vigilance, transparency, and learning about creating safety.

Safety learning occurs when work processes in the system are made transparent through reporting. Reporting offers the opportunity to gain more knowledge about the design failures and operational failures that may be contributing to and potentiating human fallibility. Such data hold the opportunity for improvements to occur before a disaster takes place. Consider an iceberg of which only a portion is visible. In health care, the tip of the iceberg reveals both beauty and danger: the beauty is the triumphs and hope provided to millions through modern medicine, and the danger is the harm suffered by thousands. Hidden below the surface are near misses, which dwarf accidents in number. These are dangerous situations caused by system vulnerabilities. Near misses, along with countless glitches (deviations and variances in practice) that occur daily, sometimes push through to the surface to cause harm. Blameless reporting systems make visible what is hidden below the surface. Figure 6.1 depicts this situation.

Reporting is a critical information source and an intellectual mainstay for creating safety. A system for reporting and learning is a powerful tool that supports the advancement of a culture of safety. The analysis and conversations that emerge from the reporting system provide the engine that drives improvement. Counting and trending incidents and adverse events is insufficient for understanding where or how to reduce risk and improve care. The reporting system that asks, "What happened?" generates information that can be transformed into knowledge for informing system changes through cycles of improvement.

The implementation of a voluntary blameless reporting system is a deep cultural intervention in an organization that legitimizes transparency of system vulnerability, nurtures an "alert field," and empowers front-line providers to expose risks. In turn, the front line learns to expect responses from managers at the blunt end to support the work of improvement. The few organizations in health care that have developed reporting systems believe that the effort is 75 percent social and only 25 percent technical (personal communication from Anne-Claire France, former director of the Center for Healthcare Improvement, Memorial Hermann Healthcare

FIGURE 6.1. ICEBERG

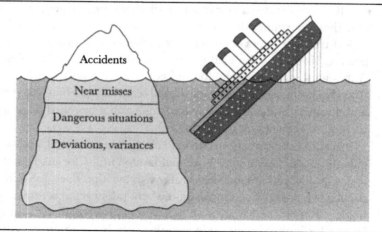

Source: J. B. Battles, H. S. Kaplan, T. W. van der Schaaf, and C. E. Shea, "The Attributes of Medical Event Reporting Systems," *Archives of Pathology and Laboratory Medicine*, 1998, *122*(3), 231–238. © College of American Pathologists. Reproduced with permission.

System, Houston, 2003). That is, the predominant feature of the work in implementing a reporting system is the engagement and education of stakeholders, balancing barriers (such as fear of reporting) and incentives (such as the desire to do the right thing), and helping participants negotiate conflicting goals (for example, the desire to complete a report versus the urgent need to complete myriad other tasks in a short time). Reporters need to see that their reporting efforts are recognized and that action to reduce risk is taken as a result. How leaders respond to near misses and accidents is paramount to the successful launch of a reporting system. Also important is the allocation of resources for infrastructure for content analysis of reports, pattern detection, and feedback to reporters. Reading panels, data entry, and databases with search capability are examples of required resources.

Lessons in Blameless Reporting from HROs

High-reliability organizations in aviation, nuclear power, petrochemical processing, military operations, steel production, and space travel, think about human fallibility and system vulnerability in particular ways. HRO reporting systems have evolved over three decades to the point of using the identified problem to understand the underlying causative factors and system vulnerabilities through focusing on near misses, providing incentives for voluntary reporting, encouraging confidentiality over **anonymity**, bolstering accountability, and emphasizing a systemic view.

Reporting systems in aviation teach that event frequency is not the only variable that determines degree of risk. Counting rates of reported events may not reflect true near-miss occurrence rates because samples are not random in reporting. However, what health care professionals see is real and needs to be fixed. Although it may be helpful to use frequency of reported risk in beginning to set priorities for interventions, leaders need to be mindful that frequency count is only a preliminary and rudimentary tool and cannot be relied on as a reliable or sole method of reducing or mitigating risk.

Health care invests considerable resources in counting and accounting for incidents. These investments have had limited utility for taking action. A more effective model is to analyze near misses, as aviation does, to create improvement. A culture has developed in aviation where safety is the central issue for all stakeholders. Reports and analyses of near misses are recognized as providing the same lessons for improvement as do actual events, but without the emotional valence that harm produces.

The History of Reporting in Aviation

The aviation reporting system began through the work of physician Charles E. Billings. In 1974, while he was with the National Aeronautics and Space Administration (NASA), Billings investigated a major aircraft catastrophe in which a crew had misunderstood the instructions given in connection with an air traffic control clearance. During the investigation, he learned that another crew had nearly perished in the same location a few weeks earlier after having made the same mistake (Billings, 1998). From this Billings understood the importance of learning from near misses rather than accidents. Billings and his colleagues developed and implemented the Aviation Safety Reporting System (ASRS). In this system, the aviation industry uses NASA as an external body to which confidential narratives about error are submitted for the purposes of learning and developing capability in resilience and prevention (Reynard, Billings, Cheaney, and Hardy, 1986).

Funded by the aviation industry, the ASRS has operated successfully for twenty-four years. The ASRS is trusted by aviation's sharp end: pilots, air traffic controllers, flight attendants, ground crew, maintenance workers, and other personnel. The system is voluntary, confidential, and nonpunitive. The purpose of the program is to collect, protect, and use incident data to improve the national aviation system. Information from the ASRS supports aviation system policy, planning, and improvement, and strengthens the foundation of human factors research in aviation by identifying deficiencies to be corrected by appropriate authorities.

More than 38,000 voluntary reports are submitted annually (L. Connell, personal communication, 2003). Anyone with knowledge of actual or potential hazards to safe operations is encouraged and able to report. In exchange for the unique and valuable information they provide, NASA guarantees reporters confidentiality and limited immunity to disciplinary action by the Federal Aviation Administration. All identifying information is removed before completed reports are entered into the database. Reports are not used for enforcement by the aviation industry but are used to create a learning system to inform changes in aviation safety. An incentive for reporting is the waiver of fines and penalties for unintentional violations of federal aviation regulations when a report is submitted within ten days of an occurrence. Accidents and criminal activities are not protected, however. They are reported through a separate, mandatory system, and there is a "firewall" between these two mechanisms.

The reports are analyzed by panels of expert readers (often retired pilots) to extract alerts, lessons learned, and trends and themes. The database of reports, with deidentified information, is available to everyone. The database contains narratives describing recognized risks, near misses, and minor accidents up to the point of a crash or significant injury. The ASRS also issues alerts and safety messages concerning potential hazards and other important occurrences in a monthly, easily read newsletter to all sharp end personnel.

Using HROs to Create a Reporting System in Health Care

The Aviation Safety Reporting System serves as the model for the reporting efforts that are emerging in health care. Medical event reporting systems all follow the ASRS model to some degree and have been used both in the United States and abroad (Runciman and others, 1993). The model has been used by anesthesia and critical care medicine as well as by transfusion medicine and blood banks. In hospital and surgical center operating rooms that analyze closed claims in a disciplined fashion, the specialty of anesthesia has reported at least tenfold reduction in mortality for healthy patients (Lagasse, 2002).

The NASA/Veterans Administration's **Patient Safety Reporting System (PSRS)** was established in 2000. It emphasises reporting close calls, and is a prototype blameless reporting system in health care. It was created through an agreement between NASA and the Department of Veterans Affairs. Strictly a tool for learning, increasing awareness, and enabling solutions, the PSRS mirrors the ASRS in that it is voluntary, confidential, nonpunitive, and contains deidentified information. Reports are submitted to NASA, which oversees all PSRS operations and maintains confidentiality of the reporting system. Reporting via the National Center for Patient Safety has increased nine hundredfold for close calls of high-priority events (Heget, Bagian, Lee, and Gosbee, 2002) and is providing information on previously undetected and under-recognized vulnerabilities, guiding predictive Failure Mode and Effects Analysis (see Chapter Five) and the development of cognitive aids to improve safety. The partnership between the VA and NASA serves five primary functions to advance health care safety:

1. Receipt, deidentification, and processing of incident and safety-related event reports
2. Analysis and interpretation of data
3. Issuance of alert messages
4. Dissemination of deidentified reports and other information
5. Evaluation and review of the program

Mandatory and Voluntary Reporting Are Different

Although mandatory systems currently exist in health care, blameless voluntary reporting systems are still the exception. Mandatory systems focus on holding medical care providers and institutions accountable for the quality and safety of the care that they provide. Mandatory systems typically focus on identifying the most serious adverse events and issues related to criminal activity, gross negligence, or professional misconduct. Public accountability, in the form of mandatory reporting to external agencies, is an important obligation that is addressed in greater depth in Chapter Eight. By contrast, voluntary reporting is an essential component of building the learning culture that is the intellectual mainstay of patient safety and a vehicle for engaging the wisdom of the front line.

How to Develop and Operate a Blameless Voluntary Reporting System

The development of a blameless voluntary reporting system builds on the assumption that accidents and near misses contain vital information about underlying systemic problems. They offer valuable information for understanding the symptoms in a system and the way the system functions. In designing a reporting system, material can be structured around key questions gathered from the recommendations of a roundtable discussion sponsored by the Kaiser Permanente Institute for Health Policy and from health care systems that are currently engaged in developing reporting systems. A one-size-fits-all approach is inappropriate for the development of a reporting system, as each organization has unique needs. However, five key questions can guide the development of a robust reporting infrastructure (Roundtable Discussion on Design Considerations for a Patient Safety Improvement Reporting System, 2000).

1. What Information Will Be Reported to Improve Patient Safety?

Reportable occurrences in the voluntary system should include any adverse event and any near miss, excluding events related to the natural course of a disease. Criminal activity, gross negligence, and professional misconduct should not be reported to a voluntary system.

Anyone should be able to report. Reports can be accepted from all parties having knowledge of the workings of the organization and should be "story based," with lots of narrative. Reports should be reviewed by clinical leaders and **risk management**.

2. How Will the Information Be Reported, and to Whom?

Reporting should be flexible and should offer several options, such as a phone line, a password-protected Web-based form, and a paper form. For example, one hospital implemented a "whoops" board on a unit where staff simply placed stickers under certain categories when they recognized that they had made mistakes. It was only after a nursing director set the tone by posting his own mistakes that other staff members began to post their mistakes as well. (This action on the part of the nursing director reinforces the point that the major work of the reporting system is social.) The information was tallied on a monthly basis and entered into the reporting system. Another hospital created the **"good catch" log**, placed in medication rooms, where staff members jotted down momentary thoughts about potential hazards or opportunities for improvement.

Reporting forms should be ubiquitous and user-friendly. The reporting format should give the reporter the option of allowing a "scrubbed" version of the report to be shared with other organizations after it is received in the voluntary system. The reporting burden should be minimized. Individuals who report should not be required to duplicate their effort in order to provide information to multiple reporting systems.

Paper forms should have limited, fixed fields and significant space for the descriptive story of what happened. For example, a Web-based reporting form that is secure and password-protected was designed at Children's Hospitals and Clinics, Minneapolis/St. Paul, Minnesota. The form asks just five questions:

1. What happened?
2. Has it happened before?
3. Could it happen again?
4. What caused it to happen?
5. Who should be told?

Refer to Appendix Six.

Information is analyzed by staff trained in content-analysis methods and is entered into a database organized by categories, called learning stacks. These stacks can be accessed by professional staff, managers, and improvement teams who want to learn about an issue. For example, members of a **safety action team (SAT)** in oncology can access the learning stack concerning chemotherapy administration, patient identification, and IV pumps. (For related information on safety action teams, see "Concept to Action: Engaging the Sharp End through Safety Action Teams," in Chapter Seven.)

The organizational home of the voluntary reporting system should be an independent, nonregulatory entity because independence mitigates reporters' fears of retribution by supervisors. The responsibility of this neutral vehicle is to collect information on adverse events, near misses, and hazards and to analyze it for the purpose of learning. The reporting entity may be internal or external to the organization. Smaller hospitals and rural areas may wish to pool their resources and develop a consortium. Children's Hospitals and Clinics, Minneapolis/St. Paul, Minnesota, established the Office of Patient Safety (OOPS) to manage and protect information. Memorial Hermann Health Care System used the department of performance improvement to perform this function.

3. How Will the Analytical Process Identify the Problems in the System, and What Expertise Will Be Needed?

The cornerstone of a reporting system is robust analysis of theme and detection of patterns within the data. After the sharp-end worker shares the narrative story about what happened, a case analysis is conducted and deidentified. The case analysis provides a window into the system to view "error-producing conditions" (Vincent, 2001). The analysis should provide a diagnosis of the problems in a system. A case analysis, performed for accidents, potential accidents, and near misses, accomplishes two goals:

1. It makes wide exploration a routine part of the culture.
2. It harnesses the expertise and knowledge of those sharp-end professionals who surround an accident or near miss.

The leverage for creating greater safety is in analyzing the story of failure and seeing the workings of the system unfold. A culture that is focused on safety is one that operates from a process-flow perspective and recognizes that there is not a single cause when things go wrong (for example, a tractable mode of failure or a single solution set).

Richard Cook (2000) challenges those who are serious about safety to focus on gaps that are revealed through reporting in systems of care. In our culture of independent departments, discipline-centric practices, divisions between labor and management, and disaggregated information flow, we do not always see gaps; rather, we view incidents in a narrow and impoverished way. It is between these entities—the gaps—that risk and safety are created.

Examining gaps requires knowing the system and its vulnerabilities from a process flow perspective that narratives can provide. According to Cook (2001), "Safety is created and maintained in the anticipation of gaps." The system, Cook continues, gradually becomes more robust and resilient as gaps are closed or bridged. The cultural challenge is that cross-functional teams must analyze and understand their work and the effects of their work, leaving behind the comfort of traditional boundaries and beliefs to take a stance of humility and learning. Cook (2000) proposes data analyses that focus on three general areas for the gaps to produce rich learning about safety:

- *Gaps in the continuity of care.* For example, patient transfers between units, to the operating room, or from the ICU or emergency department are vulnerable in terms of the continuity of information. Transfers of care between physicians, nurses, specialists, and consultants at changes of shifts and sign-out of coverage to partners also introduce risk.
- *Recovering from prior gaps.* This area is subtle and can become a factor many times in a single day. Here, the clinician recognizes the effects of discontinuity, searches into the past to recover missing knowledge, and restores continuity by partial recovery of knowledge.
- *Anticipating and bridging future gaps.* Here, the clinician recognizes probable future gaps and creates a bridge over the anticipated gaps. Continuity is maintained by the bridge, and the gap disappears from view.

Refer to Appendix Nine for further information about gaps.
Voluntary reporting exposes gaps and makes them transparent.

4. How Will the Voluntary Reporting System Align with Internal and External Existing Reporting Systems?

A successful voluntary reporting system quickly evolves into a patient safety learning center where accessible, user-friendly data are warehoused. The patient safety learning center can be enhanced when the sources of data available through other reporting systems are integrated in a single repository. Information gathered from the voluntary reporting system can be correlated with other identification systems, such as those associated with patients' complaints, patient satisfaction surveys, and internal reporting systems in specific departments (the pharmacy and the laboratory, for example). The data warehouse from voluntary reporting can be enhanced by recommendations in published literature, lessons from other health care organizations, and other authoritative external sources. Table 6.1 displays existing external reporting systems. Shaded areas indicate the type of information gathered by each system.

The voluntary system should be complementary to existing reporting systems. The goal is to integrate aggregate information from external systems to enhance the information contained in the internal reporting system. External reporting sys-

TABLE 6.1. EXTERNAL REPORTING SYSTEMS

	Adverse Events	Drugs	Devices	Vaccine	Biologics	Blood	Near Misses
State Adverse Event Tracking (Multiple States)	X						
US Food and Drug Administration		X	X	X	X	X	
JCAHO	X						
Medication Error Reporting (MER) Program		X					X
MedMARx		X				X	X
ECRI Medical Device Safety Reports			X				
US Veterans Administration PSRS	X	X	X	X	X	X	X

Source: Adapted from Roundtable Discussion on Design Considerations for a Patient Safety Improvement Reporting System, sponsored by Kaiser Permanente Institute for Health Policy, NASA Aviation Safety Reporting System, and the National Quality Forum, NASA Ames Research Center, Moffitt Field, Calif., Aug. 28–29, 2000.

tems contain valuable information, but they have not been used to their full capacity because collaboration on the part of health care organizations has been lacking.

5. How Will the Reporting System Be Used to Nurture the Safety Culture?

The reporting system provides a steady drumbeat of safety learning and continually reinforces the value of reporting. Risk identification and reporting should be recognized with thanks, timely feedback, acknowledgment of reporters' expertise, and rewards for reporting. Analysis of risk-prone conditions should be broadly communicated. These actions help to shape an alert culture that thinks critically and is heedful in its work. Team members in such an environment do not normalize deviance through acceptance of the status quo, but rather critically examine everything they do and continually seek to improve performance. Changing the frame of reference from *incident* reporting to *safety* reporting removes historic connotations of judgment, blame, and retribution and encourages front-line workers to proactively identify near misses and risks that are accidents waiting to happen. At all times, the message is one of a partnership in knowledge, with the quality of ideas more important than their source or the status of the people who have offered them. Here are a few ways to communicate lessons learned:

- *A safety database.* This database is where deidentified reports can be accessed by employees through a searchable intranet site.
- *E-mail lists.* Interested employees and physicians can opt to subscribe to an e-mail list on which internal and external alerts, case studies, and lessons are distributed.
- *Literature distribution service.* Hospital librarians can create a literature distribution service so that key lessons reported in the literature and inside the organization can be disseminated to employees working on particular areas of concern (Williams and Zipperer, 2003).
- *Report cards.* Reports into the system that have resulted in new initiatives can be reflected back to the organization through a report card. Figure 6.2 is a management report card disseminated periodically in an organization where safety reports related to medication concerns resulted in the implementation of a variety of best practices known to be effective with medication.

Lessons learned stimulate imagination and prompt ideas for improving safety as reports are gathered and analyzed, and lessons learned are reported back to the organization. Feedback and communication nurture the safety culture, and the safety culture in turn cultivates and improves the reporting system (see Figure 6.3).

Critical Principles for Success in a Blameless Reporting System

Apart from the logistical questions involved in developing the infrastructure of a reporting system, several key principles create the foundation of trust required to sustain a blameless voluntary reporting system. These principles are critical to the success of the system.

FIGURE 6.2. SAFE PRESCRIBING PRACTICES

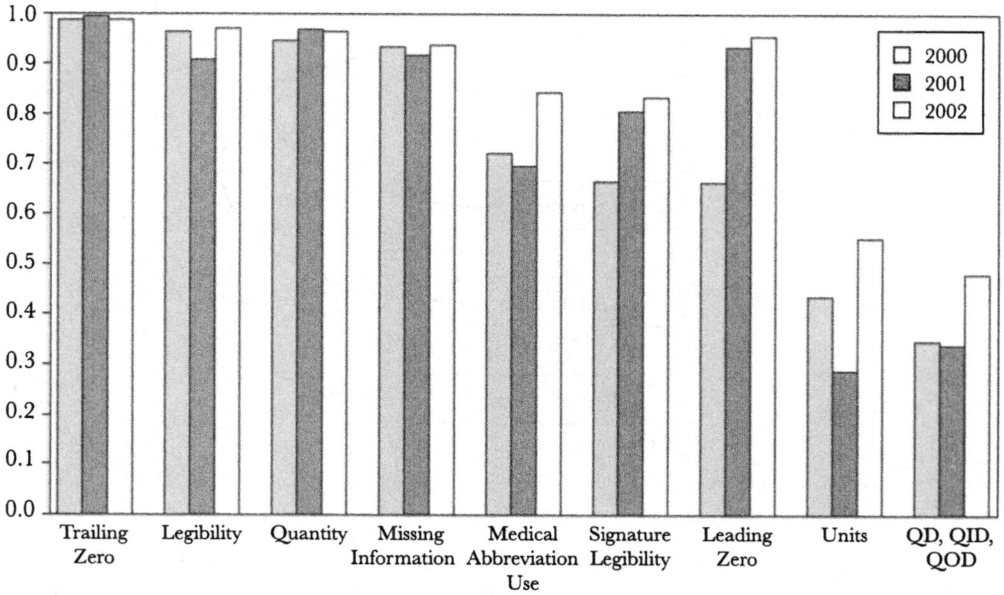

Strong Confidentiality Protections

Reporting systems in aviation were the first to confirm what seems intuitive: people are less likely to report adverse events that might be linked to them. Systems for reporting and tracking data for purposes of learning and improvement recognize that professionals need an environment of confidentiality and privileged communication. The challenge is to implement a reporting system that does not cause harm to the reporters who contribute data by keeping the data protected so that full disclosure and learning can take place. There are some risks in communicating lessons learned. However, the system makes every effort to address privacy and liability issues. Information can be "scrubbed," a process that goes beyond removal of patient identifiers and that eliminates, as appropriate, such other details as demographics, staff location, diagnosis, brand names, and patient outcome. Memorable context can be communicated securely in a separate message.

Protection and disclaimer statements should be used liberally. As with the ASRS system, where reporters must report within ten days to avoid fines and penalties for unintentional violations, incentives in a health care reporting system can promote timely reporting.

FIGURE 6.3. SAFETY LEARNING FEEDBACK

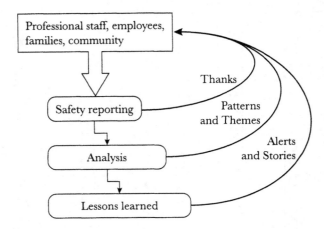

Individuals reporting to the system should be guaranteed confidentiality, but not anonymity. Follow-up with the reporter may be necessary to obtain additional information about the incident in order to gather a complete report. Information should be deidentified upon entry into the database, and the deidentification process should include removal of identifying information about the patient, the provider, and the person reporting.

A blameless, confidential system does not apply to circumstances of gross negligence, reckless or disruptive behavior, malfeasance, intentional violations, impairment due to drugs or alcohol, or inability or unwillingness to learn over time. These circumstances, although rare, pose a threat to patient safety and must be dealt with swiftly, fairly, and professionally from an administrative perspective. Blamelessness and accountability can and must coexist.

A Focus on the Story

The traditional reporting mechanism in health care has been the incident report. Incident reports rely heavily on fixed fields. For example, the user marks one option in a predetermined list of options to categorize and define an experience. Such forms simplify data entry and accounting, but they limit the effectiveness of a report because they fail to capture the complex knowledge that a front-line worker has about the system. Capturing the multiple, complex factors that may contribute to a near miss, in addition to events that reach the patient, involves capturing the rich narrative stories of front-line workers about what happened. A reporting form with limited, fixed fields and greater text allows the story of existing conditions that contributed to accident or near miss to be identified, explored, and better understood. This kind of form requires more time and analytical investment, both from the front-line provider who uses it and from the team that reads and analyzes it, but yields richer intelligence and unique insights into how systems and processes are actually operating.

Emphasis on Near Misses

Analysis of near misses is an investment in prevention. "Experience is the best teacher, but in our case the tuition is paid for by the patients. With close calls, tuition is free" (Bagian, 2002). Bagian's words challenge us to mine the rich sources of information we currently have and thereby prevent or reduce the probability of harmful or fatal medical accidents. Content analyses of more than 4,000 safety reports from a hospital system in the Midwest identified patterns predictive of medical accidents. Analysts in the hospital system found that near misses that had not been dealt with were characterized by error-prone conditions, which later reassembled to create medical accidents. This discovery jolted the organization. A question now asked on all safety reports and in all analyses of critical events analyses is "Has this event or a similar event ever occurred before? Have you seen this before?"

A near miss is alarming, but it does not carry the same sense of failure and emotional content as an incident which harms a patient. Thus it presents fewer barriers to learning because blame and fear of legal retribution are usually absent. A near miss provides two distinct opportunities for learning. The first resides in the lessons that can be gleaned from the accident that almost happened; the second resides in the interventions that prevented it. Identifying the action that prevented harm from reaching a patient is as important as identifying the changes that must be made to prevent future near misses or medical accidents. Communicating successes discovered in analysis helps build resiliency into the organization.

Near misses are far more common than adverse events. In near misses, the tendency toward hindsight bias is minimized, and the focus can be guided more easily toward how recovery took place. In this way, an organization learns about its sources of success.

The following case study involves a redesign of the reporting system at Children's Hospitals and Clinics, Minneapolis/St. Paul, Minnesota. It describes how a system was built with the knowledge of the ASRS and the work of the Veterans Administration's National Center for Patient Safety.

Concept to Action: Using Knowledge from Aviation and Safety Science to Design a Blameless, Knowledge-Centered Reporting System

When Children's Hospitals and Clinics, Minneapolis/St. Paul, Minnesota, overhauled its incident reporting process as part of a comprehensive patient safety agenda, James E. Levin, medical director of informatics, worked with the systemwide Patient Safety Steering Committee to redesign the entire reporting process based on the science of **knowledge management** and the successful reporting system created by NASA's Aviation Safety Reporting System.

Before the system was reformed, a traditional process of incident reporting had employees fill out a paper form that focused on classifying and categorizing the causes of adverse events. Each signed report, containing an array of boxes to be checked, was given to the patient care manager, who was required to document the action taken in response to the incident and to forward the original report to the Quality Resources Department. There, a single individual read each form, created a brief synopsis, and classified the incident according to the level of harm the patient, staff member, or visitor had suffered. Each month, reports were forwarded to the patient care managers, showing trends in harm levels. In addition, each incident was classified into one of five broad categories: medication, treatment, falls, behavior, and security/property. Monthly tallies were sent to the managers, and the process often ended there.

In the redesign of the reporting system, Levin incorporated three lessons from the field of knowledge management (Davenport and Prusak, 2000):

1. *The system should reward knowledge sharing, not knowledge hoarding.* Children's Hospitals and Clinics implemented incentives for filing or contributing to reports. The rewards ranged from simple notes of thanks to financial incentive plans for managers who were able to increase reporting rates in their departments.
2. *The system should package information to create knowledge in the minds of front-line staff.* The use of stories is a well-documented technique for disseminating knowledge and spurring ideas (Weick, 1995). For this reason, the new reporting forms had very few check boxes and lots of space for narrative. Patterns and themes from the narrative were coded for entry in the database.
3. *The knowledge-sharing system should be "frictionless," to ensure that communicating knowledge is not cumbersome.* To make reporting as easy as possible, the hospital system designed a paper form, prioritizing ease of use, and has worked to make use of electronic and Internet-based communication to disseminate information as widely and effortlessly as possible. The goal for safety reporting was to share two stories: the story about the potential of the system to cause harm, and, more important, the story about how the front line prevented or mitigated harm. System designers sought to create a system for collecting stories efficiently,

mining those stories for information on how systems could be improved, and sharing those stories in an anonymous format throughout Children's Hospitals and Clinics to create more potential for learning.

The Patient Safety Steering Committee incorporated elements of the ASRS into its design, such as making increased reporting a priority and emphasizing identification of themes from reports rather than counting incidents. Because the ASRS has found that reports dwindle if the information is not visibly used, dissemination of the story, and of changes that have resulted, is as important at Children's Hospitals and Clinics as is collecting the initial story.

New System at Children's

Anyone who is part of the Children's community is encouraged to report any incident or concern if there may be something to learn and share about safety. To emphasize this purpose, the incident report is now called the "Patient Safety Learning Report," and all the connotations of finding "bad apples" have been eliminated. Reports may be sent anonymously and are reviewed by the Office of Patient Safety, but staff are also encouraged to share reports with their managers. Reports can be sent via a paper form, a phone line, or through the Web site of the Children's Patient Safety Learning Center (www.createsafety.net). Children's encourages the use of Web-based reporting for several reasons:

- *The Web site collects information securely.* The Web site uses end-to-end encryption to protect the information as it is transmitted across the Internet. This is viewed as more secure than paper forms that sometimes can be casually viewed en route from the reporter.
- *The Web site ensures confidentiality.* When anonymity is important to the reporter, the Web ensures that no handwriting or voice can be recognized.
- *The Web site offers speed.* Information arrives at the Office of Patient Safety instantly, without the delays inherent in intra- and interoffice mail and in managers' busy schedules.
- *The Web site provides for better follow-up.* After collecting initial information about the seriousness of the incident, the Web site has prompts that display information for the reporter about disclosure to the family and about the need to immediately contact the department of risk management.

The Web form changes on the basis of the answers to initial information. For example, certain questions are asked only if medication was involved or if there was harm to the patient, thus minimizing the amount of time a person has to spend filling out a report.

The Safety Learning Report

Like the ASRS form, the Children's Hospitals and Clinics safety learning report asks the reporter an open-ended question about the incident: "What happened?" There is ample room for a written response. The reporter then clicks through to a new screen and is prompted with additional questions:

- What was the chain of events?
- What were the contributing factors?
- What was the work environment like at the time of this situation?
- What were the personal or team factors affecting human performance in this situation (such as inattention, perceptions, judgments, decisions, communication, co-ordination)?
- What did you learn from this situation?

In addition to this free-text narrative, boxes are checked to code information on patient demographics, event date and location, and details of specific medications or equipment involved. Then the reporter is asked a series of coded questions about the harm, or the potential harm, of the incident and the frequency with which the reporter has observed conditions for this incident in the past. The boxes and coded questions help analysts prioritize the incident on the basis of its potential harm and are used to link information to the systemwide safety database, where the data can be studied to construct a predictive model.

Other options are available for capturing the maximum possible amount of input to the database. For example, verbatim quotes, taken from patient satisfaction surveys that address safety issues, are transcribed into the safety database. Entries from a "good catch" log, often placed in the medication room of a unit for clinicians to jot down momentary thoughts or ideas about improving safety, are also entered into the database.

Processing Safety Learning Reports

Each report is reviewed the same day it is filed by at least one staff member from the Office of Patient Safety. Managers are notified immediately of reports requiring immediate action. Paper and phone reports are transcribed in full, verbatim. These deidentified transcriptions, along with the full deidentified text of reports submitted via the Web, are distributed for review to patient care units or department-based safety action teams. All reports related to the safety of medications are reviewed by a multidisciplinary medication safety reading group composed of "close to care" physicians, medical directors, and front-line clinicians. This and other kinds of reading-action groups are encouraged as a way to identify patterns and recognize themes. This wisdom is added to the original report and deployed.

Reading-action groups are instructed that the identification of themes or patterns is determined by the group's experience and expertise concerning what an event has in common with other events. To guard against hindsight bias, there is no predetermined list of categories for groups to use but rather a process that continually asks why. All reports are indexed for retrieval by Children's safety search engine, which uses commercial software designed for full-text searching.

When unit-based safety groups, policy review committees, performance improvement groups, or individual managers or executives want to tap in to the collected wisdom of the organization's safety reports, they request a topic search from the Office of Patient Safety. Accessing the safety search engine, staff members retrieve a stack of reports related to the requested topic, and these can be used to inform local innovations and improvements.

Sharing the Knowledge from Safety Learning Reports

In addition to being reviewed by interested groups, departments, or committees, the knowledge gleaned from patient safety reports is used in a variety of other ways:

- As stories of lessons learned, published in internal publications throughout Children's Hospitals and Clinics
- As case studies for periodic educational sessions that grant continuing education credits in the area of patient safety and for monthly systemwide learning dialogues hosted by members of the patient safety steering committee and devoted to relevant concepts in patient safety science
- As items for "Children's Safetylist," an e-mail distribution list edited by James Levin that also distributes stories from outside the Children's system as well as alerts and advisories from the Food and Drug Administration, the Centers for Disease Control, the National Patient Safety Foundation, and state public health departments (anyone can subscribe to the e-mail list by visiting www.createsafety.net).

Before a case study is created for a publication or an e-mail distribution list, staff members follow guidelines for deidentifying additional details to ensure confidentiality while preserving the narrative, with the help of editorial staff who also make note of actions and misunderstandings.

Results of the Children's Reporting System

In its first full year of use, the new system collected more than 3,000 reports, a sixtyfold increase from previous reporting. Although most reports were collected on paper, Web-based reporting has increased steadily each quarter. In the first full year, eighty-six alerts were sent out via the Children's Safetylist, and fifty-eight "learning stacks" were compiled from the database for committees and groups researching various safety issues, such as Foley catheter balloon deflation problems, IV and feeding tube errors, parent-sibling falls, and tracheostomy issues. More than 30,000 documents, including archival safety and incident reports and external safety-related information, reside in Children's safety search engine. Several characteristics have been identified as important elements of a reporting system's success and ongoing growth:

- *The system should be flexible.* Instead of using a one-size-fits-all approach, the system should make reporting easy and offer several options for potential reporters (see Figures 6.4 and 6.5 and refer to Appendix Six). As the Children's system continues to evolve, it is hoped that even more ways will be devised to make reporting easy and efficient for reporters.
- *The system should facilitate action.* The system should support local resolution of issues by offering rapid turnaround of reports and rapid dissemination of information, rather than waiting for a problem and its proposed solution to make its way up and down the chain of command. The goal should be to ensure that the priority is problem solving, not paperwork. Those who are reviewing the information—in unit-based safety action teams, the Office of Patient Safety, project-based committees, and other work groups—are encouraged to take initiative and share stories with anyone they

FIGURE 6.4. MODEL 1 FOR CLASSIFYING EVENTS

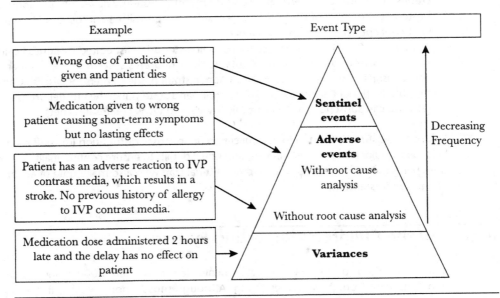

Copyright © Memorial Hermann Healthcare Systems. Used by permission.

FIGURE 6.5. MODEL 2 FOR CLASSIFYING EVENTS

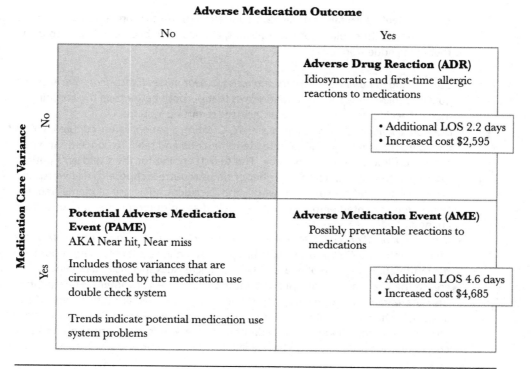

Adverse Medication Outcome

	No	Yes
Medication Care Variance — No		**Adverse Drug Reaction (ADR)** Idiosyncratic and first-time allergic reactions to medications • Additional LOS 2.2 days • Increased cost $2,595
Medication Care Variance — Yes	**Potential Adverse Medication Event (PAME)** AKA Near hit, Near miss Includes those variances that are circumvented by the medication use double check system Trends indicate potential medication use system problems	**Adverse Medication Event (AME)** Possibly preventable reactions to medications • Additional LOS 4.6 days • Increased cost $4,685

Source: Adapted from K. M. Van Voorde and A. C. France, "Proactive Error Prevention in the Intensive Care Unit," *Critical Care Nursing Clinics of North America,* Dec. 2002, *14*(4), 347–358.

think may be able to help. Readers of reports should operate with minimum specifications, or three simple rules: "Fix what you can. Tell what you fixed. Find someone to fix what you cannot." When a problem is solved, or when a safety learning report identifies a "success story" in which staff members have recovered from a potential error, the story or the solution should be celebrated for what it can teach others in similar situations.

- *The system should focus on learning.* The system should have the potential to sharpen the "safety lens" for the reporter and others, helping them detect meaningful patterns and themes in the environment and recognize when patients may be in a zone of danger. Reporters should be able to use the reporting system's structure and questions to view incidents in a new way, prospectively, through a different lens. When problems occur, exposure to the safety reporting system can help staff members and executives avoid falling into the trap of hindsight bias and focus instead on detecting meaningful patterns and themes that can help prevent future events.

Future Steps

As the Children's Hospitals and Clinics organization moves forward in its evolution toward a safety culture, plans for the following actions have been developed to glean further knowledge from data:

- *Use trending of numbers of reports and ratios of near misses to accidents.* Because the goal is to increase reporting, a ratio serves that purpose better than the counting of medical accidents as is done under incident reporting systems.
- *Use word counting as a barometer of culture.* Creating a patient safety culture involves changing the language that people use to describe and react to concerns and risk-prone conditions in the workplace. The search engine for the Children's patient safety database can track the number of times reporters choose to use words like "fault" and "error" versus "teamwork" and "accident." The use of blame-free, patient safety–oriented language will be tracked as an outcome measure of culture change.
- *Use an organizationwide data warehouse to study the epidemiology of patients at risk for accidents.* The Children's system has plans to analyze patient safety reports for the information they can offer about how characteristics specific to a patient can increase the likelihood of risk-prone conditions in the environment. For example, the data warehouse can track patients' ages, diagnoses, and admission times. Thus, if the data show that staff members report more concerns when patients who have complex, multiple diagnoses are admitted on weekends, then protocols and procedures for those patients can be modified to prevent harm.

Analyzing Medical Accidents

The predominant energy of a reporting system should be focused on uncovering risks, hazards, and near misses to prevent medical accidents from occurring, but reporting and learning can begin with a systematic analysis of accidents. Many health care facilities continue to work on fine-tuning these processes to contribute to a culture of safety. The following case study profiles how Memorial Hermann Healthcare System analyzed adverse events in order to use data and information for learning to predict and prevent future adverse events.

Concept to Action: Creating a Process of Analysis for a Medical Accident or Adverse Event

Memorial Hermann began to develop the rudiments of a reporting system by classifying and aggregating results from root cause analyses of adverse events. The first step in the process of analyzing the data collected through this beginning reporting system was to classify the events detailed in the reports and establish a common language for discussing them. Staff members found that this step in itself became an impetus for culture change.

"Often multidisciplinary teams have never met to establish consensus on critical definitions, that is, to establish a common language," says an administrative leader who took part in developing the system. "Physicians, administrators, nurses, pharmacists, and performance improvement staff created error classification schemes for medication variances together."

The performance improvement department at Memorial Hermann operated the reporting system, aggregating and analyzing the data. The decision about whether or not to conduct a root cause analysis was made jointly by the risk manager and the director of performance improvement. An internal, multidisciplinary expert panel reviewed the results of all root cause analyses on a quarterly basis and established consensus of the findings.

Figure 6.6 depicts an analysis that was conducted during the first eighteen months of development of the reporting system. It shows the common factors discovered in a rigorous process of root cause analysis. The expert review panel validated the findings.

The methodology for root cause analysis was modified as lessons emerged from experience into a structured process that could be replicated. Participants in each root cause analysis included those individuals who had been directly involved in the event, along with the medical staff, policy makers, and managers from the relevant services involved in the event. A trained facilitator guided each root cause analysis session, and a trained scribe categorized and documented the discussion.

The participants were instructed to meet once or twice, as appropriate. Facilitators were trained to focus primarily on systems and processes rather than on individual performance and to move from special cause variation to common causes in organizational processes; that is, they were trained to move from the details of the event to the area and services that were involved and finally to an identification of root causes.

"Participants were told explicitly that they would, in all likelihood, experience a tendency to place individual blame, and that the facilitator would move any attempt to place blame from an individual to a system focus," says the administrator, "and participants were informed that the root cause analysis process would repeatedly dig deeper by asking 'Why?' until no additional logical answers could be identified."

From a standardized template, an **Ishikawa diagram** (Figure 6.7) was constructed during the root cause analysis. The template was displayed during the root cause analysis as a visual aid for the participants. The exact labels for the categories were somewhat flexible and were refined over time. Participants identified as many contributing factors as possible, and the session facilitator added them to the chart as they were identified.

At the conclusion of the root cause analysis session, underlying causes of the event were summarized. Finally, participants suggested changes that could be made in systems and processes that would reduce the risk of similar adverse events occurring in the future. Methods for monitoring the efficacy of these changes were developed by the participants, and the results of the intervention were subsequently monitored.

FIGURE 6.6. SAMPLE ROOT CAUSE ANALYSIS REPORT

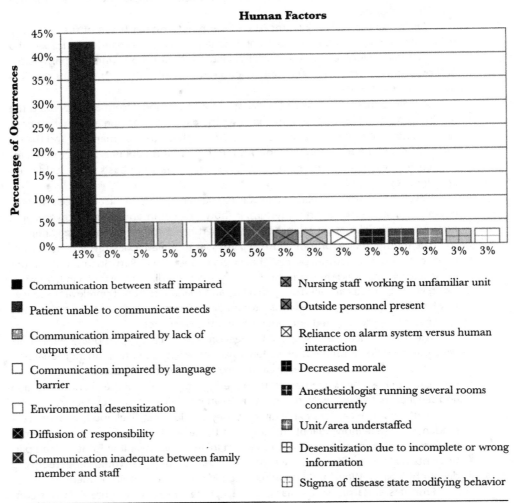

Human Factors

■ Communication between staff impaired   ⊠ Nursing staff working in unfamiliar unit

■ Patient unable to communicate needs   ⊠ Outside personnel present

▦ Communication impaired by lack of   ⊠ Reliance on alarm system versus human
   output record   interaction

☐ Communication impaired by language   ▉ Decreased morale
   barrier
                                              ▉ Anesthesiologist running several rooms
☐ Environmental desensitization   concurrently

⊠ Diffusion of responsibility   ▦ Unit/area understaffed

⊠ Communication inadequate between family   ⊞ Desensitization due to incomplete or wrong
   member and staff   information

                                              ⊞ Stigma of disease state modifying behavior

Figure 6.8 shows a reduction in medication errors that leaders at Memorial Hermann attribute to the system of reporting and analysis. The lessons from the case studies illustrate that reporting systems should be developed according to the unique needs of each organization. All reporting systems, however, should follow the auditing model depicted in Figure 6.9. As the figure shows, deaths are the least frequently reported occurrences, whereas variances in practice are the most frequently reported. The frequency of adverse event and near miss reports should

FIGURE 6.7. ISHIKAWA DIAGRAM: ROOT CAUSE ANALYSIS TEMPLATE

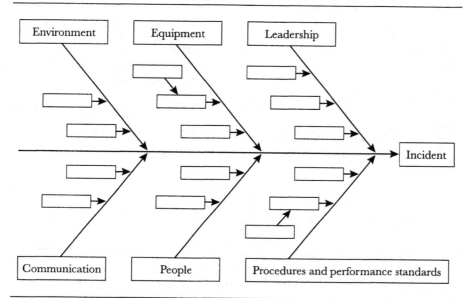

Source: K. Ishikawa, *What Is Total Quality Control? The Japanese Way* (Englewood Cliffs, N.J.: Prentice Hall, 1985).

fall somewhere between the two. In a voluntary reporting system, variances are tracked and trends are observed for the purpose of discerning patterns, but adverse events and near misses are examined in depth.

A word is in order about tracking and trending variances. Variance reporting is labor-intensive, both for front-line staff and for analytical staff. Busy professionals at the sharp end can be discouraged from reporting if feedback on their reports is not timely. To make variance tracking meaningful, Memorial Hermann rotates its variance tracking among targeted high-risk areas, using a generic Web-based form that automatically dumps reports into a database. This selected approach focuses resources on feedback and dialogue.

In the future, as legal regulations permit, a system of analysis will be able to include a network encompassing multiple centers of data analysis so that expert groups from different organizations can study the data and develop recommendations for best practices in the area of patient safety. Where a statewide reporting system exists, resources can be combined so that experts' knowledge of human factors and current medical practice is made available to analytical staff.

FIGURE 6.8. SERIOUS ADVERSE DRUG EVENTS
PER 100,000 PATIENT DAYS

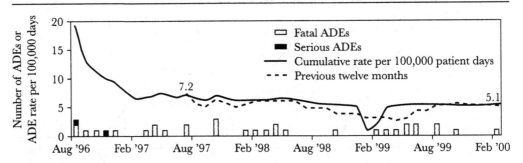

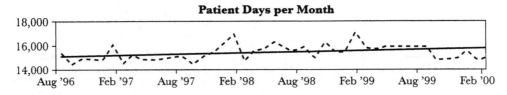

Source: J. H. Rex, J. E. Turnbull, S. J. Allen, K. Vande Voorde, and K. Luther, "Systematic Root Cause Analysis of Adverse Drug Events in a Tertiary Referral Hospital," *Joint Commission Journal on Quality Improvement,* 2000, *26*(10), 563–575. © Joint Commission Resources: *Joint Commission Journal on Quality Improvement.* Oakbrook Terrace, IL: Joint Commission on Accreditation of Healthcare Organizations, 2000. Reprinted with permission.

The purpose of data analysis is to promote learning and offer preliminary recommendations. The goal is a robust analysis that focuses on detecting meaningful patterns and identifying new themes. As the system matures, data can be augmented with reports linked to a data warehouse.

The focus is on avoiding hindsight bias, moving beyond individual error, and thus learning how safety is created by the system. The ultimate goals are to create predictive models of who is at greatest risk in order to develop prevention strategies and real-time alerts.

FIGURE 6.9. EVENT OCCURRENCE PROBABILITY

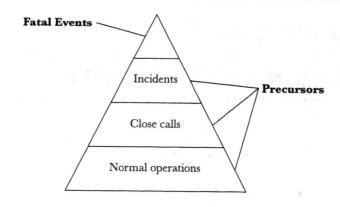

Summary Points

The success factors for a blameless, voluntary reporting system can be summarized as follows:

1. Installing a blameless voluntary reporting system is a powerful cultural intervention to create transparency of errors and latent conditions so that learning can occur and zones or margins of safety can be identified.
2. A reporting system should encourage narrative stories to understand how systems and processes are working to mitigate risk and develop resilience.
3. Reporting should be easy and reports confidential. The system focuses on understanding rather than on accounting.
4. Leaders' commitment is made evident by funding and active oversight.
5. The system's intent and goals are clear to all parties; all stakeholders are engaged.
6. Reports are analyzed by an independent party within the organization.
7. Case analyses are multidisciplinary and rigorously avoid hindsight bias by pursuing the multicausal factors that contribute to a near miss or medical accident. This information is then used to redesign processes and reduce the probability of future medical accidents.
8. Improvements are identified and a system of feedback is established so that reporters know improvement is taking place and that they are contributing to building greater safety by reporting error.

CHAPTER SEVEN

ASSIGN ACCOUNTABILITY

The well-publicized 1995 death of beloved *Boston Globe* health columnist Betsy Lehman became a call for accountability to the health care industry. Lehman died while being treated for breast cancer at one of the most prestigious institutions in the country, the Dana-Farber Cancer Institute. An anticancer drug was administered at four times the typically prescribed dose, causing her heart to stop. Although Lehman's blood and electrocardiogram readings became increasingly abnormal over the four days it took to administer the drug, failures in the system allowed the overdose to remain undetected.

The death of this well-informed thirty-nine-year-old patient, who devoted her life to humanizing medicine and improving the quality of health care through educating her readers, was a wrenching irony for her loved ones and for the entire health care community. If a fatal chain of events can be set in motion and defy detection at Dana-Farber, it can happen anywhere. The death of Betsy Lehman was a sentinel event, a call to learning and a call for action to engineer safety into every aspect of health care organizations. This goal means having eyes wide open to learn from and accept accountability for failures and learn from them. Betsy Lehman was a well-recognized person and her death put a name and face on victims of medical accidents.

Accountability to patients and families in the face of medical accident is a hallmark of a safety culture. The organization committed to creating a patient safety culture, through its board and its CEO, has in place policies, processes, and training directed toward disclosing medical accidents and significant near misses to patients and their families.

Accountability When Accidents Happen

Medical accident, especially when it harms a patient, is a defining moment for an organization. How such an event is managed both expresses and shapes the culture of the organization. When we mean to do well but harm results, we have failed the patient and the patient's family. An accident also affects the care providers at the sharp end, the point of care where technical work is done. It is a devastating event. How the organization responds can reinforce a culture of secrecy and blame, or it can advance a culture of safety, characterized by open disclosure, analysis, learning, prevention, and face-to-face accountability.

In a safety culture, executive leaders stand shoulder to shoulder with family and caregivers. This means that families are involved in all aspects of the care process and are not left out when accidents occur. The concept of disclosing medical accidents to families is a departure from the comfort zone of many executives and providers, but the greater risk lies in not communicating. Patients and their families are members of the care team and valuable partners in and contributors to creating safety. Participation in care is enhanced by information, truth telling, and disclosure in the care process.

In the rare event of an accident or near miss, the family should be brought immediately into the process. This is a departure from the traditional response of risk managers and legal counsel, who have long followed procedures that distance caregivers, families, and organizational leaders. Through focus groups, families have identified the most essential elements of communication they need after an accident or near miss (Children's Hospitals and Clinics, 1999): they want to be the first to know, they need to hear the story of what went wrong, they want to know what changes will be made to prevent the same thing from happening again, and they want to know that we are sorry.

Developing a Policy of Full Disclosure

Data from family focus groups, discussions among staff members, and professional literature were used to develop a disclosure policy at Children's Hospitals and Clinics, Minneapolis/St. Paul, Minnesota. Its creation and content are summarized here.

The board of directors endorsed a policy of full disclosure to families as part of the overall patient safety agenda. The policy states, "Children's Hospitals and

Clinics works with its professional staff to achieve complete, prompt, and truthful disclosure of information and counseling to patients and their parents or legal guardians regarding situations in which a medical accident occurred (1) when there is clear or potential clinical significance or (2) when some unintended act or substance reaches the patient." The policy title was changed from "Sentinel Events" to "Medical Accidents and Disclosure, Including Sentinel Events," reflecting the culture shift and an emphasis on patient safety, disclosure, and learning from near misses. The policy has the following purposes:

- To improve patient and staff safety by decreasing the system's vulnerability to future accidents
- To evaluate and improve the care provided to patients
- To reduce the chances for morbidity and mortality
- To restore the confidence of patients, families, employees, providers, and the community that systems are in place to ensure that accidents are unlikely to recur
- To provide emotional, professional, and legal support to staff who have been involved in events
- To ensure disclosure of accidents, near misses, and sentinel events to families, and to ensure continuous communication of system improvements to families and caregivers who have been involved in an accident

Event Analysis in the Disclosure Process

A full analysis of each accident and significant near miss is completed in the interest of understanding the multicausal components that produced the accident or near miss. The disclosure policy helps direct this analysis and sets in motion the processes and subsequent follow-up that must take place.

The human tendency to focus on a single cause often appears during a root cause analysis. To mitigate this tendency, some organizations have developed a two-step alternative process that is a variation of root cause analysis. The first step, a **sequence of events analysis**, is conducted immediately after an accident or near miss to capture the timeline of decisions and activities leading up to and surrounding the accident or near miss. This data capture serves to inform the later, second analysis, called a "focused event analysis." The focused event analysis follows the sequence of events meeting and is a causal analysis study involving all key stakeholders for the purpose of seeking knowledge about the contributing variables and the steps that can be taken to eliminate system vulnerabilities and latent conditions that could realign to produce future accidents. Formal procedures and resources are used to guard against blame, **attribution**, and hindsight bias, all human tendencies that become magnified in the context of a devastating event.

Confidentiality is maintained with respect to the patient and the providers who were involved, but a case study is created to inform others about the risks and lessons learned so that greater resilience can be introduced to prevent error from reaching a patient again. The analysis is introduced to participants through the introductory protocol shown in Exhibit 7.1. In addition, protocols (described in the following sections) have been developed for explicit guidance of the notification process after a medical accident.

Disclosure and Truth Telling. In the disclosure process, a presumption of truth telling guides all discussions. Generally, the managing physician should presume that all information that describes the specific event affecting a patient can and should be disclosed, with the exception of the identities of the specific staff members involved in the accident, if they are unknown to the family. The ultimate goal is to use a thoughtful, well-defined process that will re-establish confidence and maintain a therapeutic relationship. During initial and follow-up discussions, the following subjects are considered:

- The organization's and staff's regret, with apologies, that an accident has occurred
- The nature of the accident
- The time, place, and circumstances of the accident
- The proximal cause of the accident, if known
- The known, definite consequences of the accident for the patient, and potential or anticipated consequences
- Actions taken to treat or ameliorate the consequences of the accident
- Information about who will manage ongoing care of the patient
- Planned analysis of the accident
- Information about who else knows about the accident (in the hospital, in external regulatory agencies, and so on)
- Actions taken both to identify system issues that may have contributed to the accident and to prevent the same or similar accidents from occurring again
- Information about who will manage ongoing communication with the family
- The names and phone numbers of individuals in the hospital to whom family members may address complaints or concerns about the process surrounding the accident
- The names and phone numbers of agencies with which the family can communicate about the accident
- Information about how to obtain support and counseling regarding the accident and its consequences, both within and outside the organization
- Removal from the patient's account of charges and expenses directly related to the accident

EXHIBIT 7.1. INTRODUCTORY PROTOCOL: FOCUSED EVENT ANALYSIS

Objectives

> To support the patient, family, and caregivers
>
> To understand what happened
>
> To identify opportunities for improvement
>
> To incorporate our learning into our daily work

Rules

> Blamelessness: Refrain from passing judgment on people. We work in complex systems. We are human, and error is inherent in our work. Our goal is to eliminate harm by learning from our experience and creating safer systems.
>
> Transparency: Openly reveal all the issues. Ask yourself five "whys." Search for all contributing causes.
>
> Confidentiality: This is a peer review proceeding. We want to widely disseminate the learning, but we ask that you not reveal the patient involved, the place of occurrence, or the identity of the participants. Please leave any notes you may take.
>
> Innovation: Take on a problem-solving mind-set. Envision this patient as your child or your next patient. What systems would you want to be in place to ensure safety?

Process

- Sequence the events.
- Identify the opportunities.
- Determine the improvement action plan.
- Establish the family communication plan.

Tools for Creating Safe Systems

- Standardization (reducing variation)
- Simplification
- Redundancy (double checks, not pseudoredundancy)
- Constraint (forcing functions)
- Mapping (visual, auditory, tactile, or olfactory guides)
- Feedback loops (self-reinforcing)
- Information at point of care (Kanban)
- Defect visibility (andon cord)
- Methodical problem solving (Kaizen)
- Education
- Maintenance
- Crew resource management (standardized, redundant, constrained, mapped, and so on)

Source: C. Robison, E. Knox, and J. Morath, Children's Hospitals and Clinics, Minneapolis/St. Paul, Minnesota, 1999.

- Information about resources to which the organization can refer the family to help them obtain compensation if it is warranted by actual damages

Protecting Staff Members Who Report Accidents. Staff members who promptly and appropriately report accidents to a patient's immediate caregiver, to a manager, or to the organization's office of patient safety are not subject to retaliation, and they receive administrative support in all matters related to the accident. Nevertheless, the organization is not required to protect staff members who engage in intentional acts of malfeasance that compromise patient safety.

Concept to Action: Using a Disclosure Policy to Promote Accountability to Patients, Families, and the Health Care Team

This example combines details from actual hospital cases to describe how a disclosure policy can work in practice. Names of staff members and the patient have been changed.

12:00 P.M., July 16, 2002

Four-year-old Gunther had just been transferred from the intensive care unit to the medical-surgical unit and was sleeping in his hospital bed. His father, Jeff, would be at the hospital within the hour to help him settle in his new room.

Jennifer Causey, a registered nurse, entered the room with Keith Gliniecki, another registered nurse, who had just been hired. Causey explained Gunther's condition to Gliniecki and told him, "Dr. O'Connor wrote an order for 0.8 milligrams per hour of morphine." She showed Gliniecki how to program the electronic pump to infuse the dose. Causey needed to check on two more admissions that were about to arrive on the unit, so she left Gliniecki to manage the infusion.

Gliniecki had operated this type of pump once before, during staff training, but did not feel comfortable with his level of experience, so he found another nurse, Donna Falk, who agreed to help him program the pump. None of the nurses in this medical-surgical unit were accustomed to using the pumps, because the unit did not usually treat patients for whom continuously infused analgesics had been prescribed.

One element of programming the pump was to enter information about the morphine concentration and the appropriate rate of infusion. Gliniecki and Falk checked the label on the morphine but did not see a concentration listed, so Gliniecki watched as Falk used the other information on the label to calculate the concentration herself. Then Falk entered the rate of infusion, 0.8 milligrams per hour, using the information that Gliniecki had relayed from his conversation with Jennifer Causey.

Hospital procedure required that dosages of intravenous medications be checked by a second person, so Gliniecki himself verified the calculations that Falk had performed. Then Falk returned to her own patients, and Gliniecki went to the nurses' station to make a note in another patient's chart.

A few minutes later, when Gliniecki returned to Gunther's room, he saw that Gunther's face was blue and that the four-year-old patient was in respiratory arrest. Gliniecki called for additional staff assistance, halted the infusion, and called for an ambu bag to begin ventilating Gunther. Another nurse called Dr. O'Connor, who arrived on the floor within minutes.

O'Connor examined the pump and confirmed what the staff members already suspected: Gunther had been infused with several times the ordered dose of morphine. O'Connor administered a reversal drug. Within a few seconds, Gunther's breathing normalized.

Staff members, especially Gliniecki and Falk, were shaken. Had they been responsible for this near miss? What, exactly, had they done wrong? Who would tell the parents? They continued their care of Gunther and, for the expected upcoming review, gathered the equipment that had been involved in the near miss.

After ensuring that Gunther was out of danger, O'Connor began preparing to speak to the family. First he paged the on-call administrator and director of medical affairs, Dr. Terry Olstad, and relayed what he knew about what had happened. Then he brought Gliniecki and Falk into the medication room, a semiprivate area on the unit near the patient rooms, and, in a calm voice, asked them to walk through a detailed time sequence of exactly what had happened.

O'Connor took notes while the two told the story together, with looks of fear and concern on their faces. When they finished, he pointed out how the staff had quickly and successfully recovered from the error. He thanked them for telling their stories and reminded them that most accidents have many causes and that accidents happen even when the clinicians involved are competent. The nurses asked what would happen next, and he said that he would be disclosing the near miss to Gunther's father and that the staff members' names would be kept confidential. He also mentioned that the staff members would be involved in a meeting to capture the sequence of events, and that this meeting would take place as soon as it could be scheduled.

O'Connor reviewed the technical aspects of the near miss in his notes, anticipated the questions the family would ask, and thought about ways to describe the accident in nonmedical language. He mentally rehearsed his replies to the most common questions parents ask after hearing about a near miss: How did this happen? Who did this? How can I be sure this won't happen again to my child or another child?

2:00 P.M., July 16, 2002

O'Connor entered Gunther's room and saw the child's father sitting on his son's bed. First O'Connor verified that Jeff knew his son was stable and out of danger. Then he said, "I apologize that this terrible event has happened to your child and you. Let me tell you the sequence of events that took place." O'Connor proceeded to explain what had happened, without placing blame or using staff members' names. He talked about the currently known sequence of events, the potential long-term effects of the respiratory arrest and overdose, why he did not believe Gunther would suffer any long-term effects, and the tests that would be performed on Gunther to confirm that the brief oxygen deprivation would not have long-term effects. He gave a preliminary explanation of why staff members believed the event had happened and said that a review would take place immediately to explore the incident in greater detail.

Jeff's first question was to the point: "Who did this?"

O'Connor explained, "There were many people, including myself, involved in infusing the morphine. I wrote the order, a pharmacist drew up the medication, several nurses were involved in administering it, and many others were involved behind the scenes. We work as a team, and many of us have a role in giving a medication to a patient. What the research says about incidents like this is that most of the time, when they happen, there are many places within the system that can be improved. We will spend all the time necessary examining this case to find all the ways we can make sure it won't happen again to anyone. I want to tell you again how sorry I am and personally promise you that we will share with you all the information we find out, as we find it out."

O'Connor lingered in the room for a few minutes to check Gunther's condition and give the boy's stunned father a chance to recover and ask more questions. After asking O'Connor to explain more details about the side effects of morphine and about how an infusion pump works, Jeff had no more questions. O'Connor reminded Jeff that he could page him anytime, and he left the room.

4:00 P.M., July 16, 2002

Terry Olstad had received the call about the near miss from O'Connor a few hours earlier. After making sure that O'Connor had a copy of the disclosure policy and was comfortable proceeding with the disclosure, Olstad had let him know that he would be available to assist in any way with the needs of the family or staff members. He then called the charge nurse, explained what had happened, and reminded her that the policy encouraged the nurses who had been involved in the event to leave that day's shift if they need time to collect themselves. He then went to the medical-surgical unit and sought out Gliniecki and Falk to offer his support, tell them the time and place of the review that would take place the following day, and let them know that they could leave their shift if they wanted to.

11:00 A.M., July 17, 2002

The next day, Olstad began the review with an explanation of the process:

We have four objectives today: to support the patient and family that were involved, to support the caregivers, to understand what happened, and to identify opportunities for improvement. Today we will focus primarily on documenting the process flow of yesterday's events.

We have three ground rules for this discussion. First, this is a blameless environment. We are not here to find a scapegoat but to identify failures in our operating system. We want to reveal all of the issues and problems in an open discussion. Second, this process is confidential. Please do not reveal the name of the patient or the identity of the caregivers. Third, we ask you to think creatively about how to improve our systems and processes. Try to envision the patient as your own child and to identify systems that you would like to have in place to ensure your child's safety [Edmondson, Roberto, and Tucker, 2001, p. 2].

Olstad handed out a summary of how an event analysis is conducted. He asked Gliniecki to describe what had happened and others to contribute or clarify information. To ensure that everyone had the opportunity to contribute, he especially encouraged less verbal members to speak up. He used an overhead projector to copy down details and the information that each participant shared, periodically asking, "Have I copied things down accurately? Are we documenting the process correctly? Is anything missing?"

Together, the participants created a single process flow diagram of the sequence of events that had led to Gunther's respiratory arrest. Olstad then assembled a small team of executives, managers, and clinicians, who used the root cause analysis process chart developed by the the Veterans Health Care Administration Center for Patient Safety to analyze and study the multiple causes and latent conditions that had contributed to the event. The information gathered in this way was entered into a database containing all information about near misses, accidents, and risk-prone conditions that had been collected from staff members and families and organized for the purpose of identifying trends and themes involving safety issues at the hospital. The information was also reported to the hospital system's peer review committee (and was protected under the state's peer review statutes).

4:30 P.M., July 18, 2002

After the initial analysis of the sequences of events, O'Connor visited both of Gunther's parents and explained the main causes on which the review team was focused. He also showed them the initial list of completed and planned changes intended to prevent future near misses. The couple took notes on the information that O'Connor had shared, and they asked if Gunther could be moved to another unit of the hospital. O'Connor knew that the employees on a different unit were no less likely to make mistakes than were the employees on Gunther's current unit; in fact, the staff on the unit where the event had occurred would now be hypervigilant and unlikely to produce the same event a second time. Nevertheless, he judged that the child's transfer to another medical-surgical unit would not impede the quality of his care and would support his parents' preference and peace of mind. O'Connor shared these perceptions with Gunther's parents, and they said again that they wanted their son transferred from the unit. O'Connor arranged the transfer and asked Gunther's parents if they were interested in having the names and phone numbers of other individuals in the hospital to whom they could address complaints or concerns about what had happened or about how the review was unfolding. They assured O'Connor that they were comfortable communicating any concerns directly to him, and the parents made plans with O'Connor to get an update about the progress of the review.

After the review was completed, everyone involved was informed of the results. Several policies and procedures were changed. Tests showed that Gunther would not suffer any long-term effects from the brief oxygen deprivation and drug overdose he had experienced, and his parents continued to use the hospital as their health care facility.

Accountability Before Accidents Happen

Accountability cannot be exercised only after the fact. The work of accountability is to inculcate the science of safety and the operating practices of high-reliability organizations into disciplined performance in health care.

A safety culture is an accountable culture, and the overarching accountability is to those served. Accountability is the specific translation of responsibility. Whereas responsibility involves the authority and ability to make decisions and act independently, accountability entails the requirement of responsibility for specific conduct, behaviors, and duties. Mechanisms of accountability help create a culture of patient safety. It is the role of leaders to ensure that the following mechanisms are established:

- Patient-centered, system-centered, and evidence-based strategies must be developed and deployed.
- Specific teams must be formed and given the knowledge and resources to implement strategies.
- Monitors and measures must be in place for evaluation of effectiveness.

Before discussing specific mechanisms, it may be helpful to emphasize that accountability must be understood as a dynamic, reciprocal concept, one that is foundational in the transformation to a culture of patient safety.

Reciprocal Accountability and a Just Culture

The concept of reciprocal accountability embodies the responsibility and accountability that organizations, professionals, and regulators have to each other and that they hold collectively for patients' safe, harm-free care. In a safety culture, there is a constant state of awareness of risk and a predisposition to identify and call attention to errors, failures, risks, and hazards. Employees and providers have the responsibility of being messengers who are accountable for keeping the system's management informed about these. They do this through a robust reporting system and continuous communication. The system, through its management, listens and acts on the findings.

Reciprocal accountability, therefore, is the shared responsibility of front-line staff (at the sharp end) and management (at the blunt end) to interact for the sake of increased understanding and improved safety. Reciprocal accountability is based on trust. Managers trust that individuals at the sharp end will call out errors, failures, risks, and hazards, and individuals at the sharp end must trust that the organization's management will listen and take action without retribution or blame.

In a safety culture, where reciprocal accountability is nurtured, information about how the system operates is invited, actively sought, and rewarded. What is learned from reports is communicated throughout the organization. Changes that result from what was learned are systematically implemented and evaluated. Change is not entered into as a quick fix, but rather it leads to far-reaching reforms. The story of error is kept alive, revisited, and examined repeatedly for deeper understanding. As Reason states (2001), "You suck the marrow out of the bones of the story." Delving deeper into stories increases the level of sophistication in understanding the phenomena, and increases the capacity to learn more. This means that leaders have a responsibility to revisit safety stories, continually probe into why events may have unfolded in the way they did, and continue to learn from them as the capacity to learn becomes more developed over time. The organization, through its CEO and managers who provide active, knowledgeable direction, is accountable for knowing the perceptions of safety, the priorites for addressing safety, and improvement activities in the organization. Resources must be in place for continuous improvement of systems and for mitigation, if not elimination, of risks to safety.

The concept of reciprocal accountability includes the leader's accountability for creating a just culture. In a just culture, the leader draws a clear boundary between acceptable and unacceptable behavior. Individual malfeasance, impairment, illegal acts, intentional violation of known standards or procedures, disruptive or abusive behaviors, and the inability to learn over time are all incompatible with trust and safety. They are barriers to safety and must be dealt with fairly, definitively, and in a timely manner through management and systems for peer review. A safety culture has no tolerance for such conditions and has clear leadership and mechanisms in place to manage such issues.

The standards and mechanisms for dealing with intentional violations must be transparent to the organization so that there is a clear demonstration that rules are applied fairly. In a safety culture, there are decision supports to help the organization define and differentiate between blameworthy acts and system issues. For example, one hospital system established a strong conduct board, composed of peers, to address disruptive and disrespectful behavior that increased risk in the clinical environment. The board has the authority to affect employment, privileging status, and credentialing status, but its primary focus is facilitating successful performance.

Demonstrating That You Will Be Accountable

An organization's leaders are accountable for recognizing the nature of emerging risks and for operating a system of safety. They do this through the design and engineering of processes and through the management of those processes to eliminate or mitigate risk. The foundation for this work is the nurturing of a culture and a people system that sees, lives, and breathes safety. This is not about cautioning people to be more careful. It is about improving the systems in which people operate, and about increasing their ability to perceive, identify, and close gaps so as to eliminate or mitigate latent failures and vulnerabilities. An organization will be able to predict and prevent risk-prone conditions, near misses, and accidents only through an alert front line that perceives and reports risk.

Setting Priorities

The declaration of responsibility and accountability for patient safety must be the first powerful message from leaders. There can be no question of the priority of patient safety. The message must be clear, consistent, and concrete. There must be a steady drumbeat of messages, measures, and feedback to the organization about patient safety. The leader incorporates known practices to enhance safety into work and requires the same of others. At the same time, strategies must be implemented to remove barriers to safety as they are identified.

Charles Vincent has explored seven levels of safety as a leadership framework for analyzing risk and safety in medicine (see Raef, 2002). The seven levels are the following:

1. Patients
2. Tasks
3. Individual staff
4. Teams
5. The work environment
6. Organization and management
7. The institutional context

These seven levels help to identify patterns in risk and safety and can aid in directing the appropriate level of intervention. Vincent also suggests four diagnostic questions for choosing safety interventions (see Raef, 2002, p. 3):

1. How safe is your workplace? The most appropriate interventions are based on where your organization is now.
2. Which of the seven levels should you target? Ensure [that] foundations [are] in place before you get into some of the more subtle interventions. Identify where the major and minor problems are in your organization.
3. Stand back from what you do and ask, "Where do we rely unnecessarily on human beings?" You can improve decision making by using simple techniques, such as checklists.
4. Ask, "How can we make life easier?"

"It's a question not often asked in medicine," Vincent admits (see Raef, 2002, p. 3), "but taking the pressure off people can help improve safety."

Using Lessons from HROs

At the macro- and microsystem level, leaders must "hardwire" patient safety into the daily lifeblood and operations of the organization. Embracing and applying lessons learned from leaders in other industries, such as aviation, nuclear power, firefighting, and manufacturing, can inform and accelerate action. There are known safety principles from industry that can be incorporated into daily work (Helmreich, 2001):

- Train staff in effective teamwork, decision making, risk awareness, and error management as well as technical aspects of the job.
- Require team debriefings and simulations of high-risk processes and procedures.
- Simplify and standardize work processes and products, such as the use of a consistent monitoring system.

- Design self-correcting systems or redundant systems that make it difficult to do the wrong thing, such as verifying messages about who will take what action when, or using technical monitors to complement judgment. For example, an organization can require read-backs if staff members are taking verbal orders.
- Reduce reliance on human memory through protocols, checklists, automated systems, and checking with colleagues.
- Use automation carefully through the meticulous design of manual processes that can be converted well to automation, such as the medication record documentation process.
- Learn how each function of the organization works by studying it as a flow process. This requires a comprehensive audit of each step in a sequence, across divisions, departments, and disciplines. The technology of Failure Mode and Effects Analysis can be applied to the study of process.
- Drive out fear, and set up systems so that data can be collected for learning about error and near misses. The risk should be in failing to report, not in the act of bringing bad news.
- Find out what is going on by developing sources, asking questions, and walking around. This is accomplished by being visible and by reviewing, in person, the work activity.
- Do the obvious things one by one. When processes need correction, take action.
- Do not tolerate violation of standards or failure of staff to take available measures against error (such as getting input from a colleague or using a checklist), and hold people accountable for their actions.

Individuals in a culture open to new knowledge seek information and advice on the basis of who has content expertise rather than who is in a position of authority. Leaders and front-line workers continually question the processes of their work environment. There is a constant flow of information across departments, teams, and disciplines. Leaders and the front line are open to and sensitive to surprise in daily operations. When the unexpected happens, whether the event is noticeable to all or recognized only by one, individuals trust their sense of surprise, and they capture the moment for further learning and system improvement. New strategies are tested frequently as everyone works toward continually improving the resilience of the system. When the story of a risk, hazard, or error is told, members of the organization continually ask, "Why?" and they explore and exhaust what the story has to teach. The organization resists the human impulse toward closure, keeping the stories alive and revisiting them periodically for new lessons and insights.

Making Implicit Knowledge Explicit

Implicit knowledge is the information and know-how that individuals uniquely possess (Norman, 1988). In health care, a great deal of the work in developing care paths or clinical protocols, process mapping, structured debriefings, simulations, and best-practice models is about making explicit each provider's knowledge of how a care process works. Working to define the knowledge that people have, but do not know they have, is a critical step in understanding work flow and seeing the whole picture. It also helps in focusing on who in the system has knowledge and reinforces that everyone on the team gets to ask questions.

Experience in the aviation industry suggests that everyone has knowledge about different things and that everyone can ask questions. The leader has a responsibility to both model and set expectations for using team- and crew-based communication, explicit sharing of information and knowledge, and tools for transferring knowledge and information.

Process Auditing

Process auditing establishes a system for ongoing checks and formal audits to spot unexpected safety problems. Questions for the leader include those listed here:

- Is there an objective process for inquiry, review, and measurement of critical performance areas for the organization and its parts?
- Is there an internal function, apart from defined work groups, departments, and care units, for conducting audits and reports?
- Are critical indicators systematically measured, reported, and reviewed with frequency and regularity?
- Is a formalized framework for safety self-assessment used, such as the ones now available through the American Hospital Association, Veteran's Healthcare Administration, Child Healthcare Corporation of America, and other professional organizations?
- Are accrediting and regulatory surveys used as an opportunity for rigorous self-assessment?

Reward Systems

Questions for leaders concerning incentives or rewards include those listed here:

- How are reward systems used to drive the attention and behavior of the organization?

- Are reward systems aligned consistently with promoting safe practice and behavior?
- Are shortcuts used and rewarded to reduce costs that have potential to compromise safety?
- Is the disclosure of risk- and failure-prone practices recognized and rewarded?

Pursuit of Safety Standards

Studies of catastrophic accidents, such as the Exxon *Valdez* oil spill in Prince William Sound, the Chernobyl nuclear plant explosion in the Soviet Union, the Bhopal gas spill in India, and the incident of the Hubbell Telescope's misguided mirror, reveal a pattern of subordinating safety and quality to costs. Neither the standards for basic safety nor those for the particular industry were met in these cases. Questions for leaders concerning safety standards include those listed here:

- Do clear standards exist that differentiate safe, high-quality practices from substandard practices?
- Are monitors of performance, as measured against relevant best-in-class standards, in place and rigorously applied?
- Are data transparent, shared, and benchmarked?
- Is performance improvement required, and is it monitored to achieve best-in-class performance standards?

Perception of Risk

The perception of risk has two aspects: Is the organization aware of existing risks? If so, what measures are being taken to minimize them? This issue is related to the question of which data are collected, monitored, and acted on. In a high-reliability organization there are effective monitoring systems, and the organization acknowledges and confronts the existing reality. Questions for leaders in the area of risk perception include those listed here:

- Do you require and regularly use effective monitors?
- Are the measures used the right measures, and of sufficient sensitivity, to detect early signals of declining performance?
- Are actions for improvement required, along with ongoing follow-up, to ensure that improvement is sustained?
- Do you make ongoing safety rounds and personally inquire into accidents, barriers, risks, and latent conditions?

Staffing Resources and Support

Health care leaders are accountable for providing the environment, systems, and context of care in which clinicians and all other health care employees work. Questions for leaders in this area include those listed here:

- Are there clear expectations around communication and teamwork?
- Have human resource systems been designed to ensure proper screening and education targeted at specific learning needs and experience for the work performed, standards, and expectations?
- How are employees monitored and supervised to ensure adequate knowledge, skills, and training?
- How are employees monitored and supervised to ensure that they are performing within the appropriate scope of practice and within their job descriptions?
- Have enough nurses, pharmacists, and therapists been appropriately prepared to meet the needs of the patient population?
- Are work schedules and safety practices (such as a policy prohibiting nurses from working more than twelve hours in any twenty-four hour period, or more than sixty hours per week) consistent with the goal of eliminating or reducing error-producing fatigue?
- Is the organization complying with all relevant standards to ensure that the physical facility and equipment are in proper condition?
- Are policies, procedures, monitoring, and control functions in place to ensure that the physical facility and equipment are in proper condition?

Command and Control

Although formal rules and procedures are necessary, establishing them should not be confused with creating bureaucratic complexity. Their goal is to ensure adherence to the standards and shared knowledge of best practice. This goal implies intelligent, thoughtful application of rules and procedures, not routine compliance. The rules and procedures should foster knowledge-based decisions whereby experts can determine when a variation or innovation is required because of a unique condition. Roberts (1999) expands on this concept by outlining the following elements of command and control:

- *Migrating decision making.* The person with the most expertise makes the decision.
- *Having redundancy.* Backup systems are in place, whether they are intended to support people or technology.

- *Seeing the big picture.* Senior managers do not micromanage. Instead, they attend to patterns and systems.
- *Establishing formal rules and procedures.* There is a hierarchy, with procedures and protocols that are based on evidence.
- *Conducting ongoing training.* Investment is made in the knowledge and skills of workers on the front line. This investment includes training in teamwork, such as the team technologies involved in crew resource management.

Mechanisms for Learning

Mechanisms for learning are detailed throughout this book, but a few are listed here for extra emphasis:

- A blameless reporting system
- A new vocabulary for safety
- Focus groups
- Quarterly minicourses
- Monthly dialogues
- "Good catch" logs
- Safety action teams and complex conversations

Engaging the Organization

Assigning accountability also carries with it the requirement to actively engage employees and professional medical staff in the design and execution of the patient safety agenda. Providing care that is free of harm is a shared interest among those who have committed their careers to health care. Actively engaging all stakeholders starts with aims, goals, and associated measures that are directly relevant to patient care. The most important engagement strategy is the leader's creation of a safe environment for talking about error and asking questions. The leader's consistent nurturing of this environment, and his or her consistent follow-through on the conversations that exist within it, will eliminate skepticism about patient safety being a fad or merely a reflection of shallow rhetoric. Such actions emphasize patient safety as a long-term, never-ending pursuit. Failure of executive leaders to model the principles of safety will result in an impoverished, pale expression of patient safety that will fall far short of the aim.

There are many examples of engagement strategies. Managers can establish safety or "good catch" logs in all units, where staff can enter observations and concerns about safety. Managerial leaders and medical directors then meet regularly, with an interdisciplinary team, to review the content of the logs, set priorities, and plan actions to eliminate or mitigate the identified risks. A safety action team can be assembled at each local unit, populated by interdisciplinary and interdepartmental staff, and empowered to take the necessary actions to implement changes that increase safety and reduce the probability that accidents will occur. The teams can develop and use data sources, such as logs, safety reports, provider insights, and feedback from patients and families. They can also scan the relevant literature to gain ideas from the experience of others.

At a broad organizational level, a patient safety steering committee, with membership from across the organization and professional medical staff, clinical frontline staff, consumers, and board members, can be appointed to advise on strategy and policy. The steering committee can also monitor results, and members can act as organizational resources and emissaries for patient safety. One responsibility of leaders is to charter and chair such a forum. Doing so sends a powerful, visible message about the organization's commitment and priorities in patient safety. It provides a forum for practicing clinicians, clinical leaders, executives, communication experts, consumers, and governing directors to discuss issues and the changes that must be made for ever-increasing levels of safety to be achieved.

Further areas of engagement include leveraging information technology and the expertise of clinical staff in designing the necessary decision supports, alerts, documentation processes, information migration, and reports to enhance patient safety. Starting points are direct order entry, dose-range checking, bar coding, and alerts for incompatibilities and allergies in the medication use system. The use of information technology is just beginning to be fully realized in the domain of patient safety. Most leaders are not technical experts, but they can gain a working knowledge of what is possible and then engage experts to anticipate and build what is necessary.

The hospital librarian can also be engaged to establish a knowledge map outlining where safety expertise lies within the organization. The librarian can serve as a human bridge between the sharp and the blunt end to improve transparency and help disseminate safety lessons (Zipperer, Gluck, and Anderson, 2002).

Concept to Action: Engaging the Sharp End through Safety Action Teams

Engaging the sharp end of the organization is critical to the success of patient safety. At Children's, front-line staff members developed the concept of safety action teams (SATs) to capture the knowledge and resourcefulness of front-line providers and to better enable them to improve safety at a local level.

Casey Hooke, advanced practice nurse and creator of the Safety Action Team (SAT) concept, defines SATs as department- or unit-based interdisciplinary work groups that provide a "think tank" for staff to identify safety concerns, process them, and brainstorm new ways to address them (Hooke, 2002). Group membership varies according to individual needs, but SATs strive to include members who represent the continuum of care for the patients they serve. SATs include registered nurses, physicians, pharmacists, respiratory care practitioners, child-life specialists, unit service coordinators, and members of the management team. The group is chaired by a staff leader, or sometimes by two staff leaders who share the responsibility.

Leadership support and a strong reporting system have been identified as key success factors for SATs. At Children's, support has taken several forms:

- The Patient Safety Steering Committee is the multidisciplinary, cross-functional, systemwide group committed to directing the overall patient safety agenda. Each SAT has one representative from the Patient Safety Steering Committee as a mentor who helps the team get started, attends ongoing meetings, reports back to the Patient Safety Steering Committee about successes and challenges, and is a resource to continually deepen member understanding of patient safety.
- The Office of Patient Safety is a virtual department whose work is protected under the state peer review statutes. It serves as the central catalyst and coordinating body for the work of patient safety. All reports of potential risks, near misses, and medical accidents are processed through the Office of Patient Safety.
- A strong system of reporting, crucial to the success of SATs, includes the patient safety report. The report is a narrative, text-based report that encourages staff members to identify errors and latent conditions in the environment before they manifest in an accident. The Office of Patient Safety receives reports and screens them to identify those requiring an immediate response. Reports are entered into a database and distributed to SATs for review, discussion, and action. All safety reports are entered into a safety database, so that the data can be analyzed for detection of patterns and identification of trends. These analyses inform organizational priorities.

The SATs work with simple rules. They are: "Fix what you can. Tell what you fixed. Find someone to fix what you cannot." Local accountability and involvement is a powerful part of the safety agenda. It is the vehicle that engages and empowers the sharp end. Yet, to be effective, local work requires a broad and facilitative infrastructure so efforts are aligned throughout the organization, maintaining flexibility to work on locally relevant issues.

The design of the SATs is sensitive to the demands on sharp-end staff in a busy clinical environment. Introductory SAT meetings run three hours and communicate two main messages:

1. The safety action team focuses on systems, not people. Participants view a ten-minute video, *Beyond Blame* (see Resources), that educates staff on the basics of

patient safety and sets a tone of learning versus blame. The group learns about basic concepts such as hindsight bias, the sharp end, the blunt end, reciprocal accountability, and the Swiss Cheese Model of Accident Causation. The facilitator helps group members process a safety learning report, using systems thinking. For example, the hematology-oncology SAT meeting examined a report of a chemotherapy order that contained errors. The facilitator pointed out where vigilance and recovery by the staff had deflected the errors from reaching a patient: a near miss. The group members used a flow diagram to determine what happened, and used the Swiss Cheese Model to prompt questions about how to examine and improve the system of chemotherapy administration. They identified changes in policy, protocol, and practice to reduce the probability of the same errors in the future.

Each SAT member receives a brochure that encourages the use of language for building a safety culture.

2. The safety action team is respectful of clinicians' time and is oriented to **rapid cycle change**. Participants determine their meeting times, and staff members (nurses, for example) are replaced, as necessary, so they can attend. After the initial three-hour meeting, meeting times are sixty to ninety minutes. Meetings are scheduled in advance and are held at consistent times. Agendas are kept simple. All safety reports forwarded by the Office of Patient Safety are discussed, and actions are assigned. The goal is for improvement projects, informed by the reports, to be completed within thirty to ninety days. To maintain momentum, large projects are assigned to a task force that reports back to the SAT. When a project has been completed, SAT members encourage staff members' further engagement by broadly communicating and celebrating improvement outcomes within the organization.

The SATs use "good catch" logs as one of the options for reporting. The "good catch" log is an open, narrative notebook where staff members jot ideas and insights about how to improve safety.

The "good catch" logs are placed in the medication or break rooms for ease of access. They are reviewed regularly by SATs in order to explore and prioritize ideas and take action.

An SAT toolkit provides resources for the team. The kit includes educational resources on patient safety and information about Children's patient safety agenda. Documents, such as minutes from other SATs, give SAT members a model for their work, and serves to disseminate learnings and innovations across teams.

Typically, an SAT will review between twenty and twenty-five items culled from safety reports and "good catch" logs at each monthly meeting. To keep SATs productive and efficient, members prepare for meetings and dive into complex conversations.

The SATs have helped standardize and improve practices across the system. For example, one project targeted was managing allergic side effects of a specific new chemotherapy drug. This problem was identified through a safety report. Delayed reactions to the drug were causing families to return to the clinic. A home prescription kit was developed with medications for managing this type of allergic reaction. The parent education sheet for the drug was revised. Since implementation, all patients on both campuses have been able to manage delayed reactions at home without the need to return to the clinic.

The SAT initiative has created an environment where staff members regularly review their individual and team practices for signs of emerging risk or potentially unsafe conditions. "It's created an understanding that we all have accountability and responsibility for creating safety in our own environment," says a nurse participant. "It's created a better mechanism for regularly stepping back and evaluating: Is this a safe place to give and receive care?"

Accountability for Establishing a Reporting-Learning System

The leader is responsible for ensuring that reporting mechanisms are in place. Although this area of responsibility includes reporting both for purposes of accountability and for purposes of learning and improvement, the focus of this chapter is the leader's responsibility for establishing a reporting system for the purpose of learning.

When leaders support a learning and improvement system of reporting, and protect the environment of confidentiality, professionals gain trust that the organization seeks freedom from blame, punishment, and exposure to legal liability. When this trust is present, disclosures and learning increase.

When leaders use timely feedback to thank, recognize, and celebrate risk identification and reporting, they reinforce a culture that is alert, thinking critically, and heedful in its work. Instead of normalizing deviance through resignation to the status quo as the acceptable standard, this activated environment critically examines everything it does. Changing the frame of reference from "incident reporting" to "safety reporting" removes historic connotations of performance judgment. The learning-oriented reporting system is an information source for improvement for local teams as well as broad organization-wide efforts.

Grounding Safety in the Overall Strategic and Operations Plan

To make sure that safety is not viewed as a project grafted onto the organization but rather as an enduring effort, safety should be a prominent feature of the overall strategic operational plan of an organization. One example of incorporating safety into organization strategy comes from Children's Hospitals and Clinics, Minneapolis/St. Paul, Minnesota. The strategic operations plan, abbreviated to the acronym S.A.F.E., includes the planks of *s*afety, *a*ccess, *f*inancial stewardship, and experience. The acronym encourages all members of the Children's community to remember that safety is their primary job.

The plan is based on four promises to the community, each one the basis of a strategic plank:

- To do no harm (safety)
- To be there when you need us (access)
- To be affordable and never turn away a child because of inability to pay (financial stewardship)
- To be a partner in care (experience)

The experience plank includes promises to patients that contribute to customer service over and above the primary purpose of reinforcing safety. For example, the "nothing about me without me" policy commits the organization to partnering with patients and families in decision making and care, and the "if it looks wrong, it is wrong" policy legitimizes patients' and families' knowledge and expertise by asking them to stop an intervention if there is a concern or question about its appropriateness, accuracy, or safety.

The Work Plan for Safety

A specific work plan for safety, with ambitious aims, goals, assigned accountabilities, and measures, is an essential tool. The work plan provides a road map to achieve the aims, and a way for the organization to gauge effectiveness. The designation of the technical leader for patient safety deserves serious consideration to help the executive leaders implement the patient safety work plan. The role of a patient safety director, grounded in logistics and follow-up, can support the leader's role, through acting as a content expert, a consultative resource for managers and front-line providers, and a change catalyst for the organization to develop greater capacity at the sharp end of care. Defined and focused resources to execute the plan are essential. The plan is organized around three levels of intervention: culture, infrastructure, and focused initiatives.

1. Interventions at the cultural level include such tactics as these:
   - Educating about safety science and creating organizational awareness of risk
   - Changing responses to medical accidents and errors, including the development of disclosure policies
   - Creating a dialogue about safety, and about the expectation that there will be transparency around errors and mistakes, by embracing storytelling and

teamwork, using a new vocabulary to demonstrate attitudes toward safety, and aligning governance, executive management, and expectations regarding their role in advancing safety.

2. Interventions at the level of infrastructure include:
   - Designing and installing a blameless reporting and learning system
   - Developing an office of patient safety
   - Appointing a patient safety steering committee
   - Aligning resources for risk management and performance improvement
   - "Hardwiring" safety into job descriptions, orientation, training, and competencies
   - Establishing news and communication flows around patient safety

3. Focused initiatives are needed to prioritize and leverage resources for results. Candidates for focused initiatives include:
   - In the medication use system
   - In transitions and transfers in care, an area shown in safety sciences to be rife with potential for serious errors
   - In areas where priorities have been identified through the Failure Mode and Effects Analysis process
   - In teamwork and communication

Focus initiative(s) will be specific to the needs of each organization.

Measuring Safety Improvements

Measures serve as the gauges for determining whether desired changes are taking place and desired effects are being achieved. Increasing the frequency of measures, and providing feedback to front-line workers, can create and sustain change.

The debate about sound measures for safety is still evolving, but there are initial measures that can engage the board and the organization to focus attention on safety. For example, a starting point is to measure increased reporting. Measures could also include a goal of completing targeted improvements or implementing known best practices. Several measures that have been developed are briefly profiled in the following sections.

Using National Quality Forum "Never Again" Events

There is growing interest that mandatory reporting and measures should center on the National Quality Forum's published list of "Never Again" events. The top six priorities from this list, as identified by NQF, are as follows:

1. Surgical events
2. Product or device events
3. Patient protection events
4. Care management events
5. Environmental events
6. Criminal events

Refer to Appendix Twelve.

Using the VA Culture Survey

An exemplar of accountability is the Veterans Affairs system that, under the leadership of Dr. Ken Kizer, established the Veterans Affairs National Center for Patient Safety. Kizer chose physician and former space shuttle astronaut James Bagian to lead both the center and a relentless, evidence-based campaign to eliminate harm across the 170-hospital VA system and to test new technologies and interventions to make health care safer. While at the VA, Dr. Nancy Wilson developed a culture survey. This leadership tool evaluates whether specific tactics are in place to advance the culture of safety. The survey measures leadership and strategy, and it includes the following dimensions (Wilson, 2000):

- Demonstration that safety is a top priority
- Promotion of a nonpunitive culture for sharing information and lessons learned
- Routine organizationwide assessment of the risk of error and adverse events in the care delivery process
- Active evaluation of the competitive and collaborative environment, and identification of partners with whom to learn and share best practices in clinical care
- Analysis of adverse events, and identification of trends across events
- Establishment of rewards and recognition for reporting errors and for safety-driven decision making
- Fostering of effective teamwork and crew resource management, regardless of team members' positions of authority
- Implementation of process improvements that avoid reliance on memory and vigilance
- Engagement of patients in work flow design and feedback in the care delivery system

The specific tactics listed under strategies provide a road map to follow in the pursuit of establishing a safety culture. Evidence of the leader gaining personal knowledge related to patient safety is an important demonstration of accountability in nurturing a safety culture. Several areas have been identified as crucial to the leader's learning about safety:

1. Setting goals for the "meta-management of patient safety" (Weingart, Morath, and Ley, 2003), including not only the question of how to create an environment in which the organization can create safety improvements but also the question of a strategic vision for harm-free care, a vision shared and pursued throughout the organization and through specific initiatives

2. Designing management and governance structures in which patient safety is an explicit assignment, and where there is an experience of reciprocal accountability

3. Introducing the role of change agents to stimulate patient safety and improvements

4. Demonstrating leadership in communication by engaging the medical staff, taking the pulse of the organization, establishing trust, sharing authority to gain commitment, engaging consumers, and articulating arguments and behaviors to support patient safety and demonstrate that it is a priority

5. Monitoring and measuring patient safety activities, including the auditing of high-risk procedures and environments

6. Participating in public reporting and demonstrating accountability to consumers by sharing information about reportable events and making explicit promises to the public

7. Spreading and sustaining the safety culture amid competing priorities for resources

Using Measures of Specific Strategies

Such strategies as implementing computerized order entry, best practices in medication use, simulations for teams working under dynamic high-risk conditions, and teamwork development enable the organization to focus very specifically on improvement. One way to give an organization feedback about its successes and challenges in the area of improving safety for patients is to use a report card that tracks the implementation of specific initiatives. An example, as in Figure 7.1, shows simple measures developed from the priorities identified in the S.A.F.E. agenda and incorporated into a target plan for overall organizational performance. Exhibit 7.2 shows greater detail for key performance indicators.

Working in Complexity

A strategic and operations plan, a work plan, and measures are necessary but not sufficient to guide the work of improving safety because creating a safety culture is a complex, multifaceted endeavor. Linear processes do not easily lend themselves to work performed in conditions of complexity. Rather, multiple internal and external events, in addition to opportunities and the contributions of individuals,

FIGURE 7.1. CHILDREN'S HOSPITALS AND CLINICS Q4 2002 TARGET PLAN

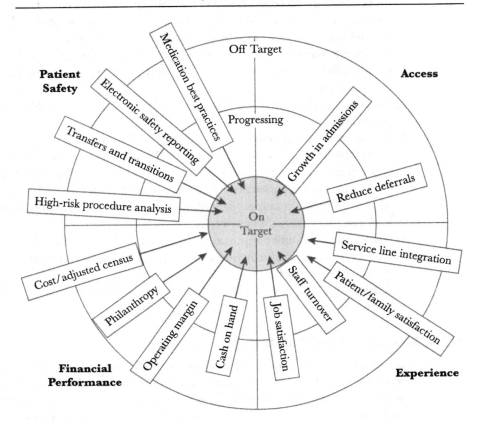

shape and advance patient safety. Figure 7.2 depicts one organization's journey in creating a culture of safety. Note the myriad inputs, some of which are planned as parts of an overall strategy, whereas others are serendipitous. Nevertheless, all inputs inform and advance the work. Indeed, serendipity—defined as "the faculty of making unexpected discoveries by accident" (Allen, 1990, p. 1105)—can create defining moments for an organization.

The ability to use the energy in an organization to shape its culture is a distinction of those organizations that have advanced safety. The patient safety agenda taps in to the most fundamental value of those who work in health care— to do no harm—and serves as an interest that is shared by even the most disparate elements of the organization.

EXHIBIT 7.2. PATIENT SAFETY INDICATORS: END OF YEAR 2002

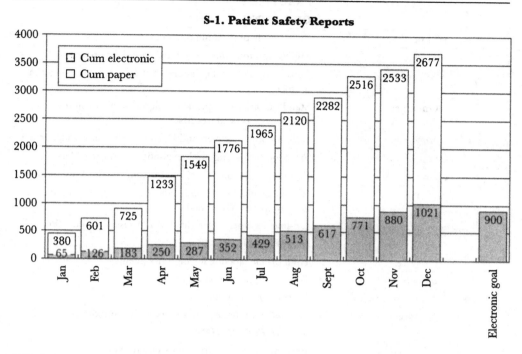

S-1. Patient Safety Reports

INDICATOR S-1: Total system-wide patient
safety reports submitted electronically.

DEFINITION—includes all locations. Includes
all types of patient safety reports.

TARGET—900

SPOKESPERSON—XXX

DATA SOURCE—XXX
COMMENTS—Goal was exceeded.

Source: Key Performance Indicator Report, Children's Hospitals and Clinics of Minnesota, October 2002.

Q4 2002	S-2. MEDICATION BEST PRACTICES
	ORDERING
Maintenance	Enforce safe prescribing practices
Maintenance	Mg/kg and total dose on all high risk drug orders
Maintenance	Restrict verbal orders, establish a standard communication protocol
On target	Standard order sets, prioritize high risk/high volume diagnosis or procedures first
Off target	Patient name, number, and DOB clearly visible on all orders
Maintenance	Protocol for nursing implementation of range orders
Maintenance	Eliminate "Continue previous or home medication" orders
Maintenance	Readily available and updated on-line drug information Lexicomp and Micromedex
Initiation/planning phase	On-line provider order entry with decision support (Phase I)
	DISPENSING
Maintenance	High profile labeling for high risk agents
Maintenance	Dispensing safety competencies
Initiation/planning phase	Barcode medications
On target	Evaluate and maximize automation to support safety
	ADMINISTRATION
Maintenance	Implement allergy wristbands system-wide
On target	Consistent labeling
On target	Patient/Parent partnership and education
Maintenance	High-risk medication double checking program
On target	Administration safety competencies
Initiation/planning phase	Review team for new technologies
Maintenance	Access to good on-line information
Initiation/planning phase	Transition from transcribed to on-line medication administration records
Initiation/planning phase	Implement a Point-of-Care Bar-Code verification system (Phase I)
	MONITORING
On target	High-risk drug—daily monitoring
Maintenance	Retroactive and proactive program for assessment of risk
Initiation/planning phase	On-line multi-disciplinary care documentation
Maintenance	I.T. Focused Event Reviews for all unexpected downtime occurrence
Off target	Maximum 12 hour shifts for all personnel

INDICATOR S-2: Medication Best Practices

DEFINITION—Implementation of
Medication Safety Best Practices in the
care environment.

TARGET—Active completion or
maintenance during 2002.

SPOKESPERSON—XXX

DATA SOURCE—XXX

COMMENTS—
- "Swiss Cheese" symbol now prints
  on all high-risk medication labels.
- Allergy Alert wristbands policy has
  been implemented.
- Medication range orders policy
  developed, approved, and education
  completed.
- Pyxis Profile software implemented
  on the Minneapolis campus.
- Pyxis stock evaluated to minimize
  "over-rides." Performance
  improvement plan implemented.
- New "Value Analysis" team to be
  established utilizing human factors
  and safety evaluations. IV pumps
  to be first project.

Q4 2002	S-3. Process Analysis of High Risk Procedures
Done	Infant Abduction
Done	Medication Administration
Done	ECMO
In progress	Suicide Attempt

INDICATOR S-3: Process Analysis of High-Risk Procedures

DEFINITION—Failure Mode and Effects Analysis or other accepted
analytic methodology to increase prospectively the safety of high-risk
procedures.

TARGET—Achieve completion of one FMEA or other high-risk
improvement per year.

SPOKESPERSON—XXX

DATA SOURCE—XXX

COMMENTS—Aggressively pursuing prospective safety practices.

FIGURE 7.2. CHILDREN'S JOURNEY TO A PATIENT SAFETY CULTURE

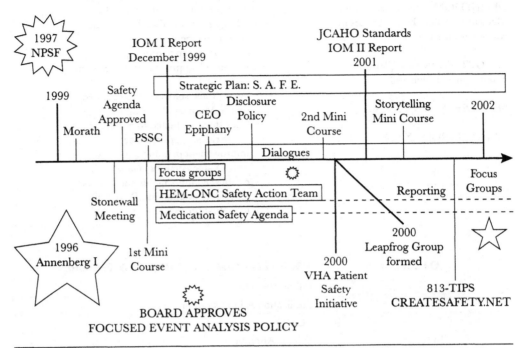

Source: J. Morath, Children's Hospitals and Clinics of Minnesota, 2002.

Accountability for Influencing the External Environment

A safety culture is created through trust, knowledge, and well-designed interventions to produce desired effects. The role of the leader is to be active in fostering these characteristics inside the organization as well as in the organization's social context.

In the broad view, the domain of patient safety encompasses three issues:

1. How society understands and talks about safety
2. How the legislative and legal systems act
3. What we do in and across health care organizations and systems, including academic and professional organizations

Although the emphasis in this book has been on what we do inside health care organizations and systems, the role of leader must encompass having an influence on public discourse about patient safety and preparing the next generation of health care executives, clinical professionals, and the broader workforce. The prepared leader who has an unflappable belief and compelling aim of harm-free care and who can recognize and orchestrate energy and events in the environment will be most successful in creating safety. An incalculable number of improvements and projects can shape a patient safety culture, but patient safety is neither a project nor the sum of multiple projects. Patient safety requires changing the whole system, not small parts within it, and this kind of change includes changes in the broader social context of health care. Chapter Eight focuses more specifically on opportunities for partnering with patients, other health care consumers, and academic and other institutions.

Summary Points

1. Accountability is a specific outcome of responsibility. Whereas responsibility in general involves authority and the ability to make decisions and act independently, accountability involves the requirement to take responsibility for conduct and duties in specific areas.

2. Reciprocal accountability is a construct based on trust. The term denotes the shared responsibility of front-line staff and management to interact in the interest of improving safety.

3. The overarching accountability of the health care system is to those served. One hallmark of a safety culture is an organization's acceptance of accountability and disclosure to patients and families in the face of medical accident.

4. Families require specific knowledge after an accident or near miss. Disclosure to families must include: timely disclosure, an apology, what happened, what will be the process to analyze what happened, what was learned, what changes are being made to prevent the same thing from happening again. Leaders also have accountability for supporting staff members who have been involved in adverse events.

5. Leaders are responsible and accountable for "hardwiring" the science of safety into their organizations' operations and performing as a high-reliability organization. An essential tool in achieving these aims and gauging an organization's effectiveness in reaching them is a specific work plan for safety, organized around three levels of intervention: the level of culture, the level of infrastructure, and the level of focused initiatives.

6. Leaders are accountable for creating a just culture by clearly marking out the boundary between acceptable and unacceptable behavior.

7. Leaders are accountable for clearly, consistently, and concretely declaring that patient safety is a priority and for reinforcing that priority with a steady drumbeat

of messages, measures, and feedback to the organization about patient safety. When the leader has become exhausted and bored with messages about patient safety, members of the organization are just beginning to hear those messages.

8. The most powerful cultural interventions is for leaders to gain personal knowledge about advancing safety learning and to change their own responses to failure in the interest of fulfilling the strategic vision of harm-free care.

CHAPTER EIGHT

ALIGN EXTERNAL CONTROLS AND REFORM EDUCATION

Patient safety is created by what we do within our organizations, by what we do in collaboration with other health care organizations, and in how the regulatory, legislative, and legal systems operate. Up to this point, we have focused on strategy, techniques, methods, and tools for building a patient safety culture in an organization. In this chapter, the focus turns outward to partners in the larger community of interest, to their needs and goals, and to ways of influencing them, learning from them, and aligning with them to strengthen and perpetuate a culture of safety. This chapter offers a discussion of aligning with consumers, with the academic community, with purchasers, and with regulators. Most important, it discusses rebuilding alignment and trust with victims of medical accidents, who are turning increasingly to the legal system and to the media to fill the void that health care organizations create when they fail to disclose information after a medical accident.

Aligning with Consumers

Consumers are asking who is responsible for the state of the health care system, and what is being done to address the gaps in safety and quality in health care, gaps that are so wide that the Institute of Medicine called them "chasms" (Institute of Medicine, 2001). *To Err Is Human*, the first of three IOM reports regarding the state of health care, exposed medical error resulting in injury and death as a daily occurrence throughout the U.S. health care system (Kohn, Corrigan, and Donaldson, 1999). This was in dramatic contrast to the idealized view of health care in the United States, and it jolted the American consumer into a stark realization: that the health care system, for all its miracles of modern knowledge and technology, has a dark side: not only is the system potentially dangerous, it is also potentially lethal (Merry and Brown, 2001). The second volume in the IOM series, *Crossing the Quality Chasm: A New Health System for the 21st Century*, clearly asserts that the nation's health care delivery system has fallen short in its ability to translate new scientific knowledge into practice and to apply that knowledge safely and appropriately. The report highlights a grave state of affairs in health care: "The U.S. health care delivery system does not provide consistent, high-quality care to all people. Americans should be able to count on receiving care that meets their needs and is based on the best scientific knowledge—yet there is evidence that this is not the case" (Institute of Medicine, 2001, p. 1). *Crossing the Quality Chasm* lists six aims that health care must meet: health care must be safe, effective, patient-centered, timely, efficient, and equitable.

A 2002 Kaiser Family Foundation survey showed the public to have mixed reactions about the heavy burden of health care injury. In fact, although 42 percent of those surveyed reported that they or a family member had experienced a medical error, and a significant number reported serious consequences of the errors, just 6 percent reported medical errors as a top concern; 38 percent reported that cost was the top problem (Blendon and others, 2002). This is a significant disconnect, and as dialogue continues with consumers, and within the health care community, the context and meaning of these results will deepen. In the meantime, however, a 2002 Harris poll has revealed that 56 percent of those Americans who responded believe that the current health care system needs "radical change" (Louis Harris and Associates, 2002). Public trust has given way to a call for expanded accountability. The consumer is becoming increasingly informed and activated as part of the system and is no longer a passive recipient of its services.

What Consumers Want

In their groundbreaking book *Through the Patient's Eyes*, Gerteis and others (1993) learned from patients and families themselves what mattered to them in their health care experience. Consumers repeatedly stated that information, choice, participation, coordination of transitions, and knowing that their preferences would be honored and respected were critical dimensions of health care for them. Table 8.1 summarizes those findings. These dimensions of care form the founda-

TABLE 8.1. WHAT IS IMPORTANT TO PATIENTS IN THEIR HEALTH CARE EXPERIENCE

Inpatients	Ambulatory Patients
Respect for preferences	Respect for preferences
Coordination of care	Access
Information and education	Information and education
Physical comfort	
Emotional support	Emotional support
Involvement of family and friends	
Continuity and transitions	Continuity and coordination

Source: Gerteis and others, 1993.

tion of a safe and healing environment in which the six aims advanced in *Crossing the Quality Chasm* can be met. Gerteis and others published their book in 1993, but the evidence suggests that few strategies have been built around improving the quality of care, beginning with the essential perspective of the patient at the center (Crawford and others, 2002).

Protecting Consumers by Anticipating Their Unique Needs

The "one size fits all" approach to health care must give way to an educated and sophisticated awareness of the differences in people who are served—their customs, beliefs, preventive health practices, social and support structures, and need for information. Berwick (1997) has discussed mass-customized stratification as a mechanism for achieving the efficient, individualized care that consumers are demanding and that clinicians want to provide. This strategy builds on the principles of population management; that is, it assesses the needs of different population groups—the elderly, various ethnic groups, women, those with different types of chronic illnesses—and builds them into care strategies. Safety strategies must be population specific. The safety concerns of the neonate in an intensive care unit are vastly different from those of the elderly person living alone. Since one-by-one, individualized care is costly, we must learn from those served to truly understand the patterns in their requirements and preferences for care. Then we can design care that is customized to the needs of specific populations, thus leaving resources for complex, resource-intensive cases and the unique exceptions of individuals.

Multicultural Solutions for Safe and Equitable Care

Patients and families bring an abundance of knowledge and a unique perspective into the care setting. They also bring their fears, their uncertainty, and their various ethnicities, religions, languages, cultures, and family histories. There are distinct issues of safety for different groups, and so leaders must be accountable for building multicultural competence into the patient safety culture.

There is ample evidence that disparities in health care exist among different groups (Smedley, Stith, and Nelson, 2003). Given the growth in multiculturalism in the United States, the ability to eliminate disparities and provide safe care will require people to think and act with informed grace across ethnic, cultural, and linguistic lines; as Hughes has remarked in the context of the American business world (1992, p. 49), "In the world that is coming, if you can't navigate differences, you've had it." Effective and safe care delivery can be achieved only in organizations that are culturally competent. Walker (2003) defines cultural competence as "individuals and organizations with the knowledge, skills and abilities required to provide high quality health care to diverse cultural groups," and he describes multiculturally competent organizations as having the following attributes:

- Bilingual and bicultural staff at all levels
- Professionally trained medical interpreters
- Providers with expertise in cross-cultural care
- Multidisciplinary care

Communication methods must serve all patients and families in the health care system if we are to achieve the Institute of Medicine's aims of safe, effective, patient-centered, timely, efficient, equitable care. Multicultural competence is not about "tolerance or polite accommodation" of differences (Chase, 1989, p. 36) but rather about awareness of and respect for cultural differences as evidenced in care that meets physical, emotional, and spiritual needs. This kind of care takes time and humility in addition to expertise.

In health care encounters that involve cultural, linguistic, and other communication challenges, one can identify several elements that may cause safety concerns and poor outcomes:

- Information may not be accurately interpreted.
- Information may be interpreted precisely, but real meanings may not be captured or conveyed.

- Social-psychological factors, role expectations, and perceived power differentials can lead to communication barriers between clinicians and families.
- Systemic and structural barriers to patients and families with limited English proficiency (difficulties with hospital directional signs, transportation, documents, prescription and treatment instructions, telephone scheduling, insurance assistance) may limit the ability of patients and families to access the system, follow instructions, and follow up on health care needs.

Preferences and opinions about the Western health care model itself has implications for safety. What many consider to be conventional medical treatment (prescription drugs, surgery, invasive procedures) may seem quite alternative to some populations (such as recent immigrants) and may create misunderstandings about risks and benefits. In addition, fear and ethical or legal dilemmas are present involving questions about when providers should seek protective custody or court orders in advocating for a minor. All these factors affect safety-oriented decisions.

Specific Strategies for Increasing Cultural Competence

Strengthening cultural competence in the health care community involves developing supportive policies, procedures, and management practices, a culturally competent workforce, and linguistic and cultural services that are integrated with care delivery systems. It is a comprehensive, collaborative effort that must include health care professionals, leaders, and patients and families from the ethnic, religious, and cultural backgrounds served and that must align with federal regulations and with mandates of the Joint Commission on Accreditation of Healthcare Organizations that are related to cultural competence. The following specific strategies can serve as examples:

- *Integration of linguistic and cultural minority families into all aspects of soliciting patient opinion and feedback.* This strategy includes interpreter-facilitated patient satisfaction surveys, patient complaints, and patient postvisit interviews; the use of up-to-date demographic and patient data in situations where the patient population is rapidly changing because of influxes of new immigrants; and formal research efforts and clinical improvement initiatives around culturally diverse patient populations.
- *Use and training of interpreters, and inclusion of interpreters in the care delivery system.* Beyond transferring words and sentences from one language to another, interpreters must act as cultural mediators who transfer meaning between speakers

and share patient care–relevant cultural information and context between speakers. Creating a responsive system of qualified and well-trained medical interpreters involves finding and training interpreters in language proficiency, biomedical concepts and terminology, cross-cultural communication, and the theory and practice of interpretation.

- *Translation of vital documents and signage.* According to federal standards, written materials for patients, such as consent forms, insurance application forms, and discharge instructions, that are routinely provided in English must be available in other languages spoken by key patient groups. For some patient populations, the materials may need to be available as videos or as audio recordings.

- *Use of interactive educational formats available to the workforce for developing cultural competence.* Educational dialogues and presentations that take place at new-employee orientations, conferences, department-specific presentations, grand rounds, and other venues can include discussion of cultural and linguistic factors in health care disparities, effects of cultural differences on the care encounter, and effective communication across languages and cultures (B. Kalanj, M. Khalif, and T. Culbert, personal communications, 2003).

Large-Scale System Improvements for Consumers and Providers

Changing the entire system around a patient's needs, as opposed to making a small change within the system, helped one child go home safely on the day he was seen. Berwick relates this story (1996, p. 619):

> I had never met either Jimmy (the six year old boy) or his mother (a single inner city teenage parent) before. His asthma attack was severe, his peak expiratory flow rate only 35 percent of normal. Twenty years ago my next steps would have been to begin bronchodilator treatment, call an ambulance, and send the boy to the hospital. That also would have been the story ten years ago, or five, or two.
>
> But today, when I entered the room, the mother handed me her up to date list of treatments, including nebuliser treatment with B2 agonists, that she had administered with equipment that had been installed in her home. It continued with her graph of Jimmy's slowly improving peak flow levels, which she had measured and charted at home, having been trained by the asthma outreach nurse. She then gave me the nurse's cellular phone number, along with a specific recommendation on the next medication to try for her son, one that had worked in the past but was not yet available for her to use at home.
>
> My reply was interrupted by a knock on my door. It was the chief of the allergy department in my health maintenance organization. He worked one

floor above me in the health center and, having been phoned by the outreach nurse, had decided to "pop down" to see if he could help. He also handed me a vial of the same new medication that the mother had just mentioned, suggesting that we try it.

Two hours later Jimmy was not in a hospital bed; he was at home breathing comfortably. Just to be safe the allergy nurse would be paying him a visit later that afternoon.

In this story, the design of a system—encompassing departmental design, use of equipment and technology, and flawless transitions—converged on one individual patient. Instead of the physician and the patient becoming encumbered by the system, the system was able to meet their needs and close gaps in care and communication where risk resides, because all were focused on the common goal of sending the patient home.

Changing Dialogues with Consumers

That knowledge will be placed in the hands of patients and consumers is a rapidly expanding expectation, and efforts to meet it are taking place at the level of the individual patient and clinician as well as at the level of the community. Many consumers, arriving for medical appointments, come prepared with Internet research regarding their concerns and have often found information through chat-line conversations with others who share their concerns. These consumers are seeking to avoid embodying the statistic described by Millenson (1997, p. 352): "From ulcers to urinary tract infections, tonsils to organ transplants, back pain to breast cancer, asthma to arteriosclerosis, the evidence is irrefutable. Tens of thousands of patients have died or been injured year after year because readily available information was not used—and is not being used today—to guide their care. If one counts the lives lost to preventable medical mistakes, the toll reaches the hundreds of thousands." Dr. John Wennberg and other researchers have shown that informed patients choose more conservative, less risky, and lower-cost options for treatment (Wennberg and Cooper, 1998). This suggests that the informed consumer can be a primary driver in increasing safety and lowering the burden of costs in health care.

Berwick (1997, p. 246) challenges the health care community with the following thought: "We persist in believing that consumers have unrealistic expectations about health care experiences—such as relief from pain, access to their doctors, desire to survive cancer, and affordable care—then we deny ourselves the opportunity to invent, innovate, and improve health care." He did not mention, perhaps, the most fundamental expectation—not to be harmed or killed.

When we are challenged by the question of how consumers will affect health care, we can consider that the real question is how health care will embrace and benefit from the consumer's perspective. The issues are difficult and broad, but the opportunities are abundant. Aligning consumers with the health care community can provide a wealth of largely untapped resources to improve our health care system.

Learning from the perspectives of patients and families and building systems around their needs is what is required; our health care routines and traditions are the first to go. As Berwick (1996, p. 619) said about Jimmy, the asthma patient, "This is what it took to send Jimmy home safely in his mother's arms; this is what it will take in the future to improve the lot of those who place themselves in our care." And it is such an approach that eliminates the gaps in the safety of care.

Aligning with the Academic Community: Implications for Education

In *Crossing the Quality Chasm,* the Institute of Medicine (2001, p. 4) highlights a grave state of affairs in health care and points to the current academic curriculum as a critical source of the problem: "Physician groups, hospitals, and other health care organizations operate as silos, often providing care without benefit of complete information about the patient's condition, medical history, services provided in other settings, or medications prescribed by other clinicians. Team practice is common, but training health professionals is typically isolated by discipline. Making the necessary changes in roles to improve the work of teams is often slowed or stymied by institutional, labor and financial structures, and by law and custom."

Safety is created in teams. Complexity is tamed through interdisciplinary and interdepartmental communication and alignment. Yet few of our academic and training institutions construct curricula or create experiences that prepare students to move beyond discipline-centric approaches to care. Expectations of teamwork, leadership, and know-how in creating safety and improving care are too often thrust upon professionals struggling to practice their professions in the face of complexity, fragmentation, clumsy systems, and production demands. Miscommunication and lack of communication are ever-present conditions as care is provided in isolated, disciplinary silos. This, too, is the framework in which students are trained and conditioned for professional life.

At the University of Minnesota Academic Health Center, there is a movement afoot to better align the educational experience with the challenges that lie ahead in building a safer and better health care system. One innovation is called CLARION, which offers an opportunity for health care students from all disciplines, along with health care administration students from the business school, to engage in dialogue and activities designed to increase interdisciplinary appreciation and collaboration. The glue that makes this effort cohesive is the quest to build world-class safety and quality in health care. Students explore concepts pertinent to leadership: interpersonal and emotional intelligence, managerial and technical skills, analytical and conceptual reasoning, and industry knowledge focused on the six aims (safety, timeliness, equitability, patient-centeredness, effectiveness, and efficiency) for the new health care system outlined in *Crossing the Quality Chasm.*

The staggering complexity of the health care system, representing a $1.3 trillion industry, is still based on a pre–Industrial Revolution craft model from about 1795—train the craftspersons (clinicians), leave clinical care to them, and create a parallel administrative process to provide resources for what the clinicians do (Merry, 2003). Our academic environments continue to train and educate according to this prescription. The legacy of this practice is huge variation in clinical practices and outcomes, harm to patients, numbing inefficiency, paralyzing misunderstandings and conflicts between clinicians and managers, and unsustainable cost escalation (Merry, 2003). And as if these effects were not enough, workforce shortages will continue as the health care industry struggles to recruit and retain qualified people.

The University of Minnesota Academic Health Center, although enthusiastic about the work and results of CLARION and its Interprofessional Education and Resource Center, has realized that it must do more. Work is currently under way on an interprofessional education model, grounded in patient safety as the overarching theme, with mastery of professional and interprofessional competencies as the outcomes. Figure 8.1 represents the movement to collaborative, team-based preparation and continuing education of health care professionals.

Aligning with Purchasers: Turning Up the Heat for Change

It is estimated that at least 30 percent of all direct health care costs today are the result of poor quality and medical errors, and the percentage is increasing (Midwest Business Group on Health, 2002). Purchasers do not want to enable or promote this level of performance and are taking action to demand higher quality and greater safety from us.

A major change is the notion that the health care system is a supplier and needs to be held accountable for the value it delivers. It is strange that health quality systems developed (or failed to develop) in total isolation from the rest of the American

FIGURE 8.1. THE TEAM

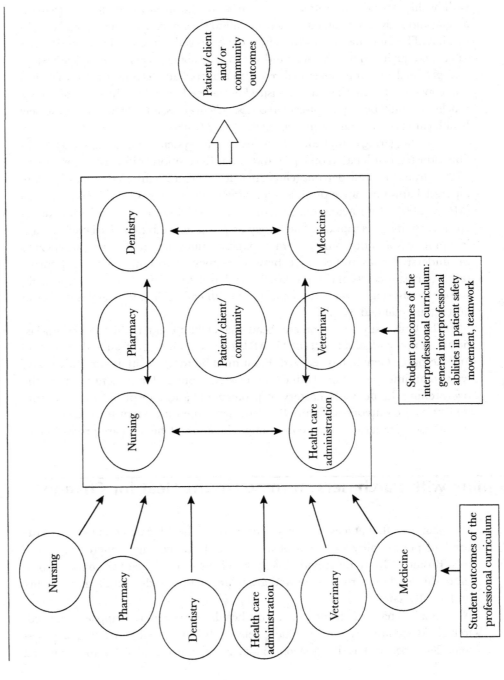

Source: Adapted from B. Brandt, "Vision for Moving Interprofessional Education Forward" presented at the Minnesota Executive Session V, March 31, 2003.

economy; a senior manufacturing executive, referring to this phenomenon, says, "For the past decade every one of our suppliers—except health care—has offered us higher quality at lower costs. Health care alone continues to offer us lower quality and ever-increasing costs" (Merry and Crago, 2001, p. 30). One respondent at the national level, the Leapfrog Group—alarmed by the growing knowledge of error and medical accident, and by the toll exacted in lives lost, pain and suffering, and a staggering economic burden—has identified a set of practices in patient safety that purchasers can use to measure the performance of the health care organizations with which they contract (Midwest Business Group on Health, 2002). These practices include computerized provider order entry, intensivist coverage in ICUs, and referral to high-volume centers for certain procedures (such as open-heart surgery) when correlations between outcome and volume have been established for them.

With more information about the poor quality of health care becoming available, consumers, purchasers, and health plans are asking questions that will change health care delivery and the practices of purchasers. Fragmented approaches—fleeting incentives, short-term transaction-based payment structures (versus outcome-based payment structures), and failure to engage the customer—are coming to an end and being replaced with collaborative and systemic views. Consumers, through their voices with purchasers of health care, are requiring new methods, new metrics, and a higher standard of accountability for all parties. Purchasers are turning up the heat for the consumer's perspective and taking the long view. Says Steve Wetzell, founding member of the Leapfrog Group and of the Buyer's Health Care Action Group, "In God we trust, all others bring data" (Midwest Business Group on Health, 2002, p. 27).

Six Sigma, a measurement and improvement system that is common in industry, has only recently been applied in health care organizations. It is a statistical control process that measures defects per million opportunities (DPMO). The six in "Six Sigma" refers to a process that produces only 3.4 defects for 1 million opportunities (Harry, Schroeder, and Linsenmann, 1999). As the sigma level increases, errors, harm, costs, and cycle times decrease, and customer satisfaction increases. In the financial services industries, for example, fewer than 5 out of 1 million financial service transactions result in error, thanks to the application of Six Sigma measurement and improvement methodologies. By contrast, most health care processes produce from 6,000 to more than 300,000 defects per 1 million opportunities (Midwest Business Group on Health, 2002). As demonstrated by Figure 8.2, the cost of poor quality with a given process declines exponentially when an industry moves from three sigma to four sigma, five sigma, or six sigma. Many health care processes are at three sigma.

Alignment between health care organizations and purchasers involves choosing meaningful performance measures and engaging the consumer in safety and quality instead of making decisions solely through cost comparisons. Purchasers

FIGURE 8.2. COST OF POOR QUALITY AS A FUNCTION OF SIX SIGMA PERFORMANCE LEVELS

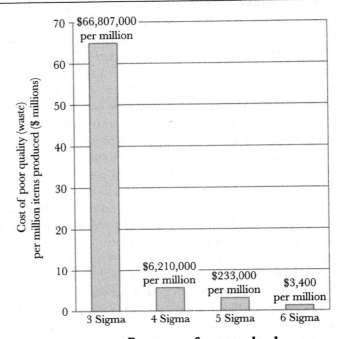

Process performance level
(number of sigmas within specification)

Source: J. A. DeFeo, "The Tip of the Iceberg," *Quality Progress,* 2001 (May), 36. Reprinted with permission. Copyright 2001 by the American Society for Quality.

are becoming increasingly informed and resolved and are appropriately turning up the heat to require measurement and evidence-based practices. Health care leaders can expect to see pay-for-performance systems in the near future, meaning that payment amounts will be tied to the quality of the care provided.

The public expects and demands near perfection in air travel, but not in health care (Chassin, 1998). This will change as the public becomes more knowledgeable. Physicians and hospitals will be held accountable to common measures of performance. Our obligation is to partner with purchasers to shape those measures (see Figure 8.3).

Aligning purchasers with health care organizations to study and define best practices is both a sound business practice and an opportunity to understand, educate for, and focus on improvement. Inherent in this effort are the rewarding and

FIGURE 8.3. A PURCHASER FRAMEWORK FOR IMPROVING QUALITY

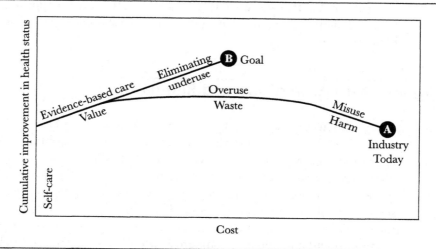

Source: Midwest Business Group on Health, *Reducing the Costs of Poor-Quality Care through Responsible Purchasing Leadership* (Chicago: Midwest Business Group on Health, 2002), 16. Used by permission.

recognition of high-quality performance (and penalties for poor-quality performance) through multiple financial incentives and selective contracting. Categories of quality problems that represent risks to safety include the following:

- Overuse (procedures, tests, medications, and treatments that expose people to unnecessary risk)
- Underuse (failure to administer known best treatments, failure to screen, failure to offer vaccines)
- Misuse (incorrect use of equipment, nosocomial infections, errors in medication administration)
- Waste (unnecessary complexity, unintended variation, faulty systems, delays and wait times)

As health care systems work to align with purchasers of care in order to make improvements in these categories, they can use many internal and external resources. An important example is offered by device and equipment manufacturers who can work with health care systems to assess device safety in the context of the work environment, redesign and customize equipment by using the principles of human factors engineering, and continually improve equipment design in ways that will reduce errors in the use of equipment (Johnson, 2003). Device manufacturers are key partners; as Bagian states (2002), "Too often the way we approach the solution is 'design the hand to fit the glove' when we should be designing the glove to fit the hand."

Aligning with Accreditors and Regulators

Accreditation surveys and regulatory reviews can be viewed as opportunities to audit the operations of an organization for expected compliance with standards and improvement, or they can be viewed as inspections to get through. How these processes are conducted, and the tone set within the organization by surveyors and inspectors, can advance patient safety or create a chilling effect, sending people scrambling to cover up. External reviews function as a vehicle for the health care organization to demonstrate accountability to society for proper operations and adherence to standards. Licensing agencies, such as health departments, have a duty to protect the public by ensuring that health care organizations are properly maintained, staffed, and operated. They also have the duty to investigate any complaints or grievances received. Although a single "bad apple" may provoke the filing of a complaint or grievance, this kind of incident is extremely rare. An investigation geared toward singling out a culprit to blame for a medical accident creates defensiveness and has a chilling effect on future disclosure and reporting—key features of creating a safety culture. Working with state health departments prospectively to educate them about patient safety aims and initiatives sets a foundation for a more effective working relationship should an investigation be required.

The JCAHO accreditation process has continued to evolve into a more robust process for focusing on safety and improvement. In recent years, the Joint Commission has made great efforts to engage the participation of all members of the interdisciplinary team, including physicians, as part of the process. Dr. William Jacott, JCAHO special advisor for professional relations, discusses the function of accreditation, citing the original 1918 hospital standardization program, whose intent was to create alignment. This intent was reaffirmed in a recent JCAHO board-approved strategic objective: "To enhance the relevance of accreditation to physicians through engaging them in the accreditation process and by assisting them to provide efficient, evidenced-based, safe, high-quality care" (Jacott, 2003, p. 10).

The JCAHO organization has initiated multiple initiatives to advance alignment among all disciplines, consumers, and health care executives. Perhaps the most interesting of these initiatives is the one called Shared Visions—New Pathways, scheduled for implementation in January 2004. The initiative focuses on looking at patient care from the perspective of process flow. Because safety is built through understanding care from this perspective, surveys trace the actual care experiences of individual patients through the organization's processes, from admission to discharge, to detect vulnerabilities and latent conditions that create risk (Joint Commission on Accreditation of Healthcare Organizations, 2002).

To encourage process auditing, another hallmark of safety and high reliability, JCAHO is implementing midpoint self-assessments, which contrast with the triennial survey preparation's "producing a contest to avoid recommendations" (Jacott, 2003, p. 11). The aim is to facilitate a more continuous and reliable audit process. These processes have the potential to create greater alignment by synchronizing JCAHO accreditation processes with high-reliability processes.

Controversy continues to surround the reporting of sentinel events to JCAHO. The lack of trust in the procedures by which such reporting will be managed has slowed the growth of reporting to a voluntary system that is still inextricably linked to the accreditation process. Although there is general agreement that such a reporting system is needed for learning and pattern detection, there continues to be debate about the design and the home for such a function. As an example of this hesitation, the percentage of self-reported sentinel events has fluctuated since 1999 (Joint Commission on Accreditation of Healthcare Organizations, 2003).

JCAHO has been instrumental in getting safety on the radar screens of all the facilities it surveys. Using information collected about serious medical errors and sentinel events, as well as consensus panels of safety experts, JCAHO has codified six patient safety goals into standards that became effective in January 2003. The goals, expressed as specific tactics in a JCAHO press release of July 24, 2002, are as follows:

1. Improve the accuracy of patient identification
2. Improve the effectiveness of communication among caregivers
3. Improve the safety of using **high-alert medications**
4. Eliminate wrong-site, wrong-patient, wrong-procedure surgery
5. Improve the safety of using infusion pumps
6. Improve the effectiveness of clinical alarm systems

An unfortunate artifact of our culture is that the primary purpose of the formal JCAHO survey has been to motivate organizations to clean up their practices every three years in preparation for the survey. The norm should be a continual readiness and state of compliance with the *intent* of the standards. That is, alignment with JCAHO standards should be embedded in the daily practices of sharp-end providers and in any health care facility's organization or management of care delivery. Organizations will have the opportunity to demonstrate such alignment with the upcoming unannounced JCAHO surveys.

Regulators and Boards

Alignment with regulators is grounded in the assumption that regulators want to use their authority to support the provision of safe care and that they recognize that health care workers approach their work with the desire and intention to provide safe care. Regulators and boards that are serious about creating safety can move from a reactive mode and toward provision of tools for professionals and organizations. Examples of such a transition would be consensus panels convened to establish best-practice guidelines for verifying surgical sites or for prescribing medications. Health care organizations have the duty to distribute these published best practices to professional medical staff and employees and to monitor their implementation. A model of this kind of activity is the Veterans Administration National Center for Patient Safety, which releases tips on published best practices to all Veterans Affairs Hospitals. The tips help in interpreting the intent of guidelines or regulatory statements. They also provide related information, discuss resources available to help implement the guidelines, and provide a clear outline of what health care professionals need to do in response to the guidelines. Organizations that monitor and measure enforcement of the guidelines and policies have the potential to produce more reliable patient safety results than do organizations that wait for the reactive external investigations that occur when things go wrong. This approach advances the ability of regulators—health departments, federal agencies, and professional boards—to fulfill their duty to the public to make sure that heath care facilities are safe. Professional boards, as vehicles of the regulatory process, can also work with facilities to create safe practice conditions and to manage unsafe professionals when they are identified.

Health Care Professionals' Job Performance

An alarming finding of a 2003 Kaiser/*New England Journal of Medicine* survey is that 40 percent of those surveyed believe that failures in care are due to "bad doctors" (Blendon and others, 2002). This public perception is fueled by the lack of a system that deals effectively with incompetent professionals. The lack of a system produces a reactive, punitive, personal, all-or-nothing approach. The current approach fails at early risk detection, intervention, and prevention of incidents creating harm to patients. At the same time, professionals fail to receive either the help they need or the opportunity to correct their performance.

Rosenthal, Booth, Flowers, and Riley (2001) write that known risks are perpetuated because it takes five to seven years to effectively address professional performance issues in physicians' practice. The myth of physicians' infallibility, together with denial of failure in the health care culture, has created the conditions that allow continued deficits in safety.

While we acknowledge the imperfections of human beings, we can proactively support the monitoring of competence as well as early intervention for professionals at risk, thus saving professionals and patients from injury. Gawande (2002) believes that physicians mirror the general population in terms of their own impairment due to substance abuse, psychological or physical illness, age-related declines in competence, and personality problems as expressed in reckless, disruptive, or abusive behavior toward other health care workers or toward patients.

Dr. Gerald Hickson has proposed that organizations and boards use a threshold number of complaints as a monitor for early detection, and that they use a broad repertoire of methods for remediation, such as education, counseling, incentives and disincentives, and restricted practice (Hickson and others, 2002). Organizational leaders are accountable for enforcing standards of performance, for ongoing monitoring as a condition of professional and medical staff appointments, and for ensuring alignment with professional boards in instances where remediation or revocation of licensure must be considered.

Aligning with the Legal System, the Media, and Victims of Medical Accident

The "blame and shame" health care culture is not just a product of health care professionals' training but also an outgrowth of a general cultural tendency to call for heads to roll when disasters occur. Catastrophes often awaken two powerful social forces, originally conceptualized as advocates for victims: lawyers and journalists.

Unfortunately, although the current legal system has been successful in delivering large monetary settlements to individual victims of medical accident, it has thwarted progress toward a safety-oriented culture. The criminalization of medical mistakes, and the subsequent penalties (including extensive monetary awards, loss of licensure, and loss of reputation), create fear-based responses to patients and families on the part of professionals. Safety could be advanced through tort reform that creates better conditions for disclosure and accountability. It would sharpen the legal focus on truly egregious events worthy of lawsuits and penalties, rather than bringing the full force of the law to bear on situations that could reach closure through mediation.

Concurrent with the increasing number of lawsuits filed because of medical mistakes has been a significant increase in media coverage of medical mistakes. The news media, which represent the interests and concerns of the public and defend the public's right to know, are aware that mistakes happen and are asking for accountability, including apologies and answers about steps that are being taken to prevent future mistakes. Consider the following excerpt from the *Los Angeles Times:*

> Medical errors happen surprisingly frequently in hospitals: An Institute of Medicine report in 1999 estimated that 48,000 to 98,000 errors occur every year. Most common are medication mistakes: giving the wrong drug or the wrong dosage perhaps at the wrong time. But doctors also have vastly misdiagnosed conditions, amputated the wrong limbs or breasts, been provided with incorrect pathology reports and left instruments or cotton at the site of the operation. In addition, an estimated 90,000 patients a year in the U.S. die of infections they acquire in hospitals, many of which are preventable, according to the federal Centers for Disease Control and Prevention.
>
> For example, in 1988, a Marin County surgeon performed bypass surgery on the wrong artery of actor/comedian Dana Carvey. The physician attached a healthy segment of Carvey's artery not to the damaged arterial section nearby but to a healthy diagonal vessel. A few months later, Carvey had to undergo an emergency angioplasty to clear the dangerously clogged artery that hadn't been repaired. He sued for $7.5 million. What he wanted, he said in a television interview describing his ordeal, was an apology from the doctor and an acknowledgment that the surgeon had erred.
>
> Said Carvey, "It is only because in his deposition he said, 'I didn't make a mistake.' Total, you know, denial. So I had to sue," Carvey said in the interview. Instead, the doctor's attorney claimed in court papers that the doctor could have been misled by the unusual anatomy of Carvey's heart. But Carvey's second surgeon said in the same interview that Carvey's anatomy was "pretty ordinary." Carvey, through a spokesman, declined to comment for this article.
>
> Jim McDonell, a Los Angeles attorney who has represented consumers in medical malpractice cases, concurs. "Clients say they never would have sued, they are just so angry when they [medical officials] deny it. Particularly in small suits. If the guy left their baby brain-dead, they probably would still sue. But in a smaller case, they figure if he can't even give me an apology, at least he can pay for his damages" [Reitman, 2003].

The traditional organizational responses of defensiveness and silence in the face of medical accidents are slowly giving way to greater cooperation and openness with the media around the issue of failures in the health care system. Positive publicity about patient safety initiatives in health care organizations has helped educate the media about the creation of a safety culture. When medical accidents happen, it is not uncommon to see leaders of health care organizations explaining what happened (within the confines of what they can say while preserving confidentiality) and issuing public apologies to the patients and families involved in the accidents.

Aligning with Victims of Medical Accident

The maelstrom of attention that comes with media stories and lawsuits creates the temptation to focus attention on journalists and lawyers instead of on the people they represent: patients and their families. Legal, risk, and media professionals can assist organizations in responding to external demands for information, but the most important question for leaders to pursue is the question of how their organizations are meeting the physical, emotional, and communication needs of the patients and families involved.

The Veterans Affairs Hospital in Lexington, Kentucky, which has had a policy of disclosure since 1987, analyzed its experiences and concluded that honest disclosure and compensation policies diminished the "anger and desire for revenge that often motivate patients' litigation" (Kraman and Hamm, 1999, p. 966). The American Hospital Association, the National Patient Safety Foundation, and the hospital accrediting body of the Joint Commission on Accreditation of Healthcare Organizations maintain that professionals and hospitals are ethically obligated to inform patients of all aspects of their care and to disclose mistakes. Nevertheless, disclosure often does not occur when the instinct for self-protection kicks in. Organizations fear legal action and public exposure, which can cripple the reputations of physicians, the involved employees, and the hospital.

Despite this growing movement for public accountability, the *Journal of the American Medical Association* has published the results of surveys, conducted with patients and physicians, showing that patients have not received the information they sought or the emotional support they needed after medical mistakes (Gallagher, Waterman, Ebers, Fraser, and Levinson, 2003). Physicians appear to have remained reluctant to provide information or to act in ways that could be interpreted as an admission of wrongdoing.

Nevertheless, more and more organizations are developing disclosure policies and preparing professionals to inform patients and their families about errors that have caused harm and about what will be done to prevent future errors. For example, Victoria Frazier, a physician and advocate of the patient safety movement in the Barnes Jewish Hospital System and at Washington University Medical Center in St. Louis, is studying accountability with respect to medical accident and is a leader in research identifying evidence-based approaches to disclosure (Frazier, 2003).

By aligning with those we serve—our patients and their families—by truly listening to them, engaging them in their care, and taking their questions, doubts, and concerns seriously, we can better meet their needs and obviate the need to turn elsewhere for advocacy. Recognizing and respecting the expertise and input being offered to us by families can further the fundamental transformation of health care necessary to provide harm-free care.

The following story is condensed from that told by Sorrel King, mother of Josie King, at the Institute of Healthcare Improvement conference on October 11, 2002 (King, 2003; see the Resources to access the full text of her speech):

Eighteen-month-old Josie died at Johns Hopkins Hospital in January 2001 with her mother at her side. First- and second-degree burns from an accident had brought her to the hospital. Throughout her hospitalization, Josie's mother had remained at her daughter's bedside, taking notes and asking questions about her child's medical care.

After ten days in the pediatric intensive care unit, Josie was healing well enough to be sent to an intermediate care unit. The family was told that she could be sent home within days, and the child's older siblings began preparing a celebration to welcome their sister home.

In the intermediate care unit, Josie began acting strangely. When she saw anything to drink, she would scream for it. When Josie's mother pointed out this behavior to staff she was told not to allow Josie anything to drink.

In the early morning of the day when Josie's condition deteriorated, fluid intake became an area of confusion, as did an order instructing that Josie not receive any narcotics.

Some hours later, in the early afternoon, a nurse came into Josie's room with a syringe of methadone. Josie's mother mentioned the earlier directive that she had heard, about no narcotics, but the nurse replied that the order had been changed, and the drug was administered.

Josie's heart stopped. As medical staff worked on the child, her mother was taken to a room where she was met by a chaplain. Two days later, back in the pediatric intensive care unit, Josie's life support was removed.

This is a story of overwhelming loss. While specific causes of death are not public knowledge, Josie's mother cites the cause as a multitude of breakdowns in communication in the complex system of care. She exhorts the health care industry to use the minds, hearts, and spirits of caregivers to solve the problem of how her daughter died and to prevent such events in the future. To this end, Josie's parents established a center for patient safety at Johns Hopkins Medical Center in memory of their daughter. The loss of Josie's life, and of the lives of other victims, obligates us to relentlessly pursue safe systems of care. As leaders, we must not refer such incidents to lawyers and risk managers, distance ourselves from the families' pain and sense of betrayal, deny the health care system's dark side, or be silent about the errors and failures of communication that occur every hour of every day. The stakes are too high, and the price of failure—paid in lives lost, and in families' wrenching sorrow—is too great. A growing segment of the patient safety movement is made up of families who have dedicated themselves to telling their stories and working with the health care community to prevent others from suffering loss. This is a partnership we cannot afford to lose. The wisdom, experience, and passion of families are critical in the work of creating safety.

Engaging the Patient through Patient-Centeredness

Paul Batalden tell us, "We should not work from an assumption of scarcity, but rather from an assumption of abundance" (cited in Berwick, 2002a). Our sources of abundance include the wisdom, resilience, and capacities of patients and families; the skill, compassion, and resourcefulness of the workforce; and the knowledge the workforce possess about what is not working for patients and the barriers to providing the best possible care. As we look to patients, families, and the health care workforce, our opportunities to bridge and ultimately close the gaps in health care are abundant.

Recognizing patients and families as active participants in the system of care brings a wealth of expertise as well as additional safety nets to the sharp end of care. Discussions around important questions—What is the right care? How is care most effectively delivered? What is important to patients and families (consumers) about their health care? What do health professionals need to know about continually improving care?—are propelling us toward a new frontier in our understanding of care delivery (Morath, 1999). The answers to these questions lead us to the conclusion that the best health care experience is achieved with an informed patient and family (consumer), and the patient's and family's (consumer's) inclusion calls for cultural changes in our health care system.

The Dana-Farber Example

The Patient and Family Advisory Council at Dana-Farber Cancer Institute was created in the late 1990s with fifteen patients and family members who agreed to one-year terms renewable for up to three years. Several members participated and shared voting privileges. Members made the commitment to attend one meeting per month and to participate in the work of at least one subcommittee, for a total commitment of fewer than ten hours per month.

Participants today are divided into several subcommittees. A communications committee works to increase visibility of the advisory council among patients and staff, and publishes a newsletter. A patients-as-educators committee works to improve physician-patient communications and the overall patient experience. A rounding committee visits patients, communicates concerns voiced by patients to the advisory council, and suggests initiatives or projects that could better meet patients' needs.

Advisory council members are participants in staff project teams and in several standing hospital committees, such as those involved with care improvement, clinical quality and safety, and facilities. Council members initiate projects to educate the Dana-Farber community about patients' viewpoints, and they participate in problem resolution when patients have concerns. The following list describes some of the advisory council's initiatives (Ponte and others, 2003):

- Creation of patient-faculty programs to help first-year medical oncology fellows understand patients' experience
- Identification of solutions to the problem of streamlining care for neutropenic patients
- Review of architectural plans as a way of building in safety and reducing patients' anxiety

Summary Points

1. Aligning with consumers includes rebuilding trust with victims of medical accidents who turn to the legal system and the media to fill the void that health care organizations create when they fail to disclose information after a medical accident.
2. Aligning with patients and families means listening to them, engaging them in their care, and taking their questions, doubts, and concerns seriously. Moreover, using the expertise and input offered by families, and recognizing them as legitimate and active partners in care, can create the fundamental transformation necessary to achieve harm-free care.
3. Alignment to advance patient safety is best served when working from an assumption of abundance. Sources include the capacities, wisdom, and resilience of patients and families; and the skill, compassion, and knowledge of the workforce on how to improve systems.
4. Aligning with academic and training institutions to construct curricula, and creating experiences (in teamwork, patient safety, improvement, ethics, complexity, and communication) that prepare students to move beyond discipline-

centric approaches to care, are mandates. In addition to mastery of professional competencies, mastery of interprofessional competency should be a primary outcome.

5. Aligning with purchasers—to create partnerships that shape performance measures for quality of care, to study and define best practices, and to engage consumers in safety and quality—is necessary to the improvement of safety performance. Pay-for-performance structures will replace transaction-based payment structures.

6. Aligning with accrediting organizations and regulatory bodies, and viewing surveys, inspections, and reviews as opportunities to audit the organization's operations for compliance with standards, can advance safety and improvement. This approach aligns high-reliability processes and the accreditation and licensing processes.

7. Aligning with regulators is grounded in the assumption that regulators want to use their authority to support the provision of safe care and that they recognize that health care workers also approach their work with the desire and intention to provide safe care.

8. Regulators and boards that are serious about creating safety can move from reactive modes toward the provision of tools for professionals and organizations to improve performance.

9. Organizations that monitor and measure enforcement of standard policies have the potential to produce more reliable results in patient safety than do organizations that initiate reactive internal investigations only after things go wrong.

10. The lack of a system to deal effectively with incompetent professionals results in reactive, punitive, personal, all-or-nothing approaches. The current approach fails in early risk detection, intervention, and prevention of incidents that create harm for patients. At the same time, professionals receive neither the help they need nor the opportunity to correct their performance.

11. The current legal system has been successful in delivering large monetary settlements to individual victims of medical accident, but has slowed progress toward a culture of patient safety. The criminalization of medical mistakes, and the resulting penalties, create fear-based responses on the part of professionals. Safety would be advanced by tort reform that created better conditions for disclosure and accountability.

CHAPTER NINE

ACCELERATE CHANGE FOR IMPROVEMENT

Change occurring in patient safety is both **threshold change**, that is moving technical performance to a higher level, and transformational change, that is changing the context and management of health care. This chapter offers ideas, tools, and methods to propel the changes forward that must take place for improving safety.

As we race to tame the complexity of today and create greater safety, new risks are being continually introduced. Such is the nature of health care, as captured by Ovid: "He who is not prepared today will be less so tomorrow." The staggering toll of harm to patients mandates that patient safety push beyond the incremental, cumulative changes that are the hallmarks of today's quality improvement and accelerate the pace of transforming health care. While methods of accelerating change can be found in many health care organizations, extraordinary measures are required to advance the widespread cultural change that patient safety entails.

It's About Leadership

Leaders must have courage, energy, and know-how to confront the reality of current performance in their organizations and demand a new level of accountability in applying safety science to all aspects of work. Successful leaders establish rigorous measures for safety and pay attention to those measures. They seek out the stories and experiences surrounding the metrics, and they keep the stories alive for learning by continually asking, "Why?" Leaders who master the discipline of effective inquiry—that is, asking the penetrating questions—will have the ability to see and understand how systems in their organizations are actually operating, as opposed to how they think or wish they were operating. In other words, they will learn the reality. Successful leaders also evaluate organizational performance against other organizations with leading-edge safety cultures. This practice provides supporting evidence to make tough decisions and focus the organization on its journey to high reliability.

The ability to align and focus the energy of an organization to take direct action, to make it clear to people "what mountain they are to climb," is what Jack Welch, former CEO of General Electric, identifies as "the edge" (cited in Tichey and Coehn, 1997, p. 153). This edge is critical to break through organizational gridlock to achieve threshold change in performance.

Urgency and impatience are necessary ingredients to achieve "the edge" that push the leader to translate information into effective focused strategies that will realize results rapidly. Accelerated improvement is better than slow improvement. It gets things done while the problem to be solved is still relevant and the team still has energy to implement. It is the leader's job to sustain and encourage the energy of teams so that they can see a clear path to desired results. Table 9.1 shows the factors that characterize the process of an accelerated team versus a slow, incremental team.

Leadership Accelerates Change

It is the leader's role to enable effective teams in order to tackle the issues of today and be prepared for the next challenge. In the work of safety, new risks continue to be introduced into the health care environment along with new knowledge, new technology, and the changing demographics of patients, providers, and the workforce. The leader's job is to insist and persist in getting results and to resist the forces that keep the energy of the organization mired in the status quo. This role cannot be delegated. The leader must unleash the blocked energy in the health care community by removing barriers and by championing strategies that accelerate forward movement. These strategies can be borrowed from sources outside health care, such as industry and the healthy communities movement, and they can also be found in the health care system itself.

Most literature on accelerating change talks about exceptional leaders who are capable of a job that seems heroic in proportion. Caldwell (1995, p. 2) calls

TABLE 9.1. FACTORS THAT CHARACTERIZE SLOW AND FAST TEAMS

Slow	Fast
Team members' mixed loyalties and commitment to outcome	Perception of common goal, enemy
Hidden agenda	Urgency, clarity, honesty
Political process	Problem and its solution perceived to be of strategic importance; data driven
Lack of clarity and accountability for results (lack of time, authority, or ability to implement solutions)	Shared vision for desired outcome and committed resources; clear charter
Unclear/absent commitment of resources to implement	Focus and committed resources
Absence of senior leadership's sponsorship; unclear messages	Senior management's visible commitment
Lack of staff support	Expert facilitation and staffing
Lack of focus (constant changes in definition of project's scope)	Clear charter
Environmental changes	Focus on aim and outcome
Changes in definition of problem	Data, not opinions, to signal change
Absence of team formation (inconsistent participation, no preparation for team members, turnover among team members)	Dedicated team and defined process
No time frame	Defined milestones
Backtracking and rework	Effective facilitation and preparation
Unmet needs for data	Well-researched issues, data, feedback
Disconnection from strategy	Clear connect to strategy

Source: Adapted from J. Morath, *The Quality Advantage: A Strategic Guide for Health Care Leaders* (San Francisco: Jossey-Bass, 1999), p. 13.

for heroic leaders who possess customer-mindedness, process-mindedness, and statistical-mindedness. Leaders play the seminal role in growing a shared vision in their organizations, creating discomfort with the current state, and asking the right questions to stimulate the curiosity of people who want change. Health care leaders have a great deal to do in fostering the will and energy of those in the industry, but these pursuits need a methodology. Armed with methods and skills, the average leaders among us can also open important doors of opportunity, learn, and define effective methods (Caldwell, 1995, p. xvii).

Studying exceptional leaders and understanding their success in executing effective and accelerated change processes are important pathways for learning. Bossidy and Charan (2002) identify essential steps for effective, accelerated change. If you are a leader in charge of designing and executing a patient safety initiative, strategies are available to help you prioritize what you do and keep you focused on the transformation instead of keeping you caught up in the details of micromanagement. Bossidy and Charan (2002, p. 57) suggest that the first and most essential step is focusing on six essential behaviors:

1. Know your people and your business.
2. Set clear goals and priorities.
3. Follow through.
4. Reward doers.
5. Expand people's capabilities.
6. Know yourself.

Paul Batalden has dedicated decades of his career considering change and improvement in health care. Learn the lessons. Batalden and associates have produced the Clinical Improvement Action Guide. Acquire and use it to achieve threshold change. It cuts through the jargon and complexity often associated with quality theorists and provides a road map, worksheets, and elegant, well-tested tools to define and focus safety issues and implement improvements that eliminate or mitigate risk. Just as a root cause analysis tool helps avoid hindsight bias and guides the uncovering of multiple factors that contribute to accidents and near misses, the Clinical Improvement Action Guide helps overcome barriers to effective change and accelerates the rate of improvement, as in the testing of rapid pilots of change (Nelson, Batalden, and Ryder, 1998).

Leadership behaviors and methodology helped one organization in its quest to reduce medication errors, as discussed in the following case study.

Concept to Action: Educating Health Care Professionals about Safe Prescribing Practices

For doctors, nurse practitioners, and other health care professionals who prescribe medications, writing a prescription easily becomes as automatic as driving a car. Unfortunately, it can be just as dangerous. Mark Thomas, director of pharmacy services at Children's Hospitals and Clinics, Minneapolis/St. Paul, Minnesota, is responsible for helping prescribers improve safety by using "safe prescribing."

"It's like reminding people to drive the speed limit," says Thomas. "Nearly everyone, at some time or another, goes over the speed limit because we're in a hurry to get somewhere or we're late for an appointment—we all understand that speed limit laws are designed for everyone's safety, but we exceed [the speed limit] because we think that accidents only happen because of the other drivers." Health care professionals, who constantly balance a busy schedule with patient safety, often take shortcuts in writing orders. The six most common errors—illegible handwriting, trailing zeros or the lack of leading zeros, dangerous abbreviations, missing essential information, illegible signatures, and orders written only in terms of quantities instead of in terms of dose strength—are the target of an ongoing safe prescribing campaign at Children's. Instead of waiting for the implementation of computerized provider entry, with rules and decision supports, Children's is acting to create greater safety in the current environment. Thomas and his colleagues have used a variety of creative methods, on-going measurement and feedback, to constantly remind prescribers to "write safe":

- A template for prescriber feedback shows prescribers how their order writing could lead to harm. Just as the police use special signs with embedded speed detectors to show drivers just how fast they are going, the feedback form gives prescribers immediate, personal feedback. Pharmacists make a copy of the prescriber's order, note the elements that are unsafe, attach the feedback form, and send it to the prescriber. Refer to Appendix Four.
- Aggregate results of findings are regularly published and sent to professional medical staff divisions to track performance over time and ensure that performance is improving in overall rate and by specific prescribing elements.
- Multilayered display boards, placed in physicians' lounges and other gathering areas, show examples of unsafe order-writing habits. An order written at the hospital is posted on a flap, and under the flap is a description of what the order writer actually intended to prescribe. "On the board is the question 'What does this say?'" says Thomas. "The person looking at the board makes a guess, then flips it up to see whether they got the right answer." This creates awareness of the issue of illegibility.
- Stickers are placed on medical charts as "road signs" for prescribers, reminding them to write out words instead of abbreviating and to avoid trailing zeros. The stickers rotate frequently to keep the messages from fading into the landscape. Other unique formats for these "road signs" include pocket reference cards, table tents, place mats in physicians' lounges, and a brochure titled "Your Role in Safe Medication Use—A Guide for the Professional Staff." A video on safe prescribing was released to all departments, top admitting physicians, and is shown during new-employee orientation. It educates staff members about patient safety, the high percentage of accidents that stem from the misinterpretation of medication orders, the six most common mistakes in prescribing, and the hospital's medication safety plan.

Thomas recommends that prior to launching a medication safety initiative pharmacy leaders identify physican champions and host focus groups with prescribers to identify leverage points that will help change behavior. He also recommends thinking beyond the organization's walls to the educational system. Medical students and residents are still being trained in risk-prone prescribing habits, increasing the difficulty in establishing new and safer prescribing practices in the practice setting. Thomas is working with local universities and the hospital residency programs to modify curricula and encourage discussion of the topic.

Formal initiatives are important, but hallway conversations can also be opportunities for learning. One executive remembers how Thomas used a dollar bill and a back-pocket stash of recent prescriptions to do hallway teaching: "He'd walk up to us and say, 'I'll give you a dollar if you can read that script.' The person guesses, and the people around him or her would demonstrate how consensus can undermine safety—they would all say, 'Yes, it does look like your guess is right.'" It was teaching, in an interactive, fun way, about **confirmation bias**—the phenomenon whereby people, in conditions of uncertainty, tend to agree with authorities.

The steady drumbeat of fresh ideas has improved safe prescribing practices in the most common error groups, from a combined average of 73.7 percent to 84.3 percent since the initiative began. In the next year, computerized order entry will effectively put speed bumps, in the form of alerts, decision support, and forcing functions, in front of busy providers to require them to clarify their orders when misunderstandings could arise.

The safe prescribing messages, Thomas believes, still will be important. Just as order writing can become a second-nature activity, so can computer entry of orders. The goal, no matter what method is used, is heedful attention to the process even when the process is a routine part of the day. Using different teaching methods, isolating specific behaviors for attention over short periods of time, and constantly rotating content, helps keep safe order writing front and center.

Leaders live their businesses, are connected to day-to-day reality, and receive information from multiple sources, such as focus groups, family advisory councils, hallway conversations, and scheduled "rounds" of departments. Realism is at the heart of effective, accelerated change (Bossidy and Charan, 2002). Many organizations, especially on the topic of patient safety, have people who avoid or distort reality. The topic of patient safety creates unease, opening a Pandora's box that can make life uncomfortable. Some leaders are in denial, focusing only on strengths of their organizations. Leaders fluent in reality are an essential ingredient, beyond any tool or method, to accelerate change.

Strategies to Accelerate Change in Your Organization

There are defined paths of accelerated change to learn from, and many of them are based on mentoring behavior, socialization of champions, and organizational engagement (Caldwell, 1995). A model can help. There are many to choose from, or the option exists to pull the best of each to create your own. Examples of such models include: FOCUS, Plan-Do-Study-Act, the Juran Quality Improvement Process, the PICOS Method, General Electric's Change Acceleration Program, Rapid Replication methodologies, and Six Sigma. The following case study discusses how one organization employed Six Sigma to accelerate improvements in safety and quality.

Concept to Action: Using the Six Sigma Improvement Methodology to Improve Patient Safety

To improve patient safety and increase efficiency and quality, Froedtert Hospital has adapted the highly disciplined improvement methodology of Six Sigma. Developed and trademarked by Motorola, and traditionally used in manufacturing and engineering, Six Sigma is data-driven. It relies on rigorous statistical analysis and follows a defined process to choose, define, measure, and maintain improvement projects.

Froedtert began its involvement with Six Sigma by forming a consortium with the American Society for Quality (ASQ) and the Medical College of Wisconsin. The goal was to pilot the application of Six Sigma to health care to reduce medical errors and enhance patient safety.

"Six Sigma hadn't been used much in health care at that point, and the few using it were applying it to improve process efficiencies and/or reduce cost," says Beth Lanham, Six Sigma coordinator at Froedtert Hospital.

The hospital initially selected two people for "black belt" training—the rigorous Six Sigma training in which participants are prepared to become the primary drivers of improvement projects at their organizations. The training, provided at ASQ, involved one intensive week per month over the course of four months. During the four months of training, participants implemented a project that put into practice what they were learning.

One Froedtert project focused on reducing errors associated with insulin. Insulin error reduction was chosen for several reasons. Insulin has been identified as a high-alert medication by the Institute for Safe Medication Practices and has been the subject of several JCAHO sentinel event alerts. Recent literature supported improved glycemic management associated with decreased mortality, complications, and infections (van den Berghe and others, 2001). Froedtert also had identified internal opportunities for improvement, and several Froedtert physician groups had expressed interest.

A multidisciplinary insulin team was formed with an endocrinologist, a certified diabetic educator, a trauma surgeon, a cardiothoracic surgeon, a pharmacist, a dietician, registered nurses representing the intensive care units and medical nursing units, a patient with a diagnosis of diabetes, and one of the Six Sigma "black belts." The acronym DMAIC (define, measure, analyze, improve, control) represents the steps in the Six Sigma model of process improvement. With the insulin improvement project used as an example of the process, the activities at Froedtert were divided in the following way:

1. Define

The Froedtert team identified the steps of the processes that preceded insulin administration:

1. Physician's initial placement of orders
2. Nurse's transcription of orders
3. Pharmacy's transcription of orders and dispensing of insulin
4. Nurse's administration of insulin
5. Technicians' monitoring of blood glucose levels

Group discussion targeted hypoglycemia as the biggest threat to patient safety in patients treated with insulin. Further discussion led to the recognition that reducing hypoglycemia was important but should be accomplished without creating additional hyperglycemia.

The team reviewed all incident reports from 2000 and 2001, downloaded and evaluated finger-stick blood glucose results from glucometers, and analyzed pharmacy data on use of insulin and 50 percent dextrose solution. A literature search was conducted, and relevant articles were reviewed.

The team constructed a map that identified variables at each step of the process. A root cause analysis tool, Failure Mode and Effects Analysis, was used to prioritize the variables that were most frequently associated with errors, that resulted in the most severe errors, and that were the most difficult to detect.

For the purposes of the project, the team had to develop operational definitions of hypoglycemia in addition to defining a target range for glycemic management. On the basis of the team's assessment, the scope of the project was narrowed, and a goal was established: to decrease the severity and frequency of hypoglycemia (defined as a glucose level lower than 70 mg/dL) and to improve overall glycemic control in hospitalized patients who were receiving insulin therapy for the treatment of hyperglycemia (defined as a target blood glucose level of 90–130 mg/dL). Excluded from the scope of this project were patients admitted with hypoglycemia, patients experiencing hypoglycemia without insulin therapy, and patients experiencing hypoglycemia after treatment for acute hyperkalemia (when treated with dextrose and insulin).

"Before Six Sigma," Lanham reports, "frequency and type of incident reports would drive the direction of improvement projects. For example, if we had chosen a direction for this project based on prevalence of incident reports, we would have focused on R.N. medication administration and brainstormed ideas for improvement in this limited area. However, it is well known that events are tremendously under-reported. Our initial analysis showed that most incident reports related to insulin were submitted by nurses and involved low-severity medication administration issues."

Few if any incident reports were written that involved other areas of the medication administration process (such as physicians' prescribing, nurses' and pharmacies' transcribing, and pharmacies' dispensing). Nevertheless, the team felt strongly that there was potential for error at each step of the process, and that if errors actually occurred, the effects could be quite significant.

2. Measure

Critical-to-quality indicators were identified to define performance standards. The team asked, "How will we know we have made an improvement in three months?" and "How will we know when we are doing a good job?" The answers became the primary or secondary metrics for monitoring the project.

Part of the Six Sigma process is searching for potential error and variation within the DMAIC process itself. For example, the project relied on bedside glucometers to create outcomes data. Froedtert participants tested the reliability and reproducibility of the glucometer results to understand variations within and between pieces of equipment.

3. Analyze

The team collected data to determine the current performance levels in the system, including how capable the system was of preventing blood glucose values under 70mg/dL and how likely the system was to maintain blood glucose values between the target ranges of 90 and 130mg/dL. The data established a baseline sigma level, baseline rates of hypoglycemia, and existing levels of glycemic control.

Key variables were measured, as identified in the process map and Failure Mode and Effects Analysis. A group of nurses was surveyed and was asked the following questions:

- At what blood glucose level do you consider your patient to be hypoglycemic?
- How do you treat hypoglycemia?
- When do you recheck a blood glucose level following hypoglycemia?

Results indicated large variability in all areas. Physicians' insulin orders showed large variations as well in the blood glucose values where insulin therapy was initiated, in the amounts of insulin used to initiate and maintain therapy, and in the ranges used for sliding scales. A review of dietary orders for patients with diabetes demonstrated opportunities for improvement in consistent ordering of qualitative diets, delivery of evening snacks, and management when patients were to receive nothing by mouth, consume only clear liquids, or have tests or other procedures.

4. Improve

The team developed and piloted protocols for treatment of hypoglycemia, continuous insulin infusions, and prescribing of subcutaneous insulin (including sliding scales). Guidelines were developed for use of oral hypoglycemia agents in hospitalized patients, for management of patients who were to receive nothing by mouth, and for diabetes management on the day of surgery.

To help improve safety, handwritten insulin orders and manual transcription of insulin orders in the pharmacy were eliminated. To reduce the likelihood that nurses might draw up incorrect doses of insulin on hospital units, an insulin dosing device was piloted on several units. The device was found to virtually eliminate the chance of a nurse drawing up an incorrect dose. Additional safety features of the device included color coding for different types of insulin, a one-patient disposable unit, and a large dial with audible clicking when a dose of insulin was dialed.

During the pilot phase, the protocols required frequent adjustments, but, along with other measures taken, they have resulted in statistically significant improvements in most areas. To date in the pilot project, all life-threatening glucose levels associated with insulin administration have been eliminated without significant increases in hyperglycemia. Improvements in overall glycemic control are steadily improving. The pilot programs are being expanded into additional inpatient areas, with plans for a systemwide rollout of the program.

5. Control

The Six Sigma program requires each project to have a plan for continuous control.

"The goal is to hold gains made and avoid slipping back into old habits," says Lanham. "You spend time at the outset, fix it right the first time, then put controls in place so you're not solving the same problem again two years later."

As the insulin program is expanded, monthly sampling is utilized to monitor the frequency and severity of hypoglycemia and overall glycemic control.

There are challenges in applying the disciplined methodology of Six Sigma to a health care environment.

"Problems in health care are very complex, with variables and a lack of obvious solutions," says Lanham. "The multiple unique individual characteristics are tremendous and can be very difficult to control. For example, even in a controlled situation, you can give two patients with the same weight, height, and diagnosis the same dose of a drug and they can have different reactions."

Additional challenges include defining and quantifying errors.

"We feel strongly, for example, that delays in communicating lab results to clinicians may impact clinical decision making," Lanham says, "but we do not have consensus on quantifying the measure."

Despite the challenges, the Six Sigma process has resulted in measurable clinical improvements. Its structured methodology and data-driven approach have helped Froedtert rethink the "brainstorm and implement" approaches of the past.

Says Lanham, "As you gain more experience with Six Sigma, you find yourself in meetings constantly asking, 'Yes, but is this idea really going to fix the problem?' or I'll think, 'Look at all the variation in that process—no wonder it is error-prone.' "

Froedtert now plans to become a "Six Sigma Organization," which involves expanding the use of the Six Sigma methodology to encompass reduction of medical errors, promotion of patient safety, cost reduction, and enhancement of process efficiency.

"Organizationally, we want it to be part of the culture" says Lanham. "It's our philosophy of doing business."

New Roles for Managers

Managers lead and manage change in organizations. It is critical that they have the knowledge and skills to tackle the changes required to improve patient safety and not be ineffectual or immobilized by the complex issues that are encountered. Middle managers in today's health care organizations live with increasing performance demands and increasing uncertainty. In contrast to the case study just presented with clear, identified problems to be solved, the field of patient safety also presents a particularly disturbing concept for managers: unsolvable problems. These are not problems difficult to solve for lack of resources; rather, they are *inherently* unsolvable. Given that a great deal of a manager's time and energy is directed toward solving problems, working in the domain of patient safety requires some new strategies and skills for managing unsolvable problems—problems of paradox, uncertainty, and polarity.

The latter term denotes sets of opposites that cannot function independently, so that a manager cannot simply choose one solution and neglect the other (Johnson, 1996, p. xviii). An example of polarity in patient safety is the competence of the individual performer, on one side, and the effectiveness of team performance, on the other. Both count. Where patient safety is concerned, there is also the need to be flexible and resilient and at the same time be clear and disciplined. Often clarity and discipline are interpreted as rigidity; whereas flexibility and resilience are interpreted as ambiguity, neither rigidity nor ambiguity is a characteristic of safety. The manager's role, then, is to manage from the perspective of both opposites—flexibility/resilience and clarity/discipline—while avoiding the outside limits of both (ambiguity and rigidity).

With development of the manager's role in leading the journey toward patient safety comes the continual repetition of polarities: individual/team, accountability/blamelessness, centralization/decentralization, disclosure/confidentiality, production/

protection, service/safety, standardization/innovation. As a result, one of the new required skill sets, and one of the greatest challenges to managers, is learning to manage polarity and paradox with conflicting views all valid, and to address conflicts in a balanced manner. The requirement to manage paradox, uncertainty, and polarity takes many leaders and managers out of the comfort zone where closure can be found, and where there is the certainty of a single set of solutions: as the saying goes, "For every complex problem there is a simple solution, and it's wrong."

Understanding and working with paradox, uncertainty, and polarity is a long-term, involved pursuit, but two skills are particularly relevant to the complex quest to develop a patient safety culture: the skill of asking **wicked questions** (Zimmerman, Lindberg, and Plsek, 1998) and the skill of practicing **appreciative inquiry** (Hall and Hammond, 1997). Wicked questions balance the tension inherent in the paradoxical work of patient safety. Examples of wicked questions are "How does focusing on systemic causes interfere with individual accountability for actions?" and "How can a harm-free culture support innovation?" Managers who are able to use appreciative inquiry with wicked questions have moved beyond their traditional roles of problem solving and control and into a method of asking questions to understand and cope with complexity.

Hall and Hammond (1997) list the following assumptions of appreciative inquiry:

- In every society, organization, or group, something is working.
- The language we use to describe reality helps to create that reality.
- People in systems move toward what they choose to study or focus on.
- The act of asking questions of an organization or group influences or changes the group in some way.
- Systems are capable of becoming more than they are, and they can learn how to guide their own evolution.
- Looking for what works well and doing more of it is more motivating and effective than looking for what does not work and doing less of it.
- People have more confidence and comfort to journey into the future (the unknown) when they carry forward parts of the past (the known).
- The collective creation of a desired future is most powerful when it is based on the best of what already exists.

With these assumptions in mind, important differences begin to emerge between the manager's traditional role of problem solving and control and the managerial role of using appreciative inquiry. Table 9.2 compares and contrasts problem solving to address complicated issues and appreciative inquiry to invite exploration and understanding of complex issues.

TABLE 9.2. DIFFERENCES BETWEEN PROBLEM SOLVING AND APPRECIATIVE INQUIRY

Basic Assumption in Problem Solving	Basic Assumption in Appreciative Inquiry
Organization as a problem to be solved	Organization as a mystery to be embraced
Felt need	Appreciating and valuing
Identification of a problem	The best of what is
Analysis of causes	Envisioning what might be
Analysis of possible solutions	Dialoguing what should be
Action planning (treatment)	Innovating what will be

Source: "A Positive Resolution in Change: Appreciative Inquiry," unpublished draft, Appreciative Inquiry Commons, Case Western Reserve University, p. 29.

The ability to ask wicked questions and use appreciate inquiry helps spur complex conversations, exploration, awareness, and collective mindfulness in an organization.

Another critical role of managers in the patient safety culture is the role of designing effective teams. The complex contexts in which today's health care is provided require relationships that are capable of generating novel solutions. Effective teams have the following characteristics (Zimmerman and Hayday, 1999):

- Members who are separate or different enough to bring distinct perspectives and training forward to challenge assumptions and explore issues deeply
- The shared perception that team members have permission to talk to and listen to each other in ways that challenge the organizational status quo, its sacred cows, and its implicit assumptions
- The members' ability to act together to co-create something new
- A reason for members to work together and share ideas, resources, thinking, and energy

Providing minimum specifications or simple rules can draw out a team's creative adaptability (Zimmerman, Lindberg, and Plsek, 1998). Giving direction and boundaries, rather than imposing detailed policies, procedures, and elaborate rules, frees teams to develop innovative solutions and question the status quo. Giving direction and simple boundaries is preferable to proclaiming the traditional detailed, maximum specifications of policies, procedures, and rules. For example, the three simple rules developed for unit-based teams that are responsible for unit-driven innovations in safety are "Fix what you can," "Tell what you fixed," and "Find someone to fix what you cannot." They contain minimum specifications that are not prescriptive; rather, they are operational guidelines for action.

If you are a manager looking at a new role in patient safety, its complexity may seem daunting, but you do not take this role on as a one-time installation. Complex systems for patient safety are assembled incrementally from simple pieces that can operate independently. Identifying the simple pieces is called "chunking." The simple pieces are used to create innovations and prototypes that can expand and spread throughout a work process, department, or organization through **plan-do-study-act (PDSA) cycles**.

Aligning with Functions of Risk Management and Performance Improvement

Aligning patient safety with risk management and performance improvement creates a focus and an incubator for patient safety efforts. Performance improvement, risk management, and patient safety each have a unique body of knowledge, and make valuable contributions to the organization's journey. Patient safety serves a distinct function and should not be coopted by performance improvement or risk management that are more familiar areas of operations in today's health care organizations.

Patient safety processes are diagnostic in nature. They are interventions to increase awareness of vulnerabilities in the system, increase resilience, offer evidence-based design principles, support patient safety research, and focus on teamwork and culture—in other words, they represent the macroergonomics and macromanagement of the system. Patient safety creates the "landing strip" on which specific improvements are made. By contrast, the performance improvement function is to help the sharp-end staff and staff at the blunt end work together to take effective action once a problem or opportunity for improvement has been identified. The risk management function, to complete the triad, makes valuable contributions to patient safety through knowledge gained in retrospective analysis of events. The primary mission of risk management is to protect the assets of the organization. Risk management efforts are moving toward prospective interventions, grounded in safety science, to educate about risk and to audit, identify, and mitigate risk and prevent adverse events. Patient safety, risk management, and performance improvement, working in interactive and aligned partnership, maximize their contributions to the organization. Without such partnership, these three functions compete independently for leaders' attention and for other organizational resources, creating gridlock and mixed messages and stalling effective change.

As organizations identify patient safety improvement activities, there is a tendency for performance improvement to constrain its activities to project management, that is, to incremental changes within the system. This approach compromises the aim of changing the whole system to focus on safety. It takes leaders' energy, creativity, and perseverance to harness performance improvement initiatives in the service of advancing the thinking of the system and not just performing maintenance work or conducting isolated projects. It is essential to build this "effector arm" of the organization so that it can help managers and front-line staff act on reported risks. Leaders must also work to help these three entities—patient safety, performance improvement, and risk management—overcome the natural tendency to "own" work in a proprietary manner, overcome their jurisdictional boundaries, and work in productive partnership.

Changes and Challenges for Physicians and Clinical Leaders

A high level of commitment, energy, and leadership among physicians is a foundation of patient safety because physician champions are a crucial ingredient in the creation of a safety culture. Edwards, Kornacki, and Silversin (2002, p. 3) offer a simple tool for assessing the current state of physicians' engagement and leadership. To be successful in creating a culture of patient safety, physician leaders, along with other organizational leaders, need to move beyond mental models of control, armed truce, and tentative trust and toward strong collaborative leadership models of mutual respect and trust. These words are easy to say, but the work of achieving such a partnership is hard. Nevertheless, the goal of safety for patients is a natural bridge between leadership domains, offering a platform of common interests and purpose.

For physicians, as has been true across all health care disciplines, many problems of the past could be described in biomedical terms and solved with the knowledge and skills with which physicians were equipped in medical school. Given the challenges of patient safety and the escalating complexities of practice, traditional Newtonian problem solving, rational deduction, and mechanistic metaphors fall short. The linear-machine metaphor is not applicable to human behavior or to organizational and system performance. Complex adaptive systems provide a better conceptual framework for dealing with the nature of patient safety. Principles to assist decision making in the complexity zone (Zimmerman, Lindberg, and Plsek, 1998) include the use of intuition and "muddle through," experimentation, minimum specifications, chunking, metaphors, and proactive questions.

Physicians' involvement and leadership are crucial, but they are not enough. Patient safety also requires great humility. It requires the shift from a self-conceptualization as autonomous operator to that of team member in a dynamic, emergent system. This shift is often difficult for physicians, but it represents an exciting intellectual challenge and learning opportunity. Creating safer care in the face of complexity is intuitively compatible for physicians. New knowledge can be an attractor to engagement. Locally relevant activities, such as incorporating safety into mortality and morbidity conferences and aligning with professional society activities, help engage physicians and call on their leadership. Examples such as that offered by the American Society of Anesthesiologists are models of how to engage interest and make a difference.

Best Practices

Specific best safety practices, adapted from aviation and industry and informed by human factors research, are being implemented in health care. These include such initiatives as the adoption of the best medication practices identified by the Massachusetts Coalition for the Prevention of Medical Error (enforcement of standardized prescribing, use of allergy-alert wristbands, removal of all concentrated potassium from floor stock, twenty-four-hour availability of pharmacists, and introduction of computerized practitioner order entry) and surgical-site verification as advanced by the American Association of Orthopedic Surgeons (Joint Commission on Accreditation of Healthcare Organizations, 1998). Attention is also being given to lessons from the aviation industry about applying crew resource management training for care teams in such high-risk areas as operating rooms, labor and delivery suites, intensive care suites, and emergency departments.

The National Quality Forum (2003) has published a report on research-based best safety practices, thirty of which—chosen for their potential impact, the strength of the evidence supporting them, and the feasibility of their implementation—rest on the establishment of a culture of safety (see Exhibit 9.1).

In addition, the report begins to articulate the minimum specifications for a health care culture of safety. These minimum specifications suggest standardized policies and operating procedures to meet the aims of harm-free care (National Quality Forum, 2003, p. 18):

- Prioritize patient safety events and situations that should be reported.
- Analyze the patient safety events and situations that are reported.
- Verify that the remedial actions identified through analysis of reported patient safety events are implemented and effective and do not cause unintended adverse consequences.

EXHIBIT 9.1. NQF-ENDORSED SET OF SAFE PRACTICES

1. Create a healthcare culture of safety.
2. For designated high-risk, elective surgical procedures or other specified care, the patient should be clearly informed of the likely reduced risk of an adverse outcome at treatment facilities that have demonstrated superior outcomes and should be referred to such facilities in accordance with the patient's stated preference.
3. Specify an explicit protocol to be used to ensure an adequate level of nursing based on the institution's usual patient mix and the experience and training of its nursing staff.
4. All patients in general intensive care units (both adult and pediatric) should be managed by physicians having specific training and certification in critical care medicine ("critical care–certified").
5. Pharmacists should actively participate in the medication use process, including, at a minimum, being available for consultation with prescribers on medication ordering, interpreting and reviewing medication orders, preparing medications, dispensing medications, and administering and monitoring medications.
6. Verbal orders should be recorded whenever possible and read back to the prescriber; that is, a health care provider receiving a verbal order should read or repeat back the information that the prescriber conveys in order to verify the accuracy of what was heard.
7. Use only standardized abbreviations and dose designations.
8. Patient care summaries or other, similar records should not be prepared from memory.
9. Ensure that care information, especially changes in orders and new diagnostic information, is transmitted in a timely and clearly understandable form to all of the patient's current health care providers who need that information in order to provide care.
10. Ask each patient or legal surrogate to recount what he or she has been told during the informed consent discussion.
11. Ensure that written documentation of the patient's preference for life-sustaining treatments is prominently displayed in his or her chart.
12. Implement a computerized prescriber order entry system.
13. Implement a standardized protocol to prevent the mislabeling of radiographs.
14. Implement standardized protocols to prevent the occurrence of wrong-site procedures or wrong-patient procedures.
15. Evaluate each patient undergoing elective surgery for risk of an acute ischemic cardiac event during surgery, and provide prophylactic treatment of high-risk patients with beta blockers.
16. Evaluate each patient upon admission, and regularly thereafter, for the risk of developing pressure ulcers. This evaluation should be repeated at regular intervals during care. Clinically appropriate preventive methods should be implemented consequent to the evaluation.
17. Evaluate each patient upon admission, and regularly thereafter, for the risk of developing deep-vein thrombosis (DVT/venous thromboembolism, or VTE). Use clinically appropriate methods to prevent DVT/VTE.
18. Use dedicated antithrombotic (anticoagulation) services that facilitate coordinated care management.
19. Upon admission, and regularly thereafter, evaluate each patient for the risk of aspiration.

20. Adhere to effective methods of preventing central venous catheter–associated blood stream infections.
21. Evaluate each preoperative patient in light of his or her planned surgical procedure for the risk of surgical site infection, and implement appropriate antibiotic prophylaxis and other preventive measures based on that evaluation.
22. Use validated protocols to evaluate patients who are at risk for contrast media–induced renal failure, and use a clinically appropriate method for reducing risk of renal injury based on the patient's kidney function evaluation.
23. Evaluate each patient upon admission, and regularly thereafter, for risk of malnutrition. Employ clinically appropriate strategies to prevent malnutrition.
24. Whenever a pneumatic tourniquet is used, evaluate the patient for the risk of an ischemic and/or thrombotic complication, and use appropriate prophylactic measures.
25. Decontaminate hands either by applying a hygienic hand rub or by washing with a disinfectant soap before and after direct contact with the patient or with objects immediately around the patient.
26. Vaccinate health care workers against influenza to protect them and their patients from influenza.
27. Keep work spaces where medications are prepared clean, orderly, well lighted, and free of clutter, distraction, and noise.
28. Standardize the methods for labeling, packaging, and storing medications.
29. Identify all high-alert drugs (e.g., intravenous adrenergic agonists and antagonists, chemotherapy agents, anticoagulants and antithrombotics, concentrated parenteral electrolytes, general anesthetics, neuromuscular blockers, insulin and oral hypoglycemics, narcotics, and opiates).
30. Dispense medications in unit-dose or, when appropriate, unit-of-use form, whenever possible.

Source: Adapted from National Quality Forum, *Safe Practices for Better Healthcare: A Consensus Report* (Washington, D.C.: National Quality Forum, 2003), p. vii.

- Ensure that organizational leadership is kept knowledgeable about patient safety issues present within the organization and continuously involved in processes to ensure that the issues are appropriately addressed and that patient safety is improved.
- Provide oversight and coordination of patient safety activities.
- Provide feedback to front-line health care providers about lessons learned.
- Publicly disclose implementation of or compliance with all NQF-endorsed safe practices applicable to the facility.
- Train all staff in techniques of teamwork-based problem solving and management.

The NQF list focuses on clinical and organizational interventions. Research is needed on such organizational interventions as computerized order entry, use of simulators, and use of crew resource management techniques.

Root cause analysis can also accelerate change by extending its use beyond medical accidents and near misses. Since 1997, when it was mandated by the Joint Commission on Accreditation of Healthcare Organizations, the systematic conducting of root cause analyses, that is, multicausal analysis, has become widespread in examining sentinel events, but it can be taken farther. For example, when root cause analysis is conducted by mental health professionals or other specially trained practitioners, it can serve as a way of debriefing the stress associated with critical incidents, allowing professionals to overcome trauma more quickly and return sooner to optimal work productivity. Experience with root cause analysis also teaches problem-solving skills via modeling.

In addition, the value of root cause analysis has been demonstrated beyond medical accidents. Root cause analysis has proved useful for some organizations outside clinical areas and can serve as the beginning for decision support tools. For example, one hospital, when it implemented its program of root cause analysis, established "significant defection of key personnel" as one of the criteria for a sentinel event. This criterion was shown to be an effective indicator when the vice president for human resources contacted the vice president for performance improvement and alerted her that seven pharmacists had resigned within one week. The discovery allowed a significant management problem to be rapidly resolved.

Optimizing Information Processes

Perhaps one of the greatest barriers to accelerated change is the inability of any collective of individuals to work cooperatively. Designing safety into the health care system requires increased cooperation, decreased delays and backlogs, and the optimization of information processes. Systems with optimized information processes engage in the following practices:

- Use of concurrent data collection and feedback to staff
- Customization of care on the basis of variations in risk
- Performance of work intended to mitigate the unintended side effects of change
- Review of abbreviations used in prescription orders and charts, to increase standardization and reduce the possibility of confusion or of multiple interpretations
- Incorporation of multidisciplinary rounds at the bedside
- Use of guidelines and protocols with variance analysis, which involves observing where front-line staff vary from written protocols and then "paving where the path is worn" rather than devoting resources to establishing compliance with poorly designed systems
- Use of control charts

An example of using these design principles to accelerate the pace of change is the work of Dr. Jim Espinosa, director of emergency services at Overlook Hospital, Summit, New Jersey, who is using a system of reports given by staff at fifteen-minute intervals in order to monitor the state of safety and quality in the emergency department. Espinosa and his team designed eight measures to be monitored. Staff members report real-time data against those measures every fifteen minutes. When any two measures exceed a predetermined threshold, immediate course corrections are made (for example, slowing down), and information is gathered on how to improve the design of the patient flow system. In this example, design of the system serves three purposes: to make failure visible, to prevent failure, and to improve processes for mitigating risk and harm.

Another application of these principles primarily involves the question of how an organization can create a system to mitigate the unintended side effects of change—for example, by making prospective use of FMEA or a protocol for simulations to anticipate failure modes in new procedures and equipment, thereby identifying and mitigating risk before it presents. This is sometimes called "thinking dirty," or anticipating gaps in the system, including potential new gaps that may be created in process, knowledge, and skill through the introduction of change. This patient safety tactic can be accomplished with the root cause analysis protocol of the Veterans Administration National Center for Patient Safety, and it is used as a prospective framework to prompt questions that should be asked before new equipment, procedures, or patient care services are introduced into the workplace. Whether a formal FMEA process is conducted or another tool is employed, a disciplined technology needs to be used to assess readiness for change and the likely impact of change, and to reduce risk, turbulence, and rework. The following example illustrates how the use of a structured tool can be used to accelerate change.

Concept to Action: A Pilot and Prototype for Eliminating Medication Error

This case study is adapted from the work of Moen and Provonost (2003). A local ICU team identified medication errors in transfer orders when patients left the ICU environment for continuing care or for other hospital units. They determined that the transfer of medication orders presented a significant opportunity for improving patient safety.

Because there was no objective standard against which to measure error, the team created a tool for data collection: the medication reconciliation form. This tool provided a means for evaluating the extent to which medication discrepancies or gaps in information were present in a patient's discharge orders at the time of the patient's discharge and transfer. The team reduced the amount of work involved in reviewing charts and orders for each transferred patient by randomly selecting fifteen patients each week and evaluating their charts and orders with the following three questions:

1. Are the medications listed in the discharge orders the same as the ones the patient is currently receiving?
2. Are the allergies listed correctly in the discharge orders?
3. Is the prescribed medication the same as the patient's home medication?

If the answer to any question was no, the team member (that is, the nurse) was instructed to ask the prescribing physician whether the change that had been made was intended. Medication error was defined as anything in the discharge and transfer process that caused a physician to change the discharge medication order.

The medication reconciliation tool was then pilot-tested and revised. On the basis of its findings, changes were made, and this tool was incorporated into the ICU discharge process. As all nurses became trained and engaged in the reconciliation of medications at the time of a patient's discharge and transfer, the form was further revised.

The process for data collection is now integrated into this local ICU's standard operating procedures, and the data are routinely reported to staff. The hospital has thus eliminated medication errors associated with patients' transfer from the ICU. The focus now is on holding the gains that have been made and spreading this methodology to other ICUs in the hospital. To that end, the original team of research nurses is disseminating this patient safety improvement.

Creating Internal Collaboratives

Don Berwick and his colleagues at Boston's Institute for Healthcare Improvement (IHI) have advanced the concept of "collaboratives," a methodology that is widely recognized as an approach to accelerate improvement. The IHI model gathers teams of professionals from different organizations, but the same model can be applied within an organization as an effective way to disseminate innovation and create alignment. To implement the collaborative model in an organization, teams are gathered in one place from throughout the organization and given a time-limited mandate to select an area for improvement. The model uses small interdisciplinary teams backed by senior leaders. Each team selects a project relevant to their area, sets clear, appropriate, yet ambitious goals, and then chooses interventions that are implemented to achieve them. In this procedure, called "small tests of change," the results are measured, and the change cycle, with any needed modifications, is repeated in an iterative fashion until the goal is reached. Factors identified as critical to the success of this model of rapid cycle change (see "Using Rapid Cycle Change," below) include solid leadership backing, the presence of a physician as a team member, selection of appropriate projects, and freedom from excessively complicated measurement schemes. As teams share results and challenges, lessons in change unfold. The process blasts open entrenched ways of thinking and doing, and liberates new ideas, allowing innovation to emerge.

One hospital distributed safety information to the front line while also gathering information from front-line experts on what changes would be most effective. The hospital held a ten-week collaborative, challenging every service line to form a team and tackle a meaningful safety project. Each project was required to include the critical success factors identified through IHI collaboratives (a physician as member, administrative support, measurable goals, and meet with other teams to share learning). Two hours were set aside each week for the teams to obtain expert consultation. Newsletters of results were posted weekly. At the end of the experience, participants' comments revealed experiences of mastery ("I learned that you did not have to have a Ph.D. to get involved in patient safety"), new insights into the organization ("I learned that goals we had on the trauma unit conflicted with those on the intermediate care unit"), and new appreciation for co-workers ("Here I am, the medical director of the lab, and I found it too complicated to enter data").

Using Rapid Cycle Change

Rapid cycle change is an approach that offers several tools for accelerating improvement. Rapid Replication (Caldwell, 1995) and plan-do-study-act (PDSA) cycles (Langley, Nolan, Nolan, Norman, and Provost, 1996), for example, are demonstrated best practices for accelerating change and improvement. The leader's urgency, focus, and skills in this area are critical to improving patient safety. Leaders must set the tone, first by requiring that changes be made and then by providing mentoring to make them happen. PDSA cycles are driven by three questions (Langley, Nolan, Nolan, Norman, and Provost, 1996):

1. What are we trying to accomplish?
2. How will we know that a change is an improvement?
3. What changes can we make that will result in an improvement?

Progressive cycles of experimentation, informed by data and measurement, create the pathway between initial hunches, theories, and ideas and changes that result in improvement. Figures 9.1 and 9.2 depict the model for improvement and repeated use of the cycle.

FIGURE 9.1. REPEATED USE OF THE CYCLE

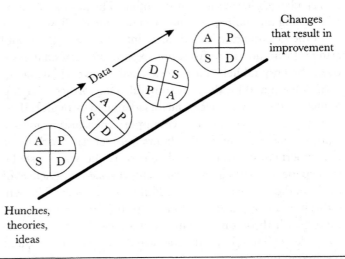

Changes that result in improvement

Data

Hunches, theories, ideas

Source: G. L. Langley, K. M. Nolan, T. W. Nolan, C. Norman, and L. P. Provost, *The Improvement Guide: A Practical Approach to Enhancing Organizational Performance* (San Francisco: Jossey-Bass, 1996). Copyright © 1996 by Jossey-Bass. This material is used by permission of John Wiley & Sons, Inc.

Memorial Hermann Hospital, Houston, used rapid cycle change and a collaborative structure to realize significant, measurable goals in safety and quality, including decreased infection rates, increased standardization, and decreased length of stay in the institution's nine ICUs. Team members studied together, tested potential solutions, and implemented them in a continuous cycle throughout a period lasting between six and eight months.

For example, Memorial Hermann used nine measures developed by the Institute for Healthcare Improvement as a starting point for reducing ventilator-acquired pneumonias (VAPs) and increasing safety and quality of care for ventilated patients. Individuals traveled to an IHI collaborative meeting and then returned to Memorial Hermann and passed on what they had learned to multidisciplinary teams from each of the hospital system's ICUs.

The nine teams began their work with assessments for VAP reduction against the nine measures. Then the ICUs chose their own measurable and actionable ideas for improvements at the patient level (elevating the head of the bed, frequent suctioning), at the staff level (team communication changes), and at the environmental level (ensuring that staff had the equipment and supplies they needed,

FIGURE 9.2. MODEL FOR IMPROVEMENT

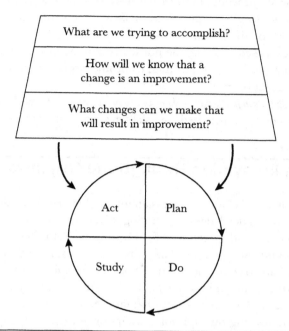

Source: G. L. Langley, K. M. Nolan, T. W. Nolan, C. Norman, and L. P. Provost, *The Improvement Guide: A Practical Approach to Enhancing Organizational Performance* (San Francisco: Jossey-Bass, 1996). Copyright © 1996 by Jossey-Bass. This material is used by permission of John Wiley & Sons, Inc.

working with families to involve them in infection prevention). The collaborative framework included the following characteristics:

- *Locally based decision making.* Each of the nine ICUs individually decided which ideas to use in attempting improvements on the nine measures. A critical care council and senior hospital leaders provided resources, support, and new information.
- *No single solution set.* The teams and units were free to test multiple strategies and regularly re-evaluated whether ideas were working as expected or whether new ideas should be attempted.
- *Open flow of communication about lessons learned.* At each meeting, a different ICU team presented its data and ideas about what was and was not working. Experts in the field, ICU staff who had made improvements, and ICU staff who had experienced failures all became teachers.

- *Ambitious aims.* Leaders of the organization were clear that they believed improvement would occur. Measures were used to inform the improvement cycles. Units were expected to make a 50 percent gain in each measure over the course of six months.
- *Reciprocal accountability.* Senior leaders made investments and changes in infrastructure as necessary, when front-line workers identified a need for change at the point of care.
- *Investments in people deep in the organization.* Training of middle-level managers and front-line clinicians increased their skills in systems thinking and change management.

Spreading Innovation through the Organization

The spread of change remains an intractable issue in health care. There is a growing body of knowledge surrounding this issue; notable are the early writings of Argyris (1991) and Rogers (1995). The lessons from these and other scholars is that myths and legends in organizations are stories, rooted in actual events, that have been adapted over time and made part of the cultural structure. These stories come alive usually in the informal leadership and communication structures.

Fraser (2003) reminds us that failure to discover and understand relevant stories, by seeking out opinion leaders or asking new employees what they have learned, will limit both the understanding of things that have worked well and the sharing of stories about how changes came about. Through such stories, insights can be gained in the interest of understanding barriers and making use of past successes. Fraser's work (2003, pp. 130–132) is helpful in planning and executing the spread of change in clear and practical ways: through adoption of SMART (*s*pecific, *m*easurable, *a*chievable, *r*ealistic, *t*ime-based) goals, identification of motivators and adopters, and construction of a completeness-and-coverage matrix to ensure communication to all key stakeholders in all internal media avenues.

Although there are many ways to disseminate safety information throughout the organization, such as newsletters, didactic presentations, printed materials, and e-mail lists, interactive methods tend to be more effective at creating change. Face-to-face learning sessions, like those that occur for participants in internal collaboratives and safety action teams, are culture-building tools. Health care is not transformed through rhetoric about safety. Rather, frameworks like safety action teams and unit briefings create an infrastructure for cross-fertilization and acquisition of new knowledge. All teams want to be successful. Accordingly, friendly competition becomes a motivating factor. Successful teams become role models for other teams, demonstrating that success is achievable.

To spread success throughout the organization, teams focused on safety issues should include an "early adopter," first mentioned in Chapter Two (Rogers, 1995). Early adopters are individuals who are willing to take risks and try new things. More important, they are the social and opinion leaders in an organization. Early adopters become key messengers on teams and are critical to the development of a network for spreading innovation.

Leaders can support the spread of innovation throughout an organization when they are certain that it is a sound practice and that it will be successful in moving the organization toward a culture of safety. Using incentives to provide motivation, leaders make certain that someone is accountable for owning the entire project. Leaders' energy must provide a relentless drumbeat to move safety forward by repeating messages of hope: "Together we can reduce harm." Leaders should recognize that passionate innovators and early adopters often face fierce resistance. At this stage of the patient safety journey, they can feel beat up and bloodied, and need support and skills to deal with resistance.

Strategies for Accelerating Change in the Health Care Community

Executive Session Technology: Changing Leadership

The Harvard Executive Session, first described in the Introduction, had a profound personal effect on its participants. This section provides insight into the methodology used to create the environment for such personal transformation to occur. The executive session is a method for creating change in leadership. The executive session model has been replicated in a variety of ways to challenge conventional wisdom and quicken the pace of cultural change in health care and other fields.

This model has its origins in Harvard's John F. Kennedy School of Government and was conceptualized as a change model for seemingly intractable social problems. The initial sessions focused on the judicial and law enforcement systems and examined how failures in existing models could be changed to create greater value to society. For example, despite continual law enforcement investments, the public felt less safe. Leaders from all aspects of law enforcement confronted their reality and, through structured facilitation and deliberations, community policing was born. Saul Weingart, a physician familiar with the emerging research on medical error, had attended the law enforcement sessions as a student of criminal justice. Concerned about the scope of medical error, he asked leaders at the Kennedy School, and the patient safety researcher Lucian Leape, whether the executive session model might be an effective vehicle for raising the profile of safety with CEOs of leading U.S. health care organizations.

An environmental scan revealed medical error as a large and looming social issue. A session was planned, designed, and convened semiannually from 1997 to 2000, with CEO attendees invited from a wide range of major health care organizations and institutions. Participants agreed on four design concepts: that the sessions were to be a confidential working group composed of members and guests only, that all members would personally attend all sessions with no substitutes, that the sessions required a long-term commitment, and that the objectives of participation were to develop important ideas and to motivate change among member organizations and beyond. Rules for the session were few: confidentiality, casual dress, honest disclosure, and active participation. Members met for two days at a time over the course of several years. The format included sharing of leadership successes and failures, "conversation starters" where experts made presentations on focused topics, carefully facilitated and researched sessions, assignments and reports by members, and case studies.

These sessions are now being replicated in Minnesota, where leaders came together with the support of Harvard University, the National Patient Safety Foundation, and the Minnesota Hospital Association to create "a threshold improvement in patient safety." The results of the session are summarized as follows (Weingart, Morath, and Ley 2003):

- Shared commitment and vision
- Public statements and policy leadership
- Establishment of corporate priorities and adoption of innovative practices
- Accelerated pace of improvement
- Work products (surveys, papers, case studies, collaborative projects)

Perhaps the greatest contribution has been the dismantling of the myths, namely that harm is an unavoidable by-product of care, that harm-free care is impossible, and that physicians are infallible.

The leaders able to change their reactions to error are the ones able to advance a culture of safety. The Minnesota Alliance for Patient Safety (2002) defined reduction of medical error as a leadership imperative and an executive responsibility that cannot be delegated. These leaders identified the following requirements to advance safety:

- Public commitment and corporate goals
- Resources
- Executive accountability

- A moral mission
- Personal involvement
- Regional collaborations

Leaders around the country are forming broad-based community coalitions on behalf of patient safety. In addition to the Minnesota Alliance for Patient Safety, coalitions are Virginians Improving Patient Care and Safety, the Wisconsin Patient Safety Institute, the Michigan Health Safety Coalition, the Georgia Partnership for Health and Accountability, the Massachusetts Coalition for the Prevention of Medical Error, the Pittsburgh Regional Health Initiative, and the Pennsylvania Patient Safety Collaborative.

These partnerships recognize that the creation of safe health care requires a broad constituency that goes beyond a single health care system. The partnerships build on innovative, collaborative strategies such as those fostered by the healthy communities movement, and on the assets of the contributing members, as opposed to seeking outside expertise. The Massachusetts Coalition for the Prevention of Medical Error brings together stakeholders from the state department of health, hospitals, health systems, health plans, professional associations, unions, peer review organizations, the hospital association, the Board of Registration in Medicine, the state legislature, academic institutions, and insurers. The group has promulgated a set of best practices in medication safety, surveyed hospitals about their compliance, and reported the results in the newspaper. The Pittsburgh Regional Health Initiative includes representatives from universities, industry, foundations, and health care and has applied the Toyota production system model to hospitals throughout the area as a way to bring safety improvements to health care.

A promising powerful new perspective on health care improvement is that the health of the community is the litmus test for patient safety. Because patients pass only briefly through episodes of care in acute care facilities, the quality of outpatient care and the safety of patients in their homes may be a more comprehensive lens through which to view the quality of care. Leaders beginning the journey can contact leading-edge patient safety organizations, as they are pleased to share their best practices, their successes, and their failures.

Reporting and Learning Collectives: Safety in Numbers

The University Healthcare Consortium is one example of a national organization that has created a reporting network among its member organizations. Premiere has a patient safety institute. In New England, Jeff Brown of the System Safety Group is leading the development of a patient safety learning system. The system, called the CoreLab, supports organizational learning through members who will contribute de-identified occurrence/incident reports to a regional database. Education, training, and applied research in patient safety will be supported through a distance-learning infrastructure that uses multiple learning methods. The same communication infrastructure will contain a system for distributing alerts by participating hospitals, outpatient facilities, and residential care centers. A goal of the CoreLab is to provide real-time decision support and hazard capture to improve safety.

Engaging the Mind and Emotions

The greatest challenge in moving beyond gridlock and toward a culture of safety is to confront denial. Some organizations have shown the video *Beyond Blame,* showing interviews of actual individuals involved in patient deaths due to medical accidents. Others have used the one-act play *Charlie-Victor-Romeo* to provoke dialogue from the intense visceral experience of watching reenactments of the cockpit in aviation disasters. (See Resources for both works.) Still others have engaged improvisational drama companies to work with their organizations. As health care audiences witness these enactments, they awaken to the dangers buried in the culture's dysfunction. The media cuts through analytical defenses, stripping away denial, and speaks straight to heart. These experiences create a new level of consciousness.

Leaders are accountable for motivating individuals, units, entire health care systems, and communities to act in an effective, coordinated way to improve safety. Individual health care professionals are experts at problem recognition, but they are caught in the current bureaucratic culture, and so have difficulty mobilizing for action. Consistent focused leadership that facilitates teamwork can help sharpend individuals move beyond problem identification and into action. Leaders must champion the spread of patient safety innovations throughout the organization. As leaders recognize that the current system is broken and champion innovations to inculcate the patient safety into the very DNA of the culture, transformational change will occur.

Summary Points

1. The scope of change must be broadened and the velocity of change must be accelerated to achieve a threshold from which health care culture can be transformed. Given the magnitude of the problem, incremental change is insufficient.
2. Rapidly prototyping a replication from known successful models can bring new ideas to the organization, and models can accelerate improvements.

3. Leaders must have courage, energy, and skill to break through gridlock and align and focus the energy of the organization to create "the edge."
4. Strategies to accelerate change in the organization include those that follow:
   - New roles for middle managers
   - Aligning rather than integrating patient safety, risk management, and performance improvement
   - Implementing evidenced-based best practices
   - Expanding the use of root cause analysis and Failure Mode and Effects Analysis methods to all areas of operations and functions
   - Creating internal collaboratives
   - Using data and feedback to front-line staff to fuel performance change
5. Leaders must participate in and support change activities in the broader health care community, such as these:
   - Executive sessions
   - Regional collaborations that include community representatives beyond health care
   - Intellectual-emotional learning experiences

CHAPTER TEN

THE END OF THE BEGINNING

Unsafe health care is not an option. Catastrophes can destroy an organization's reputation and profitability. They cause untold harm and suffering to patients, families, and involved staff. Health care cultures—national, professional, and organizational—must come together to define and advance a consistent culture of patient safety. The alternative is unsafe operating environments through conflicting and disparate goals. A safety culture extends beyond a single organization's quest for world-class performance. Patient safety must become a value in the health care industry. What this will take is a collective belief in the aim of harm-free care and a shared understanding of what it will take to move beyond competence to creating capability in patient safety. The leadership role is pivotal in initiating and deepening the dialogue, identifying and removing the barriers to safety, and recognizing attractors for change. To accomplish this, leaders need to embrace the complexity of patient safety and gain knowledge of complex adaptive systems.

Providers and leaders in health care are adept at making changes in complicated domains of work, such as when they implement quality improvement projects or perform open-heart surgery. Unfortunately, the multiple steps of analysis and the multiple perspectives necessary to design and control complicated systems pose limitations for those who work in the area of patient safety. Patient safety is beyond complicated. It is complex.

At its center health care is caring for people. The work is people-intensive. This reality contains unpredictability, emotions, subjective responses, paradoxes, and polarities. This constitutes complexity. These systems in which people give and receive care are fragmented, complex, and constantly changing in the face of new knowledge, technology, and shifting demographics. "Nobody should be surprised that [health care systems] can be difficult to reform and that 'sensible' changes may have unpredictable and adverse consequences" (Smith, 2001). This understanding leads us to reject reductionistic and mechanistic methods of improvement and error reduction and to embrace the science of complex adaptive systems for working in the domain of patient safety.

The work of patient safety involves negotiating the complexity of clinical care delivery and health care reform. Successful operations require new skills and a deepened capacity to live inside tension and polarity and paradox. Negotiating complexity also requires skill in recognizing and appreciating the emergence of order and innovation within such systems.

These new skills move away from "fixing" parts of a system, by applying localized remedies that provide relief from disagreement and uncertainty, and toward managing the tensions inherent in living with polarity and paradox.

The new skills include creating deep conversations, defining simple rules or minimum specifications for general direction, using experimentation and simulation, and multiple approaches. The skills also include paying attention to how the system performs and to the adaptations that take place at the sharp end of care. Control and measurement of patient safety are less important than harnessing the energy and intellect of the organization. What is required is increasing organizational awareness and deepening the organization's capacity to respond and adapt to continually changing circumstances (Fraser and Greenhalgh, 2001). Tools include storytelling, continuous communication and feedback, and cycles of action, reflection, and learning. Such tools pull us from zones of comfort, but also lessen the familiar frustration of failed or short-lived solutions. The new world is one of great interest and creativity. This world is intuitive, compatible with the uncertainty and messiness known to those who work in health care. And so the challenge of creating a culture of patient safety and high reliability involves complexity, that is, ambiguity, continual trade-offs, negotiation, dynamic change, and the ability to live with the uncertainty of not having a single set of solutions. Dynamic and changing interactions in one part of the system will often lead to unpredictable and nonlinear effects in other parts. Small parts of the system will combine and propagate new risks and, sometimes, effects that ripple beyond the immediate situation and make waves, distant in time and place, in the larger system.

Leadership in a complex environment involves understanding the organization in order to determine the most effective approach to patient safety. Different environments require different approaches. For example, an undisciplined, unaware, and dysfunctional organization may require a normative approach that is rule-based and uses simple tools. In contrast, a mature high-reliability organization that has pervasive literacy in patient safety science, understands safety as a constantly emerging state, and enjoys an ambience of trust can use the tools of understanding and modeling (Amalberti, 2001).

The journey to the high reliability of a safety culture is in incremental stages. Table 10.1 displays the approaches and tools for the journey. Each organization is somewhere along the way on this journey, but the journey itself is nonlinear and continually changing.

The preceding nine chapters have emphasized that medical accidents, when experienced, are unique and astonishing, and that they can be prevented only if the dynamics that combine to create them can be known in advance. A medical accident that harms a patient develops from multiple conditions and failure points that combine in a unique way to create the trajectory on which the accident occurs. There is no singular cause sufficient for such an accident; causes are dynamic, and appear in changing combinations.

Tools for developing capacity for an error-tolerant organization include understanding the system, small-team conversations and feedback, reporting, near miss analysis, risk awareness, simulations, and experimentation. Misguided actions intended to create greater safety have included training, automating people out of a process, adding more rules and regulations, and adding greater and stiffer sanctions for those who have been involved in medical accidents. Such actions encourage organizations and communities to operate inside an illusion of safety. Figure 10.1, offered by Cook (2001), illustrates this point. The ability to work in conditions of uncertainty, to predict, to innovate, and to increase resilience in the face of risk is what builds greater safety.

TABLE 10.1. APPROACHES TO SAFETY AND TOOLS FOR THE JOURNEY

Approach	Tools
Normative	Rules and controls
Use-centered	Tolerance, early warnings
Complexity-centered	Ecological design, performance control, simple organization
Negotiated	Safety clubs
Emergence-oriented	Understanding and modeling

Source: Adapted from Amalberti, 2001.

FIGURE 10.1. COMPLEX SYSTEM FAILURE: CYCLE OF ERRORS

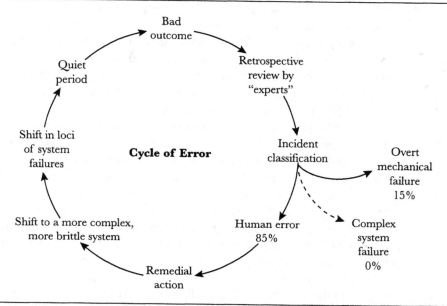

Source: R. I. Cook, Cognitive technologies Laboratory, Department of Anesthesia and Critical Care, University of Chicago, 1997. Copyright © by Richard I. Cook, Cognitive technologies Laboratory, University of Chicago. Used by permission.

Knowledge that can prevent or reduce the probability of medical accident or harm comes from educating for capability. This concept encompasses the extent to which an individual can adapt to change, generate new knowledge, and continually improve performance. This approach goes beyond competency training; rather it involves the capacity to learn in any situation and know when to improvise (Fraser and Greenhalgh, 2001).

An event that occurred in February 2003—the breakup of the space shuttle *Columbia*—demonstrates the need for constant and deep cultural change and vigilance around the work of safety. In January 1986, the *Challenger* space shuttle had been destroyed as a result of a serious problem with one of its components, the O ring. Analysis of that disaster revealed that leaders at NASA minimized previous close calls involving components, characterizing them as maintenance headaches rather than understanding them to be potentially lethal variables in a complex chain of events (Vaughan, 1996). NASA leaders ignored the warnings of expert engineers who had advised them that the O ring would fail in certain conditions. In a painful manifestation of the "blame and shame" culture, NASA leaders felt the pressure to put a human face on the cause of the catastrophe, and a senior officer was dismissed. Seventeen years later, the destruction of the *Columbia* was under review, with echoes of the past. The growth of a culture of transparency at NASA and a new focus on systems rather than on individuals were two positive developments, but it appears that several elements of high reliability did not materialize with respect to risks that were known before the *Columbia* broke up. Vaughan (cited in Schwarz and Wald, 2003, p. A15) states the lesson succinctly: "You change the cast of characters, and if you don't change the organizational context, a new person can be under the constraints and conditions they were under before." Vaughan goes on to say that "as the chain of events look[s] now, hard-numbers analysis of componentry appears to trump the gut feelings of the engineers who communicated a sense of unease and a warning before the tragedy occurred." Vaughan observed what she believes to be NASA management's "incremental descent into poor judgment" and normalization of deviance—specifically, the minimization of highly risk-prone conditions and the discounting of front-line workers' concerns. Both are markers of a culture that may have subordinated safety to other priorities.

Only the outcome of the *Columbia* disaster findings will reveal whether the lessons contained in the *Challenger*'s destruction were forgotten or never learned at all. Both disasters are sobering examples of the leadership gulfs described by Norman (1988) as the gulf (gaps) of evaluation (What is actually going on?) and the gulf (gaps) of execution (What can we do about it?). These are questions for health care leaders to pursue each day, in the interest of nurturing a safety culture and developing organizational capability to prevent medical accidents and harm. Even as analysis of the *Columbia* accident continues, lessons have been emerging. Here is an important one: safety is a fragile, transient state whose sustenance requires a culture of uncompromising vigilance and investment in preventing harm.

As leaders, we must focus on the processes as well as the systems we are trying to improve and gain leverage by focusing on the gaps between processes and systems. Through reporting and conversations, leaders can learn about the performance of the system and about gaps in process flow, both between departments and between and among disciplines. Overcoming labor-management disputes, departmental silos, and disagreements between disciplines will free us to focus on process flow, understand how systems play out, and create greater resilience and flexibility in the system. The *Challenger* and *Columbia* lessons bear directly on health care as the industry begins the safety journey.

As patient safety initiatives increase, we must be wary of getting caught up in the delusion that we are making great progress. The disasters reported in the mid-1990s that began the patient safety movement are history. An incident in the spring of 2003 at Duke University, where a young girl lost her life when she was given an incompatible heart, speaks this truth loudly.

The year 2003 produced this and other examples as potent reminders that advances are being made in patient safety but health care is still at the tip of the iceberg in addressing accident causation. The telephone still rings with news that provokes disorienting dilemmas across our organizations. In the most prestigious of our medical institutions, such as Johns Hopkins, Duke University Medical Center, and Boston Children's, events have occurred that challenge all of us working in health care, and those entering the field, to change our consciousness and subordinate our pride, in the service of a safer, more reliable system of care.

We envision a time in the near future when regulators and internal teams "under siege" will be replaced by expert teams assembled from multiple sciences to conduct external reviews of health care accidents and near misses in pursuit of high reliability. These teams will share lessons learned publicly and end forever the conspiracy of silence. And no longer will valuable learnings be lost to combat the epidemic of our time: medical accident. After all, if lethal medical accidents can occur in our best institutions, accidents can happen anywhere, and no organization is immune.

Patient Safety: A Rapidly Advancing Field

The field of patient safety is burgeoning. The National Patient Safety Foundation posts a minimum of twenty published articles twice a month, culled from the professional literature. Exciting advances in the field of patient safety are taking place. And yet there is growing awareness of how far health care still has to go. A report of research on patient safety in the United States recognizes that some effective strategies for reducing medical accident may exist, but there is still much to learn about system failure, including unique characteristics of the health care industry that are barriers to improvement (Cooper and others, 2001).

Medication error is the most frequently studied subject. But other areas of practice (anesthesia, pharmacy, surgery, and nursing) are also being studied.

Barriers to research include insufficient funding, lack of experts, legal constraints, complexity and fragmentation of the health care system, the culture of blame surrounding error and patient safety, lack of consensus in definitions, and lack of priority for patient safety in the health care arena as a whole (Cooper and others, 2001).

Basic research about the causes of error and system failure, human factors, and event reporting, including processes for accident investigation, are in order. Interdomain analyses and applications from other domains in science and industry are also needed to increase understanding (Cooper and others, 2001). Studies of culture and leadership are imperative. The existing culture of blame, shame, and embarrassment, with accompanying fear of litigation, creates a disincentive for reporting and transparency, and works against research studies in patient safety.

Insufficient information about the causes of errors and system failures in health care, and insufficient understanding of barriers create uncertainty and imprecise knowledge about the state of patient safety, and about the best ways to interpret the effects of actions undertaken to improve safety. Many participants in the patient safety movement have different ideas about what paths will be most productive. What is clear, however, is the growing recognition of the need for research in patient safety.

We hope that this primer will help open doors to new considerations of the leader's work in creating a health care culture where inquiry into patient safety can emerge more fully. We need to understand and overcome the barriers in order to advance our understanding of complex adaptive systems and build our capability in safety.

Understanding the Journey

To paraphrase Winston Churchill, *we are at the end of the beginning.* This primer was written to provide an introduction, invite deeper inquiry, and enroll you in learning what is known and being learned in the field. This book provides lessons, examples, and tools that can be applied to your health care organization. The most important lesson is that an organization serious about patient safety needs leadership grounded in the belief that harm-free care is possible. Without leaders' commitment to pursuing the vision of harm-free care and the discipline to understand complex systems, the best intentions will not be enough to reduce harm. Traditional efforts will not create patient safety. They are too restrictive. The field of patient safety requires broad, systemic interventions that have to do with leadership, communication, human factors, ergonomics, process and system design, complex adaptive systems, preparation and coordination of teams and crews, and continuous reflective learning. One mandate is the revision of academic programs so that physicians, nurses, and those working in other clinical disciplines can learn together about patient safety in health sciences education. Another is the reform of the health care system.

Leaders Create the Culture

Leadership actions are required to build the culture for transparency and learning, prerequisites for safety to be successful and sustained. These actions are in pursuit of a patient safety culture, which is an accountable culture, a just culture, a learning culture, and a culture of partnership.

Accountable Culture

An accountable culture has no room for blame or shifting the responsibility. It is a culture in which leaders accept full responsibility for patient safety, and in which all members and external partners share the obligation to continually create conditions for advancing patient safety. Although safety is everyone's responsibility, the leader is accountable. Accountability is more than acceptance of personal responsibility. It requires an accountability system at the individual, system, and governance levels, and it includes design and implementation of a work plan with measures, monitors, and reporting that can encourage learning and innovation. An accountable culture demonstrates the characteristics of high reliability throughout its performance. These characteristics include understanding the boundaries of safe practice and anticipating and planning for unexpected events and future surprises. The organization knows that conditions are dynamic and always changing. In an accountable culture, leaders are continually exploring ways to compensate for the unintended negative side effects of change. For this reason, the organization continually monitors the changing landscape of potential paths to failure. The organization and its members are accountable to patients and families when there is an event that causes harm. Accountability is expressed by apology, disclosure, and understanding of what happened and why, and taking appropriate action to reduce the probability of recurrence. Another aspect of accountability is credibility. We need to educate and inform the public and calibrate public expectations concerning the fact that accidents and errors do happen. To evade or cover up in interactions with the media, often under the cloak of confidentiality, damages credibility. The organization that attempts to obstruct the public's need to know is like the person who stands in front of a speeding train, thinking that he or she can slow it down. Being accountable means telling the truth even when the truth is complex and painful.

A Just Culture

A just culture requires timely, fair, and appropriate actions that are carried out equitably when blameworthy behaviors or actions have occurred. Blameworthy behaviors and actions are those that, with the actor's knowledge, violate standards of conduct and, in line with the actor's intentions, violate standards of practice, with no intention of following such standards. A corollary of this definition is that in unique circumstances, extraordinary actions must be confirmed by evidence, as when knowledgeable colleagues are consulted so that the safety and reasonableness of an action can be confirmed. The category of blameworthy actions includes acts carried out by individuals who are impaired, as when someone reports for work under the influence of drugs or alcohol, or when an individual's capacity is diminished by illness or by changes due to aging. This category also includes the acts of individuals who engage in reckless behavior, or who demonstrate a failure to learn over time. Unintentional actions that result in error are not considered blameworthy, and no penalties are levied in such cases.

A Learning Culture

A learning culture has a deep appreciation and insatiable quest for understanding how the system operates and why events occur. It has a robust reporting system as its intellectual foundation and encourages voluntary text-based reporting. It is clear that the purpose of reporting is for understanding and improvement. Complex, continuing conversations take place about the stories that emerge. There is continual learning about latent conditions, system vulnerabilities, and sources of success. New ideas and lessons from other domains of science and industry are brought forward and presented as examples from which to learn. New applications are tested in cycles of action and reflection. In a learning culture, gaps are made visible so that team members can learn from them and bridge or eliminate them. Interventions for taming complexity require innovation, or learning and understanding systems in new and unique ways. An important lesson for everyone in a learning culture is that hindsight does not produce the same knowledge as foresight. In hindsight, the path for avoiding an accident seems clear. In foresight, learning is created, and resilience is built, through reciprocal cycles of giving accounts and taking account of risk-prone conditions and accidents, and the organization becomes able to anticipate multiple scenarios. There is learning through the open flow of information about the changing face of the potential for failure.

A Culture of Partnership

A culture of partnership respects, values, and invests in effective teamwork and communication. This aspect of the organizational culture includes the patient and the patient's family as team members and recognizes multicultural competence as a mandate for an effective care encounter. The rights of the patient to be safe, to be informed, and to choose are protected and honored. A culture of partnership recognizes that "How the system performs, and how it is experienced, is based on the interactions of the people in that system" (Uhlig 2002).

Lessons Learned along the Way

We have learned important lessons in our journey toward creating safety for patients, and we hope that we have been able to impart many of those lessons to you. Working in the field of patient safety has changed our thinking and beliefs. For example, we used to think that error reduction was the focus. We learned instead that eliminating harm is the goal, and that error is an important data source in the pursuit of harm-free care.

We used to think that accounting for errors and monitoring the data were tools for creating safety. We learned instead that data points, without a surrounding story, lead to a diminished understanding of both the system of care and the system of safety. Storytelling and complex conversations reveal knowledge about both systems.

We used to think that studying medical accidents could create harm-free care. We learned instead that risks, near misses, hazards, and the wisdom of front-line workers teach equally important lessons about improving safety, without all the emotion and trauma of accidents. Recovery from error and resilience in a system are as important as prevention in creating safety for patients.

We used to think that well-trained, competent, careful clinicians were sufficient to create safety. We learned instead that safety requires prepared and effective teams and crews whose members share a systemic view and perspective on process flow as well as an understanding of their roles and responsibilities.

We used to think that discipline-based competence, knowledge, skills, and attitudes were sufficient to create safety. We learned instead that capability—or the extent to which individuals can, collectively and across disciplines, adapt to change, generate new knowledge, and continually improve performance—is critical.

We learned that concepts pertinent to complex adaptive systems offer a better framework than Newtonian problem solving for dealing with the nature of patient safety. This framework includes the use of such tools as storytelling, intuition, experimentation, minimum specifications, chunking, metaphor, and provocative questions.

We learned that policy, protocol, and checklists are helpful when a problem is already understood, but that it takes imagination and intuition to appreciate and understand the problem in the first place.

We used to think that creating safety for patients was the sole responsibility of those who deliver patient care. We now know that the creation of safety for patients must also include systemic design and decision making from boardroom to front office to point of care, and that an activated patient and family create a greater safety net.

We used to think that safety was created through establishing and following rules. We have learned that safety is about emergence. Safety is not just about making rules but also about breaking rules when front-line experts, after discussion with informed colleagues, judge that innovation is required. Keeping track of migrations from the rules provides information about local adaptive strategies that the front line uses both to create safety and to herald the need for testing and changing the rules. We learned that few minimum specifications that are simple and flexible, and that provide direction and permission, are more valuable tools for safety than are complicated plans.

We used to think that individual human error was a major cause of medical accidents. We learned that this is rarely the case. The human tendency to assign error as cause and place blame is universal and cross-cultural, a tremendous barrier to safety. When an accident does occur, all the victims—the patient, the family, and the providers—need support, disclosure, and accountable leadership. The focus of investigating accidents is on system breakdowns, not on individual error.

We used to think that safety for patients could become a steady state. We now believe that the state of safety is dynamic, emerging, and adaptive. We learned that safety is a cultural value requiring constant attention and investment. We learned that past success is no reason for confidence, because the knowledge base of safety is insufficient to face the still unknown hazards and risks that are continually emerging in the environment.

We were reminded that focusing on attractors is far more powerful than focusing on challenging resistance to change. Attractors are the compelling evidence, champions, and stories of success that draw people to the work of patient safety. As the critical mass of attractors develops, those who resist change either become marginalized, change themselves, or leave the field.

We learned that safety requires leadership and the belief that harm-free performance is possible. This kind of leadership, and this unflinching belief, requires study and analysis of all levels of the system's architecture, including the overall system design, the midlevel design, and the level of the microsystem.

We learned that the work of building a sustainable health care community, in which harm-free performance can be achieved, begins when we stop thinking about what we need and start thinking about how to help each other attain our shared vision of safety.

We have gained an ever-increasing appreciation for the contributions of patients and families, and for the potential power of aligning governance, regulators, industry, legal systems, and those in the academic community who share the desire to improve patient safety.

We were humbled to study from other domains of science and industry, and we are excited by the potential of what we can learn from them.

We have been inspired by generous mentors in the health care community and by our work with committed national and international health care leaders who continually renew their commitment to do no harm.

Because of all of them, and for the sake of those just beginning the work of patient safety, and all the people we care for, we are honored to have had the opportunity to contribute this book.

Our final thought for you on creating more reliable systems of patient safety is this: If not now, when? If not us, then who?

REFERENCES

Alkov, R. A., Borowsky, M. S., Williamson, D. W., and Yacavone, D. W. "The Effects of Trans-Cockpit Authority Gradient on Navy/Marine Helicopter Mishaps." *Aviat Space Environ Med.*, 1992, Aug.: *63*(8), 659–661.

Allen, R. E. (ed.). *Concise Oxford Dictionary of Current English*, 8th edition. Oxford, U.K.: Clarendon Press, 1990.

Amalberti, R. "Human Error in Medicine." Paper presented at the Salzburg International Seminar on Patient Safety and Medical Accident, Apr. 25–May 2, 2001.

American Society for Quality. *Quality Glossary*. 2000. [www.asq.org]

Andrews, L. B. *Medical Error and Patient Claiming in a Hospital Setting*. American Bar Foundation (ABF) Working Paper Series, no. 9316. Chicago: American Bar Foundation, 1993.

Andrews, L. B., and others. "An Alternative Strategy for Studying Adverse Events in Medical Care." *Lancet*, 1997, *349*(9048), 309–313.

Argyris, C. "Teaching Smart People How to Learn." *Harvard Business Review*, 1991, *69*(3), 99–109.

Bagian, J. Acceptance speech, John Eisenberg Patient Safety Award, Washington, D.C., Oct. 2002.

Barker, K. N., and others. "Medication Errors in Nursing Homes and Small Hospitals." *American Journal of Hospital Pharmacy*, 1982, *39*(6), 987–991.

Bates, D. W., and others. "Incidence of Adverse Drug Events and Potential Adverse Drug Events: ADE Prevention Study Group." *Journal of the American Medical Association*, 1995, *274*(1), 29–34.

Bates, D. W., and others. "The Costs of Adverse Drug Events in Hospitalized Patients." *Journal of the American Medical Association*, 1997, *277*(4), 307–311.

Becher, E. C., and Chassin, M. R. "Improving the Quality of Health Care: Who Will Lead?" *Health Affairs*, 2001, *20*(5), 164–179.

Belkin, L. "Who Is to Blame? It's the Wrong Question." *New York Times Magazine,* June 15, 1997, pp. 28–33, 44, 50, 63, 66, 70.

Berwick, D. M. "A Primer on Leading the Improvement of Systems." *British Medical Journal,* 1996, *312*(7031), 619–622.

Berwick, D. M. "The Total Customer Relationship in Health Care: Broadening the Bandwidth." *Journal on Quality Improvement,* 1997, *23*(5), 245–250.

Berwick, D. M. "Taking Action to Improve Safety." In A. L. Scheffler and L. A. Zipperer (eds.), *Enhancing Patient Safety and Reducing Errors in Health Care.* Chicago: National Patient Safety Foundation, 1999.

Berwick, D. M. "Patient Safety: Lessons from a Novice." *Focus on Patient Safety,* 2001a, *4*(3), 3.

Berwick, D. M. "Patient Safety and Medical Error." Paper presented at the Salzburg International Seminar on Patient Safety and Medical Accident, Apr. 25–May 2, 2001b.

Berwick, D. M. "Plenty." Plenary address, 14th annual National Forum on Quality Improvement in Health Care, Orlando, Fla., 2002a.

Berwick, D. M. "A User's Manual for the IOM's 'Quality Chasm' Report." *Health Affairs,* 2002b, *21*(3), 80–90.

Berwick, D. M. *Escape Fire: Designs for the Future of Health Care.* San Francisco: Jossey-Bass, 2003.

Billings, C. E. "Some Hopes and Concerns Regarding Medical Event–Reporting Systems: Lessons from the NASA Safety Reporting System." *Archives of Pathology and Laboratory Medicine,* 1998, *122*(3), 214–215.

Blendon, R. J., and others. "Views of Practicing Physicians and the Public on Medical Errors." *New England Journal of Medicine,* 2002, *347*(24), 1933–1940.

Blumenthal, D. "Making Medical Errors into 'Medical Treasures.'" *Journal of the American Medical Association,* 1994, *272*(23), 1867–1868.

Bogner, M. S. (ed.). *Human Error in Medicine.* Hinsdale, N.J.: Erlbaum, 1994.

Boodman, S. G. "No End to Errors: Three Years after a Landmark Report Found Pervasive Mistakes in American Hospitals, Little Has Been Done to Reduce Death and Injury." *Washington Post,* Dec. 3, 2002, p. HE01.

Bosk, C. *Forgive and Remember: Managing Medical Failure.* Chicago: University of Chicago Press, 1981.

Bossidy, L., and Charan, R. *Execution: The Discipline of Getting Things Done.* New York: Crown, 2002.

Brassard, M. *The Memory Jogger: A Pocket Guide of Tools for Continuous Improvement,* 2nd ed. Salem, N.H.: Goal/QPC, 1988.

Brennan, T. A. "The Institute of Medicine Report on Medical Errors: Could It Do Harm?" *New England Journal of Medicine,* 2000, *342*(15), 1123–1125.

Brennan, T. A., and others. "Incidence of Adverse Events and Negligence in Hospitalized Patients: Results of the Harvard Medical Practice Study I." *New England Journal of Medicine,* 1991, *324*(6), 370–376.

Caldwell, C. *Mentoring Strategic Change in Health Care: An Action Guide.* Milwaukee: ASQ Quality Press, 1995.

Canale, S. T., and others. *Report on the Task Force on Wrong-Site Surgery.* (Rev. ed.) Rosemont, Ill.: American Academy of Orthopedic Surgeons, 1998.

Caranasos, G. J., Stewart, R. B., and Cluff, L. E. "Drug-Induced Illness Leading to Hospitalization." *Journal of the American Medical Association,* 1974, *228*(6), 713–717.

Carthey, J., de Leval, M. R., and Reason, J. T. "Institutional Resilience in Healthcare Systems." *Quality and Safety in Health Care,* 2001, *10*(1), 29–32.

Centers for Disease Control and Prevention. "National Nosocomial Infections Surveillance (NNIS) Report, Data Summary, October 1986–April 1996, Issued May 1996: A Report from the National Nosocomial Infections Surveillance (NNIS) System." *American Journal of Infection Control*, 1996, *24*(5), 380–388.

Chantler, C. "The Role and Education of Doctors in the Delivery of Healthcare." *Lancet*, 1999, *353*(9159), 1178–1181.

Chase, W. M. "The Language of Action." *Wesleyan*, 1989, *62*(2), 36.

Chassin, M. R. "Is Health Care Ready for Six Sigma Quality?" *Milbank Quarterly*, 1998, *76*(4), 565–591.

Children's Hospitals and Clinics. *Focus Groups with Families*. Minneapolis: Children's Hospitals and Clinics, 1999.

Cohen, M. R. "Medication Error Reports." *Hospital Pharmacy*, 1975, *10*(5), 202–203.

Cohen, M. R. "Medication Errors." Washington, D.C.: American Pharmaceutical Association, 1999.

Conway, J. *Strategies for Leadership: Hospital Executives and Their Role in Patient Safety*. Chicago: American Hospital Association, 2001.

Cook, R. I. *How Complex Systems Fail*. Chicago: Cognitive technologies Laboratory, Department of Anesthesia and Critical Care, University of Chicago, 2000.

Cook, R. I. "Operating at the Sharp End: The Complexity of Human Error." Paper presented at the Salzburg International Seminar on Patient Safety and Medical Accident, Apr. 25–May 2, 2001.

Cook, R. I. *Brief Look at the New Look in Complex System Failure, Error, and Safety*. Chicago: Cognitive technologies Laboratory, Department of Anesthesia and Critical Care, University of Chicago, 2002.

Cook, R. I., and Woods, D. D. "Operating at the Sharp End." In M. S. Bogner (ed.), *Human Error in Medicine*. Hinsdale, N.J.: Erlbaum, 1994.

Cooper, J. B., and others. *Current Research on Patient Safety in the United States*. Chicago: National Patient Safety Foundation, 2001.

Crawford, M. J., and others. "Systemic Review of Involving Patients in the Planning and Development of Health Care." *British Medical Journal*, 2002, *325*(7375), 1263–1267.

Darley, J. M., and Latane, B. "Bystander Intervention in Emergencies: Diffusion of Responsibility." *Journal of Personality and Social Psychology*, 1968, *8*(4), 377–383.

Davenport, T. H., and Prusak, L. *Working Knowledge*. Boston: Harvard Business School Press, 2000.

Davis, K., and others. *Room for Improvement: Patients Report on the Quality of Their Health Care*. New York: The Commonwealth Fund, 2002. [http://www.cmwf.org/programs/quality/davis_improvement_534.pdf]

Delbanco, T., and others. "Healthcare in a Land Called Peoplepower: Nothing About Me Without Me." *Health Expectations*, 2001, *4*(3), 144–150.

Denham, C. "The Economics of Honesty: Is There a Business Case for Transparency and Ethics?" Presentation at the National Patient Safety Foundation Congress, Washington, D.C., March 2003.

Donchin, Y., and others. "A Look into the Nature and Causes of Human Errors in the Intensive Care Unit." *Critical Care Medicine*, 1995, *23*(2), 294–300.

Dovey, S. M., and others. "A Preliminary Taxonomy of Medical Errors in Family Practice." *Quality and Safety in Health Care*, 2002, *11*(3), 233–238.

Edmondson, A., Roberto, M. A., and Tucker, A. "Children's Hospitals and Clinics." Harvard Business School case N9-302-050. Boston: Harvard School Publishing, Nov. 15, 2001.

Edwards, N., Kornacki, M. J., and Silversin, J. "Unhappy Doctors: What Are the Causes and What Can Be Done." *British Medical Journal,* 2002, *34*(7341), 835–838.

Emergency Care Research Institute (ECRI). "Educational Videos on Surgical Fires." *Health Devices,* 2000, *29,* 7–8.

Ernst, F. R., and Grizzle, A. J. "Drug-Related Morbidity and Mortality: Updating the Cost-of-Illness Model." *Journal of the American Pharmaceutical Association,* 2001, *41*(2), 192–199.

Fischhoff, B. "Hindsight ≠ Foresight: The Effect of Outcome Knowledge on Judgment Under Uncertainty." *Journal of Experimental Psychology and Human Performance Perception,* 1975, *1,* 288–299.

Fisher, E. S., and Welch, H. G. "Avoiding the Unintended Consequences of Growth in Medical Care." *Journal of the American Medical Association,* 1999, *281*(5), 446–453.

Fiske, S. T., and Taylor, S. E. *Social Cognition.* Belmont, Calif.: Addison-Wesley, 1984.

Flinchbaugh, J. "Beyond Lean: Building Sustainable Business through New Ways of Thinking." *Center for Quality Management Journal,* 2001, *10*(2), 37–50.

Flynn, E. A., Pearson, R. E., and Barker, K. N. "Observational Study of Accuracy in Compounding I.V. Admixtures at Five Hospitals." *American Journal of Health-System Pharmacy,* 1997, *54*(8), 904–912.

Forster, A. J., Murff, H. I., Peterson, J. F., Gandhi, T. K., and Bates, D. W. "The Incidence and Severity of Adverse Events Affecting Patients After Discharge." *Annals of Internal Medicine,* 2003, *138*(3), 161–167.

Frankel, A., and others. "Patient Safety Leadership WalkRounds™." *Joint Commission Journal on Quality and Safety,* 2003, *29*(1), 16–26.

Fraser, S. W., and Greenhalgh, T. "Coping with Complexity: Educating for Capability." *British Medical Journal,* 2001, *323*(7330), 799–803.

Frazier, V. "Patient Safety Research Initiatives." Paper presented at the Patient Safety Forum, St. Louis, Mo., Feb. 2003.

Gallagher, T. H., Waterman, A. D., Ebers, A. G., Fraser, V. J., and Levinson, W. "Patients' and Physicians' Attitudes Regarding the Disclosure of Medical Errors." *Journal of the American Medical Association,* 2003, *289*(8), 1001–1007.

Gandhi, T. K., and others. "Drug Complications in Outpatients." *Journal of General Internal Medicine,* 2000, *15*(3), 149–154.

Gawande, A. *Complications: A Surgeon's Notes on an Imperfect Science.* New York: Metropolitan Books, 2002.

Gerteis, M., and others. *Through the Patient's Eyes: Understanding and Promoting Patient-Centered Care.* San Francisco: Jossey-Bass, 1993.

Gladwell, M. *The Tipping Point: How Little Things Can Make a Big Difference.* Boston: Little, Brown, 2000.

Grabowski, M. R., and Roberts, K. H. "Risk Mitigation in Large-Scale Systems: Lessons from High-Reliability Organizations." *California Management Review,* 1997, *39*(4), 152–162.

Gurwitz, J. H., and others. "Incidence and Preventability of Adverse Drug Events in Nursing Homes." *American Journal of Medicine,* 2000, *109*(2), 87–94.

Haley, R. W., and others. "The Nationwide Nosocomial Infection Rate: A New Need for Vital Statistics." *American Journal of Epidemiology,* 1985, *121*(2), 159–167.

Hall, J., and Hammond, S. "The Thin Book of Appreciative Inquiry." *Thin Book* series. *OD Practitioner,* 1997, *29*(2), 2–3.

Harry, M. J., Schroeder, R., and Linsenmann, D. R. *Six Sigma: The Breakthrough Management Strategy Revolutionizing the World's Top Corporations.* New York: Doubleday, 1999.

Heget, J. R., Bagian, J. P., Lee, C. Z., and Gosbee, J. W. "System Innovation: Veterans Health Administration National Center for Patient Safety." *Joint Commission Journal of Quality Improvement*, 2002, *28*(12), 660–665.

Heider, F. *The Psychology of Interpersonal Relations.* New York: Wiley, 1958.

Helmreich, R. "On Error Management: Lessons from Aviation." *British Medical Journal*, 2000, *320*(7237), 781–785.

Helmreich, R. "Applying Aviation Safety Initiatives to Medicine." *Focus on Patient Safety*, 2001, *4*(1), 1–2.

Hickson, G. B., and others. "Patient Complaints and Malpractice Risk." *Journal of the American Medical Association*, 2002, *287*(22), 2951–2957.

Hooke, C. "Safety Action Teams: Improving Care for Children with Cancer." *Journal of Pediatric Oncology Nursing*, 2002, *19*(2), 59.

Hughes, R. "The Fraying of America." *Time Magazine*, Feb. 3, 1992, pp. 44–49.

Institute of Medicine. *Crossing the Quality Chasm: A New Health System for the 21st Century.* Washington, D.C.: National Academy Press, 2001.

Jacott, W. "Shared Visions, New Pathways." *Minnesota Physician*, 2003, *16*(11), 1, 10–11.

Johnson, B. *Polarity Management: Identifying and Managing Unsolvable Problems.* Amherst, Mass.: HRD Press, 1996.

Johnson, J. A., and Bootman, J. L. "Drug-Related Morbidity and Mortality and the Economic Impact on Pharmaceutical Care." *American Journal of Health-System Pharmacy*, 1997, *54*(5), 554–558.

Johnson, T. R. "Medical Device Safety: New Roles for Purchasing and Users." Unpublished paper, Scottsdale Patient Safety Interest Group, 2003.

Joint Commission on Accreditation of Health Care Organizations. *Conducting Root Cause Analysis in Response to a Sentinel Event.* Oakbrook Terrace, Ill.: Joint Commission on Accreditation of Healthcare Organizations, 1996.

Joint Commission on Accreditation of Healthcare Organizations. *Sentinel Events: Evaluating Cause and Planning Improvement.* Oakbrook Terrace, Ill.: Joint Commission on Accreditation of Healthcare Organizations, 1998.

Joint Commission on Accreditation of Healthcare Organizations. "Shared Visions—New Pathways." *Joint Commission Perspectives*, 2002, *22*(10), 1, 3.

Joint Commission on Accreditation of Healthcare Organizations. *Sentinel Event Glossary of Terms.* 2003. [http://www.jcaho.org/accredited+organizations/ambulatory+care/sentinel+events/glossary.htm]

King, S. Sorrel's Speech to IHI Conference, October 11, 2002. Presented at Institute for Health Improvement National Conference. [http://www.josieking.org/speech.html], 2002.

Kohn, L. T., Corrigan, J. M., and Donaldson, M. S. (eds.). *To Err Is Human: Building a Safer Health System.* Washington, D.C.: National Academy Press, 1999.

Kotter, J. P. *Leading Change.* Boston: Harvard Business School Press, 1996.

Kraman, S. S., and Hamm, G. "Risk Management: Extreme Honesty May Be the Best Policy." *Annals of Internal Medicine*, 1999, *131*(12), 963–967.

Kübler-Ross, E. *On Death and Dying.* New York: Macmillan, 1969.

Lagasse, R. S. "Anesthesia Safety: Model or Myth." *Anesthesiology*, 2002, *97*(6), 1609–1617.

Lakshmanan, M. C., Hershey, C. O., and Breslau, D. "Hospital Admissions Caused by Iatrogenic Disease." *Archives of Internal Medicine*, 1986, *146*(10), 1931–1934.

Langley, G. J., Nolan, K. M., Nolan, T. W., Norman, C., and Provost, L. P. *The Improvement Guide: A Practical Approach to Enhancing Organizational Performance.* San Francisco: Jossey-Bass, 1996.

Leape, L. L. "Error in Medicine." *Journal of the American Medical Association,* 1994, *272*(23), 1851–1857.

Leape, L. L. "Institute of Medicine Medical Error Figures Are Not Exaggerated." *Journal of the American Medical Association,* 2000, *284*(1), 95–97.

Leape, L. L. "The Epidemiology of Patient Safety." Paper presented at the Salzburg International Seminar on Patient Safety and Medical Accident, Apr. 25–May 2, 2001.

Leape, L. L., Brennan, T. A., and Laird, N. "The Nature of Adverse Events in Hospitalized Patients: Results from the Harvard Medical Practice Study II." *New England Journal of Medicine,* 1991, *324*(6), 377–384.

Leape, L. L., Kabcenell, A., Berwick, D. M., and Roessner, J. *IHI Breakthrough Series Guide: Reducing Adverse Drug Events.* Boston: Institute for Healthcare Improvement, 1998.

Leape, L. L., Lawthers, A. G., Brennan, T. A., and Johnson, W. G. "Preventing Medical Injury." *Quality Review Bulletin,* 1993, *19*(5), 144–149.

Leape, L. L., and others. "Systems Analysis of Adverse Drug Events." *Journal of the American Medical Association,* 1995, *274*(1), 35–43.

Libuser, C. B., and Roberts, K. "Risk Mitigation through Organizational Structure," *Organizational Management Theory,* 1998, 1–27.

Louis Harris and Associates. *Public Opinion of Patient Safety Issues: Research Findings.* Chicago: National Patient Safety Foundation, 1997. [http://www.npsf.org/download/1997survey.pdf]

Louis Harris and Associates. "Attitudes toward the United States Health Care System: Long-Term Trends." *Health Care News,* 2002, *17*(2), 1–6.

Luther, K. *Zone Strategy: Knowing Your Zone Keeps Patients Safe.* In National Patient Safety Foundation, *Spotlight on Solutions: Patient Safety Initiative 2000.* Chicago: National Patient Safety Foundation, 2001.

Margolis, J. D., and Clark, J. B. *Workplace Safety at Alcoa.* Boston: Harvard Business School Press, 1991. HBS Case Study 9–692–042.

Marx, D. *Patient Safety and the "Just Culture": A Primer for Health Care Executives.* New York: Columbia University, 2001. [http://www.mers-tm.net/support/Marx_Primer.pdf]

McCandless, K., and Zimmerman, B. *Simplicity on the Other Side of Complexity.* Chicago: Patient Safety Fellowship, Health Forum, American Hospital Association, 2002.

McDermott, R. E., Mikulak, M. J., and Beauregard, M. R. *The Basics of FMEA.* Portland, Ore.: Resources Engineering, Inc., 1996.

Merry, M. "Healthcare's Need for Revolutionary Change." *Quality Progress,* 2003, *36*(9), 31–35.

Merry, M., and Brown, J. P. "From a Culture of Safety to a Culture of Excellence: Quality Science, Human Factors, and the Future of Health Care Quality." *Journal of Innovative Management,* 2001, *7*(2), 29–41.

Merry, M., and Crago, M. "The Past, Present, and Future of Health Care Quality." *The Physician Executive,* 2001, *27*(5), 30–35.

Meziroff, J. *Learning as Transformation.* San Francisco: Jossey-Bass, 2000.

Midwest Business Group on Health. *Reducing the Costs of Poor-Quality Care through Responsible Purchasing Leadership.* Chicago: Midwest Business Group on Health, 2002.

Millenson, M. L. *Demanding Medical Excellence: Doctors and Accountability in the Information Age.* Chicago: University of Chicago Press, 1997.

Minnesota Alliance for Patient Safety. *A Call to Action: 2002.* St. Paul: Minnesota Alliance for Patient Safety, 2002. [http://www.mnpatientsafety.org/pdfs/A%20Call%20to%20Action.pdf]

Minnesota Hospital and Healthcare Partnership and Minnesota Medical Association. *Redefining the Culture for Patient Safety.* Minneapolis–St. Paul: Minnesota Hospital and Healthcare Partnership and Minnesota Medical Association, 2000.

Moen, R. D., and Provonost, P. J. *Quality Measurement: A Practical Guide for the ICU.* Marblehead, Mass.: HCPro, 2003.

Morath, J. *The Quality Advantage: A Strategic Guide for Health Care Leaders.* San Francisco: Jossey-Bass, 1999.

Morath, J., Malone, G., and Anderson, A. *The Patient Safety Learning Packet.* Minneapolis: Children's Hospitals and Clinics of Minnesota, 1999a.

Morath, J., Malone, G. and Anderson, A. *The Patient Safety Resource Guide.* Minneapolis: Children's Hospitals and Clinics of Minnesota, 1999b.

Moray, N. "Error Reduction as a Systems Problem." In M. S. Bogner (ed.), *Human Error in Medicine.* Hillsdale, N.J.: Erlbaum, 1994.

Moser, R. H. "Diseases of Medical Progress." *New England Journal of Medicine,* 1956, *255,* 606–614.

National Center for Patient Safety. *NCPS Triage Cards™ for Root Cause Analysis.* Ann Arbor, Mich.: National Center for Patient Safety, 2001.

National Patient Safety Foundation. *Talking to Patients about Health Care Injury: Statement of Principle.* Chicago: National Patient Safety Foundation, 2000. [http://www.npsf.org/html/statement.html]

National Quality Forum. *Safe Practices for Better Healthcare: A Consensus Report.* Washington, D.C.: National Quality Forum, 2003.

Nelson, E. C., Batalden, P., and Ryder, J. *Clinical Improvement Action Guide.* Oakbrook Terrace, Ill.: Joint Commission on Accreditation of Healthcare Organizations, 1998.

Nelson, E. C., and others. *Microsystems in Health Care: The Essential Building Blocks of High Performing Systems.* 2001. [http://www.dartmouth.edu/~cecs/hcild/downloads/RWJ_MS_Exec_Summary.pdf]

Norman, D. A. *The Design of Everyday Things.* New York: Basic Books, 1988.

Northern New England Cardiovascular Disease Study Group. *Electronic Second Opinion Summary Data, 1998–2001.* Lebanon, N.H.: Clinical Research Division, Dartmouth-Hitchcock Medical Center, 2001.

Office of the Auditor General. *Report of the Auditor General of Canada to the House of Commons.* Ottawa: Minister of Public Works and Government Services, 2002.

Osbon, D. K. (ed). *The Joseph Campbell Companion: Reflections on the Art of Living.* St. Helens, Ore.: Perennial, 1995.

Perrow, C. *Normal Accidents: Living with High-Risk Technologies.* Princeton, N.J.: Princeton University Press, 1999.

Pierce, E. C., Jr. "40 Years Behind the Mask: Safety Revisited." *Anesthesiology,* 1996, *29*(4), 965–975.

Plsek, P. E., and Greenhalgh, T. "Complexity Science: The Challenge of Complexity in Health Care." *British Medical Journal,* 2001, *323,* 625–628. [http://bmj.bmjjournals.com/cgi/content/full/323/7313/625]

Ponte, P. R., and others. "Making Patient-Centered Care Come Alive." *Journal of Nursing Administration,* 2003, *33*(2), 82–90.

Poole, R. "When Failure Is Not an Option." *Technology Review,* 1997, *100,* 38–45.

Prager, L. O. "Safety Bills Take Voluntary Tack on Reporting Errors." *American Medical News,* July 3, 2000. [http://www.ama-assn.org/amednews/2000/07/03/gvsb0703.htm]

Press Ganey Associates. *Satisfaction Measurements, Concord Hospital Inpatient Reports, 1998–2002.* South Bend, Ind.: Press Ganey Associates, 2002.

Quality Interagency Coordination Task Force. *Doing What Counts for Patient Safety: Federal Actions to Reduce Medical Errors and Their Impact.* Report of the Quality Interagency Coordination Task Force (QuIC) to the President. Washington D.C.: Quality Interagency Coordination Task Force, 2000.

Raef, S. "Exploring 7 Levels of Safety." *Focus on Patient Safety,* 2002, *5*(2), 1–3.

Rasmussen, J. "Market Economy, Management Culture, and Accident Causation: New Research Issues?" Address presented to the Second International Conference on Safety Science, Budapest, 1993.

Rasmussen, J. "Risk Management, Adaptation, and Design for Safety." In N. E. Sahlin and B. Brehmer (eds.), *Future Risks and Risk Management.* Dordrecht, Netherlands: Kluwer, 1994.

Rasmussen, J. "Merging Paradigms: Decision Making, Management, and Cognitive Control." In R. Flin, E. Salas, M. E. Strub, and L. Marting (eds.), *Decision Making Under Stress: Emerging Themes and Applications.* Hampshire, England: Ashgate, 1998.

Reason, J. T. *Human Error.* Cambridge, England: Cambridge University Press, 1990.

Reason, J .T. *Managing the Risks of Organizational Accidents.* Brookfield, N.Y.: Ashgate, 1997.

Reason, J. T. "Human Error: Models and Management." *British Medical Journal,* 2000, *320*(7237), 768–770.

Reason, J. T. "The Basics of Human Factors." Paper presented at the Salzburg International Seminar on Patient Safety and Medical Accident, Apr. 25–May 2, 2001.

Reason, J. T., Carthey, J., and de Leval, M. R. "Diagnosing 'Vulnerable System Syndrome': An Essential Prerequisite to Effective Risk Management." *Quality in Health Care,* 2001, *10*(suppl II), 1121–1125.

Reitman, V. "Healing Sound of a Word: 'Sorry'; Doctors and Hospitals Are Learning to Disclose Their Mistakes. Patients Often Respond with Lowered Demands for Damages." *Los Angeles Times,* Mar. 24, 2003, p. F1.

Reynard, W. D., Billings, C. E., Cheaney, E. S., and Hardy, R. *The Development of the NASA Aviation Safety Reporting System.* Houston: National Aeronautics and Space Administration, 1986.

Risser, D. T., and others. "The Potential for Improved Teamwork to Reduce Medical Errors in the Emergency Department." *Annals of Emergency Medicine,* 1999, *34*(3), 376.

Roberts, K. H. "Five Ingredients for Patient Safety." *Ambulatory Outreach,* Fall 1999, pp. 10–13.

Rogers, E. M. *Diffusion of Innovations,* 4th ed. New York: Free Press, 1995.

Rosenthal, A. M. *Thirty-Eight Witnesses: The Kitty Genovese Case.* (Rev. ed.) Berkeley: University of California Press, 1999.

Rosenthal, J., Booth, M., Flowers, L., and Riley, T. *Current State Programs Addressing Medical Errors: An Analysis of Mandatory Reporting and Other Initiatives.* Portland, Me.: National Academy for State Health Policy, 2001.

Roundtable Discussion on Design Considerations for a Patient Safety Improvement Reporting System, sponsored by Kaiser Permanente Institute for Health Policy, NASA Aviation Safety Reporting System, and the National Quality Forum, NASA Ames Research Center, Moffitt Field, Calif., Aug. 28–29, 2000.

Runciman, W. B., and others. "Errors, Incidents, and Accidents in Anesthetic Practice." *Anaesthesia Intensive Care,* 1993, *21*(5), 506–519.

Runciman, W. B., and others. "A Comparison of Iatrogenic Injury Studies in Australia and the USA. II: Reviewer Behavior and Quality of Care." *International Journal of Quality in Health Care,* 2000, *12*(5), 379–388.

Sagan, S. *The Limits of Safety: Organizations, Accidents, and Nuclear Weapons.* Princeton, N.J.: Princeton University Press, 1995.

Schein, E. H. *Organizational Culture and Leadership,* 2nd ed. San Francisco: Jossey-Bass, 1997.

Schwarz, J., and Wald, M. "Echoes of *Challenger:* Shuttle Panel Considers Longstanding Flaws in NASA's System." *New York Times,* Apr. 13, 2003, p. A15.

Senge, P. M. *The Fifth Discipline: The Art and Practice of the Learning Organization.* New York: Doubleday, 1990.

Shapiro, J. P. "Taking the Mistakes Out of Medicine." *U.S. News & World Report,* July 17, 2000, pp. 50–53, 56, 58, 62–64, 66.

Sharpe, V. A., and Faden, A. I. *Medical Harm: Historical, Conceptual, and Ethical Dimensions of Iatrogenic Illness.* Cambridge, England: Cambridge University Press, 1998.

Slovic, P. "The Perception and Management of Therapeutic Risk." Fourth Annual Lecture, Center for Medicine Research, Carshalton, Surrey, England, June 1989.

Smedley, B. D., Stith, A. Y., and Nelson, A. R. (eds). *Unequal Treatment: Confronting Radical and Ethnical Disparities in Health Care.* Washington D.C.: Institute of Medicine, 2003.

Smetzer, J. L., and Cohen, M. R. "Lesson from the Denver Medication Error/Criminal Negligence Case: Look Beyond Blaming Individuals." *Hospital Pharmacy,* 1998, *33*(6), 640–657.

Smith, R. "Foreword." *British Medical Journal,* 2001, *323,* n.p.

Studdert, D. M., Brennan, T. A., and Thomas, E. J. "Beyond Dead Reckoning: Measures of Medical Injury Burden, Malpractice Litigation, and Alternative Compensation Models from Utah and Colorado." *Indiana Law Review,* 2000, *33*(4), 1643–1686.

Tai, D. Y., and others. "A Study of Consecutive Autopsies in a Medical ICU: A Comparison of Clinical Death and Autopsy Diagnosis." *Chest,* 2001, *119*(2), 530–536.

Tennen, H., and Affleck, G. "Blaming Others for Threatening Events." *Psychological Bulletin,* 1990, *108,* 209–232.

Thomas, E. J., and others. "Incidence and Types of Adverse Events and Negligent Care in Utah and Colorado." *Medical Care,* 2000, *38*(3), 261–271.

Tichey, N., and Coehn, E. *The Leadership Engine: How Winning Companies Build Leaders at Every Level.* New York: HarperCollins, 1997.

Trunet, P., and others. "The Role of Iatrogenic Disease in Admission to Intensive Care." *Journal of the American Medical Association,* 1980, *244*(23), 2617–2620.

Uhlig, P. N. Acceptance speech, John Eisenberg Patient Safety Award, Washington, D.C., Oct. 2002.

Uhlig, P. N., Brown, J., Nason, A. K., Camelio, A., and Kendall, E. "John M. Eisenberg Patient Safety Awards: System Innovation-Concord Hospital." *Joint Commission Journal of Quality Improvement,* 2002, *28*(12), 666–672.

Uhlig, P. N., and others. "Reconfiguring Clinical Teamwork for Safety and Effectiveness." *Focus on Patient Safety.* 2002, *5*(3), 1–2.

van den Berghe, G., and others. "Intensive Insulin Therapy in the Critically Ill Patient." *New England Journal of Medicine,* 2001, *345*(19), 1359–1367.

Vaughan, D. *The Challenger Launch Decision: Risky Technology, Culture, and Deviance at NASA.* Chicago: University of Chicago Press, 1996.

Vincent, C. "Framework for Analyzing Risk and Safety in Clinical Medicine." *British Medical Journal,* 1998, *316*(7138), 1154–1157.

Vincent, C., Young, M., and Phillips, A. "Why Do People Sue Doctors? A Study of Patients and Relatives Taking Legal Action." *Lancet,* 1994, *343*(8913), 1609–1613.

Vincent, C. A. (ed.). *Clinical Risk Management: Enhancing Patient Safety.* London: British Medical Journal Publications, 2001.

Walker, P. F. "Eliminating Health Disparities: The Journey to Cultural Competence." Paper presented at the Lawrence Singher Memorial Lectureship, Minneapolis, Apr. 23, 2003.

Wears, R. "The Science of Safety." In L. A. Zipperer and S. Cushman (eds.), *Lessons in Patient Safety.* Chicago: National Patient Safety Foundation, 2001.

Weeks, W. B., and Bagian, J. P. "Making the Business Case for Patient Safety." *Joint Commission Journal of Quality Improvement,* 2003, *29*(1), 51–54.

Weick, K. E. *Sensemaking in Organizations.* Thousand Oaks, Calif.: Sage, 1995.

Weick, K. E. *Making Sense of the Organization.* Malden, Mass.: Blackwell, 2000.

Weick, K. E., and Sutcliffe, K. *Managing the Unexpected.* San Francisco: Jossey-Bass, 2001.

Weingart, S. N. "Patterns and Causes of Medical Error." In L. A. Zipperer and S. Cushman (eds.), *Lessons in Patient Safety.* Chicago: National Patient Safety Foundation, 2001.

Weingart, S. N., Morath, J. M., and Ley, C. A. "Learning with Leaders to Create Safe Health Care: The Executive Session on Patient Safety." *JCOM,* 2003, *10*(11), 597–601.

Weingart, S. N., Wilson, R. M., Gibberd, R. W., and Harrison, B. "Epidemiology of Medical Error." *British Medical Journal,* 2000, *320*(7237), 774–777.

Weinstein, R. A. "Nosocomial Infection Update." *Emerging Infectious Diseases,* 1998, *4*(3), 416–420.

Wennberg, J. E., and Cooper, M. M. (eds.). *The Dartmouth Atlas of Health Care.* Chicago: American Hospital Publishing, 1998.

Wenzel, R. P., and Edmond, M. B. "The Impact of Hospital-Acquired Blood-stream Infections." *Emerging Infectious Diseases,* 2001, *7*(2), 174–177.

Westrum, R. "Cultures with Requisite Imagination." In J. A. Wise, V. D. Hopkin, and P. Stager (eds.), *Verification and Validation of Complex Systems: Human Factors Issues.* Berlin: Springer-Verlag, 1992.

Wickens, C. D., Gordon, S. E., and Liu, Y. *An Introduction to Human Factors Engineering.* New York: Longman, 1998.

Williams, L., and Zipperer, L. "Improving Access to Information: Librarians and Nurses Team Up for Patient Safety." *Nursing Economics,* 2003, *21*(4),199–201. [http://www.npsf.org/download/NEJulAug03.pdf]

Wilson, N. *An Organizational Approach to Patient Safety.* Irving, Tex.: VHA Health Foundation, 2000.

Wilson, R., and others. "The Quality in Australian Health Care Study." *Medical Journal of Australia,* 1995, *163*(9), 458–471.

Woods, D. D., Johannesen, L., Cook, R. I., and Sarter, N. *Behind Human Error: Cognitive System, Computers, and Hindsight.* Dayton, Ohio: Crew Systems Ergonomics Information Analysis Center, Wright-Patterson Air Force Base, 1994.

Zimmerman, B., and Hayday, B. "A Board's Journey into Complexity Science." *Group Decision Making and Negotiation,* 1999, *8,* 281–303.

Zimmerman, B., Lindberg, C., and Plsek, P. *Edgeware: Insight from Complexity Science for Healthcare Leaders.* Irving, Tex.: VHA Health Foundation, 1998.

Zipperer, L., Gluck, J., and Anderson, S. "Knowledge Maps for Patient Safety." *Journal of Hospital Librarianship,* 2002, *2*(4), 17–35.

Zipperer, L. A., and Cushman, S. (eds.). *Lessons in Patient Safety.* Chicago: National Patient Safety Foundation, 2001.

GLOSSARY

In this glossary, we have collected terms and definitions used in the emerging field of safety science; most of these terms are also used in this book. Some are technical and come from the various disciplines that comprise safety science. Many will be new to the health care professional who is learning about safety science in order to create a culture of safety. Other terms may be familiar from other contexts, but they are explained here as they relate to patient safety. This list is not meant to be comprehensive, and the definitions are not meant to be official. Rather, our intent is to provide helpful operational definitions, and we have based some of them on the use of these terms in the current literature on patient safety. When formal definitions do exist and are helpful, we have used them and provided their sources in the literature.

The patient safety movement is growing and is in a state of flux. Experts from all arenas—clinical, administrative, academic, regulatory, and governmental—debate not only which definitions are most important but also the meanings and applications of even the most basic terms. Therefore, we have worked to create a glossary that builds on existing definitions. The creation of a conventional taxonomy of patient safety, with definitions that are recognized and accepted by the health care industry, is crucial to moving the field forward. We hope the definitions offered here will contribute to this effort. Even more, we hope they will aid you on your journey to a culture of safety.

The first time we (rather than sources we cite) use a term in the text, it appears there in bold type, and its listing here includes a reference to the chapter in which we first use it.

accidents (Introduction) Unplanned, unexpected, and undesired events, usually with one or more adverse consequences (Bogner, 1994, p. 166).

accountability (Introduction) The obligation to demonstrate, review, and take responsibility for performance, both for the results achieved in light of agreed expectations and for the means used (Office of the Auditor General, 2002, p. 1).

active failures (2) Direct operational errors that occur at the delivery level of the organization. Active failures may be the results of action, inaction, or faulty decision making (Reason, 1997, p. 15).

adverse drug events (2) Like adverse events, adverse drug events are unplanned, unexpected, and undesired. The term is limited to events related to medication use, but at the same time it is broader than both of the other terms because it includes such things as allergic reactions.

adverse events (Introduction) Unplanned, unexpected, and undesired outcomes that result from medical care rather than from the natural course of disease. Adverse events often result in extended hospitalization, disability at the time of discharge, or death (Brennan and others, 1991).

ambient listening (5) Purposeful listening that is done to detect anything unusual in the noise or nature of communications in the work area.

andon cord (4) Cord that hangs near employees on an assembly line. When an employee on the line spots a quality problem or needs assistance from another team member, the employee pulls the cord, and the line shuts down (Flinchbaugh, 2001, p. 39).

anonymity (6) Refers to reports of events or near misses in which the reporter is unknown. The assurance of anonymity encourages reporting by reducing fear of retribution. Anonymous reporting systems contrast with blameless reporting systems, which protect the reporter with confidentiality but allow the reporter to be contacted for further information if it is needed.

appreciative inquiry (9) A way of thinking, seeing, and acting for powerful, purposeful change in organizations. Appreciative inquiry works on the assumption that if more of something is desired, it already exists in the organization and can be discovered if questions are asked in a positive, focused way. Appreciative inquiry engages the entire system in inquiry about what works by uncovering information that is analyzed for common themes (Hall and Hammond, 1997).

attribution (7) The imputing of a cause when an accident occurs. Human beings search for reasons behind behavior, especially when an accident occurs. The cause may be assigned to situational factors (that is, the environment is seen as a strong influence or primary cause) or to dispositional factors (that is, something unique to a particular person is believed to have caused the event). Hindsight bias (see definition below) influences attribution so that when an accident occurs, outside observers are likely to assign the cause to the individuals involved, whereas the individuals involved in the event are likely to pin the cause on environmental influences (Heider, 1958).

authority gradient (Introduction) Refers to a relationship of perceived power in which the an individual is reluctant to give negative information to a person in a position of higher status and to question that person's decisions. Organizational rank contributes to the creation of the authority gradient (Alkov and others, 1992).

Aviation Safety Reporting System (ASRS) (4) Developed by the National Aeronautics and Space Administration (NASA) for the aviation industry. NASA, external to the industry, accepts confidential narratives about near misses and accidents up to the point of a crash (Reynard, Billings, Cheaney, and Hardy, 1986). The system is voluntary, confidential, and nonpunitive, and its purpose is to collect and use incident data to improve the national aviation system. The ASRS supports aviation system policy, planning, and improvement and strengthens the foundation of human factors research in aviation by identifying deficiencies for correction by appropriate authorities. The Veterans Administration is the only health care entity to contract with NASA for a blameless reporting system at this time.

best practices (2) Actions, protocols, or guidelines considered, on the basis of the current state of knowledge in given field, to be the best in their class, having demonstrated effectiveness in carrying out processes or subprocesses. Best practices can be identified inside or outside an organization. They can be stored in electronic repositories for sharing throughout the organization, and thus they can become the nucleus of a knowledge management initiative (Davenport and Prusak, 2000, p. 167).

blameless environment (4) A nonpunitive approach achieved in a culture of safety. In a blameless environment, the front line is comfortable and feels compelled to report errors, failures, and near misses so they can be studied for system improvement.

blameless reporting (Introduction) A process of collecting information in order to learn and design fail-safe care delivery processes that stop errors before they can harm a patient.

blameworthy actions (4) Individual actions that are purposefully negligent and can cause or could cause harm to patients and do not result from flaws in the system. Blameworthy actions include alcoholic or other chemical impairment, felonies, malfeasance, reckless behavior, and failure to learn over time. Blameworthy actions are not covered by blameless reporting systems and need to be dealt with through administrative processes that are timely and fair.

blunt end (1) The work of management. The blunt end of the system generates the resources, constraints, and conflicts that shape the world of technical work. Blunt end decisions and actions can produce latent failures (that is, system vulnerabilities that are hidden in work processes). The blunt end contrasts with the sharp end (that is, direct care delivery on the front line).

boundaries of excediency (4) The limits of safe performance, beyond which individuals, teams, or organizations move into zones of intolerable risk. The boundaries of excediency are revealed by increased error, surprise, fatigue, and communication and technical glitches. Crossing these boundaries serves as a warning to pull back, slow down, and reassess action.

bureaucracy (4) A system of administration marked by adherence to fixed rules, red tape, and authority based on position rather than expertise. Work in bureaucracies tends not to be team-based but instead is specialized and takes place in isolated "silos." Political decision making tends to obscure the flaws in work processes and protects the status quo.

bureaucratic culture (4) Refers to an organizational culture that handles safety-related issues through compartmentalization. In a bureaucratic culture, safety information and safety management are not integrated throughout the organization.

Accidents and near misses are dealt with in an isolated, local fashion, and lessons from failures are not shared across the organization. Bureaucratic cultures differ from pathological cultures in that reporters are not punished, but organizations with bureaucratic cultures do not know what to do with new ideas. Most health care organizations are bureaucratic (Westrum, 1992).

causation (Introduction) The act by which an effect is produced (also known as "causality"). In epidemiology, the concept of causation is used to relate certain types of influences (predisposing, enabling, precipitating, or reinforcing factors) to the occurrence of disease. The doctrine of causation is important in determining negligence and thus is an important concept in the field of criminal law (Joint Commission on Accreditation of Healthcare Organizations, 2003).

cognition (3) Processes and structures that have to do with perception, recognition, recall, imagination, conceptualization, and thought as well as with supposition, expectation, planning, and problem solving.

collaborative structure (5) Describes a highly interactive way of working in which positional authority gives way to expertise for the sake of safety.

command and control (5) Refers to formal procedures that create adherence to the shared experience of a best practice. Command and control, as distinguished from bureaucracy, is an intelligent, thoughtful application of rules and procedures, not routinized compliance. The elements of command and control are migrating decision making (the person with the most experience makes the decision), creation of redundancy (backup systems are in place), seeing the big picture (senior managers do not micromanage but rather attend to patterns and systems), establishment of formal rules and procedures (hierarchy as well as procedures and protocol are based on evidence), and training (investment is made in the knowledge and skills workers at the front line; see Roberts, 1999).

complex (Introduction) *Complex, simple,* and *complicated* are terms that refer to domains of work within organizations. The idea of complexity, better understood through illustration than through definition, takes us into a domain of ambiguity involving dynamic and changing interactions of parts that combine and propagate in unpredictable ways, with nonlinear effects. Disagreement is high. Continual trade-offs and negotiations are required. Examples of complex domains are those involved in raising a child and creating a culture of safety. Solving a complex problem requires more individual freedom, with reminders and alerts and sharing and understanding of deviations from protocol. Complexity-inspired approaches are likely to have the highest probability of success in complex systems. Small changes can have big effects in complex systems because of the attribute of non-linearity: a single event can engender big results, whereas big initiatives can effect very little change. There is no single strategy for decision making; rather, multiple sources of information—people, events, and relationships—continually provide input into decision making (McCandless and Zimmerman, 2002).

complex adaptive system (5) A collection of individual agents having freedom to act in ways that are not always totally predictable, and whose actions are interconnected so that one agent's actions change the context for other agents. Examples of complex adaptive systems include the immune system, a colony of termites, the financial market, and just about any collection of humans (a family, a committee, or a health care team; see Plsek and Greenhalgh, 2001, p. 625).

complexity (Introduction) Characteristic of systems where nonlinear interactive components, emergent phenomena, continuous and discontinuous change, and unpredictable outcomes are found. Although there is at present no single accepted definition of complexity, the term is applied across a range of different yet related system features, such as chaos, self-organized criticality, adaptivity, neural nets, nonlinear dynamics, and far-from-equilibrium conditions (Zimmerman, Lindberg, and Plsek, 1998).

complicated (Introduction) Describes certain types of domains of problems or work. Complicated problems require multiple steps of analysis and multiple perspectives for system design and control. A complicated problem introduces greater variability, less certainty, and a broader zone in which agreement must be negotiated. Examples of complicated problems include conducting open-heart surgery or a quality improvement project. In a complex system, a complicated approach may use resources and effort yet have little impact or sustainability (McCandless and Zimmerman, 2002).

computerized provider order entry (CPOE) (Introduction) A networked system that allows health care professionals to enter orders via computer. Uses of CPOE include but are not limited to orders for medications and diagnostic tests (clinical laboratory, imaging), nursing orders, and special types of orders (dietary, for example). Sometimes also called "computerized physician order entry" or "computerized practitioner order entry."

confidentiality (2) The condition of not disclosing identifying information, such as names of the reporter and the patient and location of the incident. In blameless reporting systems, confidentiality is preferred over anonymous reporting so that the reporter can be contacted to provide further information if it is needed.

confirmation bias (9) The tendency to select pieces of information that substantiate one's currently held view. Confirmation bias tends to be strong in experiences of failure as evidence contradicting one's current view prompts one to seek confirmation of what is likely to have been a preliminary hypothesis based on insufficient information.

constraining function (3) An interruption of automatic action, creating a pause for deliberation.

continuous quality improvement (Introduction) Ongoing betterment of products, services, and processes through incremental and breakthrough refinements (American Society for Quality, 2000). Sometimes called "continual improvement."

crew resource management (Introduction) A process of training, used in the airline industry, that considers human performance limitations (such as fatigue and stress) and designs countermeasures to combat them (for example, briefings, monitoring and cross-checking, decision making, and review and modification of plans) along with instruction in confronting the authority gradient (see definition above). Sophisticated simulators allow full crews to practice dealing with accident-inducing situations without jeopardy and to receive feedback on both individual and team performance (Helmreich, 2000).

culture carrier (Introduction) An enduring intervention that both defines and shapes the actions of an organization. Policies are strong culture carriers because they codify expectations and give guidance to behavior.

culture of safety (Introduction) A culture in which safety is the top priority. A culture of safety is characterized by vigilance and by authority based on expertise rather than on position. A culture of safety constantly seeks to learn, not only from failure but also from anticipation of failure and from mental simulations of possible failure scenarios. Transparency of error and failure and an ambience of trust are hallmarks.

default hierarchy (5) Characteristic of organizations that operate reliably by transferring the basis of decision-making authority in conditions of emerging risk from hierarchy and position or rank to technical expertise and collaboration, immediately deferring to predetermined, understood, well-rehearsed roles for taking action in an emergency.

diffusion of responsibility (3) A term borrowed from social psychology and used to name the phenomenon of ignoring a need or not performing a task because one assumes that someone else will take care of it.

disclosure (Introduction) The act of informing others that an event has occurred. Disclosure of errors and accidents in a health care setting should include a prompt and compassionate explanation of what is understood about what happened and about the probable effects; information about what is being done to ensure safety; assurances that a full analysis will take place and that the findings of the analysis, as they are known, will be communicated; information about changes that are being made, on the basis of the analytical findings, to reduce the likelihood of a similar event; and an acknowledgment of accountability (National Patient Safety Foundation, 2000). When an accident occurs, disclosure to patients and their families is in order.

early adopters (2) A group of individuals in an organization who adopt innovations soon after they are introduced; said to constitute 13.5 percent of the organization's population (Rogers, 1995, pp. 262, 264). Early adopters are well integrated into large social systems. As social leaders in organizations, they have a great degree of opinion leadership; that is, they are respected, and others listen to them. They are key messengers on teams and are crucial to the development of a network for spreading innovation and for speeding the process of diffusing an innovation. Potential adopters look to early adopters for advice and information about innovations.

epidemiology (2) A field of study concerned with determining the causes, incidence, and characteristic behavior of disease outbreaks affecting human populations. It includes the interrelationships of host, agent, and environment as these pertain to the distribution and control of disease (Joint Commission on Accreditation of Healthcare Organizations, 1996).

ergonomics (3) The field of equipment design and, more broadly, the design of equipment. Ergonomics includes studies of task-related movement patterns, studies whose findings are used to reduce errors and injuries when equipment is used by humans (Bogner, 1994, pp. 59, 69).

error (Introduction) Failure in the intended completion of a planned action (an error of execution), or use of the wrong plan to achieve an aim (an error of planning). A single error rarely leads to an accident; rather, it is the concatenation of errors that produces accidents (Kohn, Corrigan, and Donaldson, 1999, p. 179).

errors of omission (2) Errors that result when a necessary step is left out of a process (Bogner, 1994, p. 168).

error-tolerant culture; error-tolerant system (5, 3) A culture or system that accepts errors as a fact of life and creates strategies and work processes designed to mitigate errors. Nevertheless, an error-tolerant culture or system does not accept the violation of formal rules, especially those that have been validated as having strategic value for avoiding or mitigating errors (Helmreich, 2001).

Failure Mode and Effects Analysis (FMEA) (5) A systematic method of identifying and preventing product and process problems before they occur. FMEA focuses on identifying and removing defects, enhancing safety, and increasing customer satisfaction (McDermott, Mikulak, and Beauregard, 1996).

forcing function (3) A technique for making it impossible to complete a work process that may cause danger to a patient. An example of a forcing function would be using, for oral doses of liquid medication, an oral syringe that does not fit with intravenous tubing, and to which needles cannot be attached, to prevent the medication from being administered in a potentially lethal manner. Another example would be using a computerized order entry system that forces physicians to place orders in a standardized way.

foresight (3) The ability of human beings to see or anticipate, when looking ahead, parallel paths of action that can lead to a desired outcome, by contrast with seeing the single simple, obvious path of action revealed as an effect of hindsight bias (see definition below).

formal rules; formal rules and procedures (4, 5) In the context of patient safety, written protocols that purposely create an environment of thoughtful, intelligent adherence as opposed to thoughtless, blind routine or ritualistic compliance.

fundamental attribution error (3) An outcome of the pervasive human tendency to explain a bad result as the product of an actor's personal inadequacies (dispositional causes) rather than explaining it as the product of situational factors, such as role or context, that are beyond the actor's control (situational causes; see Fiske and Taylor, 1984).

generative culture (4) Characteristic of an organization that encourages workers to actively bring observations related to important aspects of the system to the attention of higher management (Westrum, 1992, p. 402).

"good catch" log (6) A simple tool used at the sharp end of care delivery to capture thoughts, suggestions, and perceptions of risk for the purpose of improving safety. Staff who work in the care environment make entries in a notebook reserved for this purpose. The log entries are regularly reviewed by interdisciplinary safety teams as they set priorities for actions that will be taken to mitigate risk.

harm (Introduction) A category of adverse effects that includes a patient's death, or any temporary or permanent impairment of the patient's bodily functions or structure that requires medical intervention. Harm stems from system flaws that go unchecked and are allowed to affect a patient.

Harvard Medical Practice Study (HMPS) (2) A 1991 study of medical records from fifty-one hospitals in New York State. The study found that almost 4 percent of all patients whose records were studied had suffered adverse events as a result of their medical care (Brennan and others, 1991).

heedful procedures (4) Actions or tasks designed to be performed with proper attention. They include steps that require the actor to maintain situational awareness and obtain verification of previous steps in a process (for example, by verifying an order) before taking action. In heedful procedures, individuals exercise a high degree of vigilance and judgment while conducting even repetitive actions over time. There is intelligent and thoughtful application of rules and procedures rather than ritualized, automatic compliance with them.

hierarchy; structure of hierarchy (1, 5) A system of formal rules, structures, procedures, training, and decision making in the service of organizational mission and values. In a safety culture, the meaning of the term differs from what it means within a bureaucratic organizational structure in that a hierarchy is flexible and can be modified when organizational conditions so warrant. A hierarchy provides a clear chain of command so that people working at the sharp end know where to go for help. This arrangement is distinct from bureaucracy, which implies politics, red tape, and a reliance on positional authority.

high-alert medications (8) Medications that carry a heightened risk of causing injury if they are misused. Errors may or may not be more common with high-alert medications than with other drugs, but the consequences of these errors may be more devastating. Examples of high-alert medications include heparin, warfarin, insulin, chemotherapeutic agents, concentrated electrolytes, intravenous digoxin, opiate narcotics, neuromuscular blocking agents, thrombolytics, and adrenergic agonists (Cohen, 1999, p. 5.1).

high-reliability organizations (HROs) (Introduction) Organizations in which the performance of high-risk activities is the norm but rates of accident or harm are low. In HROs, failure is not an option, because lives are at stake. Performance of tasks is highly disciplined, and creating safety is everyone's practice and first priority. HROs are characterized by communication, training, default hierarchy (that is, in conditions of emerging risk, the basis of decision-making authority moves from rank to technical expertise), continual process auditing, standards that establish quality, reporting, learning, and an ambience of trust.

hindsight bias (Introduction) Hindsight bias comes into play when human performance is judged in the context of accidents or near misses (Cook and Woods, 1994). Hindsight bias, always present when a situation is evaluated in retrospect, has two aspects: observers of past events exaggerate what others should have been able to foresee, and they are unaware of how much their own perceptions are influenced by their retrospective knowledge of the situation's outcome.

human factors (Introduction) A field concerned with understanding and enhancing human performance in the workplace, especially in complex systems. Among this field's significant contributions to patient safety is the notion that creating safety requires changing the conditions in which human beings work.

implicit knowledge (7) Information and know-how that individuals uniquely possess (Norman, 1988). In health care, working to define the knowledge that people have but are unaware of possessing is a critical step in understanding work flow and seeing the whole picture.

Ishikawa diagram (6) Diagram developed to represent the relationship between some effect and all possible causes influencing it (also known as a "cause and effect diagram" or "fishbone diagram"). The Ishikawa diagram is drawn to clearly illustrate the various possible causes affecting a process by sorting out and relating the causes. For every effect there are likely to be several major categories of causes. From a defined list of possible causes, the most likely are identified and selected for further analysis (Brassard, 1988).

judgment (2) Assessment of the likelihood of uncertain events. In making such assessments, people rely on a few limited principles (heuristics) that make this complex task simpler but that also can lead to severe, systematic errors (Reason, 1990, p. 40).

knowledge management (6) The collection of information about staff members' experiences, and the coordination of efforts to make this information available for the betterment of the organization and its clients. According to Davenport and Prusak (2000, p. 62), the principles of conducting such an effort include the following imperatives:

1. Foster awareness of the value of knowledge sought and be willing to invest in the process of generating it.
2. Identify key knowledge workers who can be effectively brought together in a fusion effort.
3. Emphasize the creative potential inherent in the complexity and the diversity of ideas, seeing differences as positive rather than as sources of conflict, and avoiding simple answers to complex questions.
4. Make the need for knowledge generation clear so as to encourage, reward, and direct it toward a common goal.
5. Introduce measure and milestones of success that reflect the true value of knowledge more completely than simple balance-sheet accounting.

knowledge-based activities (3) Activities that occur in new, unfamiliar situations in which clinicians must make judgments by relying on what they already know. A diagnostic judgment is an example of a knowledge-based activity.

lapses (3) Errors that result from some sort of failure in the execution or storage phase of an action sequence. Lapses differ from slips in that they are not visible.

large-scale complex systems (5) Systems that have the following characteristics: (1) tightly coupled work processes that frequently create situations in which individuals who may be socialized to be independent operators must rely on each other in order to succeed; (2) many distinct cultures that operate simultaneously; (3) intended and unintended consequences whereby every intended consequence of an action may also have unplanned outcomes; (4) long incubation periods during which risk can arise; and (5) risk that can be mitigated in one part of the system only to move to another (Grabowski and Roberts, 1997).

latent conditions (3) Hidden factors, rooted in the work processes of the organization, that can provoke operational errors in certain circumstances or present hazards of their own accord. Examples of latent conditions for failure include inadequate training, unworkable procedures, poor or inadequate technology, undue time pressure, understaffing, and fatigue (Reason, 1997).

leadership (Introduction) A set of processes that create organizations in the first place or adapt them to significantly changing circumstances (Kotter, 1996, p. 25). Without sustained leadership from the top of the organization, patient safety is impossible.

Leapfrog Group (2) A body formed by the Business Roundtable, a coalition of prominent business leaders who purchase health insurance for 25 million Americans. Organized to confront the problem of medical accident, the Leapfrog Group established a voluntary program that rewards the health care industry for breakthrough improvements ("big leaps") in patient safety.

learning organization (4) An organization that continually expands its capacity to create its future by moving beyond adaptive learning (that is, learning that has survival value alone) and toward generative learning (that is, learning that enhances the capacity to create). A learning organization is a place where people are continually discovering how they create their reality and how they can change it. In a safety culture, the term denotes an organization that actively pursues continuous learning to create safety, where the goal is to learn from failure as well as from successes. The learning organization that has a safety culture is characterized by seeking information, rewarding messengers, and discovering improvements that lead to far-reaching innovation and change (Senge, 1990).

medical accident (Introduction) Patient death or injury, usually caused by multiple systemic flaws.

metaphor (4) Language used in such a way as to suggest parallels between the situation at hand and a markedly different experience in order to make sense of phenomena of interest. The metaphor directs thinking by framing situational awareness, identifying appropriate goals, and flagging relevant pieces of information. Researchers have found that metaphors structure thinking and condition emotional reactions, thus governing the way people think about issues. Computers and biological processes serve as bases for good metaphors.

microsystem (4) A group of people and resources formed in response to specific patterns of patient need. For example, a clinical microsystem in an open-heart surgery unit includes surgeons, nurses, pharmacists, therapists, nutritionists, social workers, and others who routinely interact to care for patients. This microsystem also includes the resources necessary for them to do their work.

mindfulness (3) In high-reliability organizations, the quality of organizing in a way that enables people to notice and halt unexpected developments. According to Weick and Sutcliffe (2001), mindfulness is a process, a constant "struggle for alertness," in which HROs continually revise and update their information as events unfold. Mindfulness is characterized by five key features: preoccupation with failure, reluctance to simplify interpretations, sensitivity to operations, commitment to resilience, and deference to expertise. These key features must be present at all levels of an organization in order for a collective state of awareness to develop.

mistakes (Introduction) Deficits or failures in judgment, either in selecting an objective (such as a treatment goal) or in specifying the means to achieve it (such as formulating a treatment plan; see Reason, 1990).

multicausal (Introduction) Having many interacting variables that come together to create the conditions for an event. Medical accidents usually result from multiple causes rather than from a single cause.

near miss (Introduction) An event or situation that might have resulted in an accident, injury, or illness but did not, either by chance or through timely intervention (Quality Interagency Coordination Task Force, 2000). Near misses are valuable tools for learning about system vulnerability and resilience.

normalization of deviance (Introduction) The acceptance of, or failure to recognize, faulty and risk-prone processes, and the minimization of serious deficiencies so that they become familiar, pervasive, and entrenched in the culture of the work environment and are accepted as normal.

pathological culture (4) The culture of an organization that does not want to know about safety problems. Pathological cultures punish reporters of accidents and those involved in the accidents; they cover up failures and discourage new ideas (Westrum, 1992).

patient safety (Introduction) A condition in which patients are protected from medical accidents and other types of harm. Patient safety is achieved through the disciplined and aggressive creation and maintenance of systems that take account of safety science, accident causation, and human factors.

patient safety officer (2) An appointed officer who reports to the chief executive. The patient safety officer is responsible for orchestrating patient safety–related activity and importing new knowledge into the organization.

Patient Safety Reporting System (PSRS) (6) A prototype blameless reporting system established in 2000 by NASA and the Veterans Administration. The PSRS emphasizes the reporting of near misses (see definition above).

patient safety science; safety science (Introduction) An emerging discipline that integrates knowledge from fields outside health care, such as human factors and organizational sociology, as well as lessons from high-reliability organizations, and applies them to the delivery of health care services. Cognitive psychologists, human factors engineers, sociologists, and organizational scientists have contributed to safety science by studying accidents and near misses in aviation, the nuclear power industry, military operations, and, occasionally, health care delivery (Wears, 2001).

patient safety steering committee (Introduction) A committee whose members come from across the organization, including professional staff, clinical front-line staff, health care consumers, and board members. The committee is appointed by the organization's leadership to import new knowledge, study applications, and advise on strategy and policy. Reporting to the chief executive, the patient safety steering committee also monitors results and serves the organization as a resource and emissary on patient safety.

performance improvement (Introduction) A movement encompassing a philosophy and attitude dedicated to analyzing the organization's capabilities and processes and repeatedly making them better in order to achieve the objective of improving the organization itself.

plan-do-study-act (PDSA) cycles (9) Elements of a method for discovering assignable causes and correcting them in order to improve the quality of processes (Joint Commission on Accreditation of Healthcare Organizations, 2003). The acronym PDCA (plan-do-check-act) is also used, as are the phrases "Deming cycle" and "Shewhart cycle."

process auditing (5) An activity that establishes and uses a system for performing ongoing checks and formal reviews of work processes in order to spot unexpected safety problems.

process failures (4) Instances of faulty or absent completion of one or more steps in an ordained sequence.

process flow (1) The orderly progression of a goal-directed series of interrelated actions, events, mechanisms, or steps to achieve a defined outcome. Ordering medication entails a process flow, as does administering anesthesia, points discussed at Institute for Healthcare Improvement National Congress on Reducing Adverse Drug Events and Medical Errors, held Mar. 26–27, 1997.

process flow diagram (3) A pictorial representation that shows all the steps of a process and uses easily recognizable symbols to represent how various steps in a process are related to each other. Also known as a "sequence of events diagram."

punitive or retaliatory environment (4) An environment that punishes workers in close proximity to an accident as well as individuals who report potentially hazardous situations. The organization with a punitive or retaliatory environment creates an atmosphere where staff members at the sharp end are afraid to disclose failures and near misses. The organization thus eliminates the opportunity to learn from mistakes.

rapid cycle change (7) A structured methodology of conducting progressive cycles of experimentation based on plan-do-study-act (PDSA) cycles of improvement, informed by data and measurements to gauge whether change is achieving the desired results.

reciprocal accountability (Introduction) Responsibility that front-line staff and management have to each other, and that they hold collectively to patients, for providing safe, harm-free care. Front-line staff are accountable for informing management about dangerous situations, and management is accountable to front-line staff for creating the environment that allows this reporting activity to occur. Reciprocal accountability is based on mutual trust: trust on the part of management that the front line will report error and vulnerability, and trust on the part of the front line that management will respond appropriately to what is reported. This definition extends to the power and responsibility that regulators have to see that organizations and boards support safety systems.

redundancy function (3) An action that builds double checks into a work process. The requirement for countersignatures on a procedure is an example of a redundancy function.

risk management (6) Clinical and administrative activities undertaken to identify, evaluate, and reduce the likelihood of injury to patients, staff, and visitors and the likelihood of loss to the organization itself (Joint Commission on Accreditation of Healthcare Organizations, 1996).

root cause analysis (RCA) (Introduction) A process for identifying the basic or causal factor(s) underlying variations in performance, which may include the occurrence of a sentinel event (see definition below; see Joint Commission on Accreditation of Healthcare Organizations, 1996).

root causes (Introduction) The most fundamental reasons for the failure or inefficiency of a process (Joint Commission on Accreditation of Healthcare Organizations, 1996). The vast majority of medical accidents have more than one cause.

routine procedures (4) Procedures performed so many times that they can become automatic and thus introduce greater risk because vigilance is reduced.

rule-based activities (3) Activities that rely on a plan, a guideline, or a protocol that organizes a sequence of steps known from prior experience to lead to success.

safety action team (SAT) (6) A department- or unit-based interdisciplinary work group that discusses safety issues and develops ways to address those issues to increase safe care. The group's membership depends on individual needs, but efforts are made to include people who represent the continuum of care for patients.

safety science (Introduction) See **patient safety science**.

sensemaking (Introduction) The process by which individuals in organizations take the time to understand a complex situation thoroughly before making a decision. By creating understanding and informed action, sensemaking allows managers to deal properly with unforeseen events while they are still issues, before they become problems or crises (Weick, 2000).

sentinel event (Introduction) An unexpected occurrence involving death or serious physical or psychological injury, or the risk thereof. Serious injury specifically includes loss of limb or function. The phrase "or the risk thereof" includes any process variation whose recurrence would carry a significant chance of a serious adverse outcome. Such events are labeled "sentinel" because they signal the need for immediate investigation and response (Joint Commission on Accreditation of Healthcare Organizations, 1996).

sequence of events analysis (7) An activity that convenes stakeholders to create and recreate a timeline of events and actions prodromal to an accident or near miss.

sharp end (1) Points of vulnerability in the care delivery system where expertise is applied, and where error is experienced. Health care workers who provide direct patient care are working at the sharp end (Reason, 1990).

simple (Introduction) Describes certain types of domains of problems or work. Simple problems can be managed with recipes or protocols that bring stakeholders close to agreement and certainty. Following a recipe to bake a cake is a simple procedure. A simple approach may not use many resources or require much effort but may still have great impact in a complex system (McCandless and Zimmerman, 2002).

simulations (3) A training and feedback method in which learners actually practice tasks or processes in lifelike circumstances, using models or virtual reality, with feedback from observers, other team members, and video cameras to assist improvement of skills (Leape, Kabcenell, Berwick, and Roessner, 1998, p. 177). Teamwork and communication are a focus in simulations pursuing patient safety. Use of electronic equipment designed to reproduce characteristics of a process are potential hazards used in training programs to improve pilot and crew skills (Oster, Strong, and Zorn, 1992, p. 192).

single-point failures (3) Missteps by a single human being; extremely rare occurrences.

situational awareness (Introduction) Vigilance applied to a specific context, such as a dangerous work situation. Situational awareness can be observed in specific behaviors, such as constant communication and eye contact among members of a team as they watch each other, or listening for what is unusual so problems can be rectified before intolerable risk emerges.

Six Sigma (8) A measurement and improvement system that involves attaining an error rate equivalent to no more than 3.4 errors per 1 million opportunities for error.

slips (3) Errors that result from some failure in an action's execution phase or storage phase, or in both phases; the plan guiding the actions may or may not have been adequate to achievement of the desired objective. Examples are slips of the tongue, slips of the pen, and slips of action (Reason, 1990).

stop-the-line (Introduction) In a safety culture, describes a work policy by which any member of a team may stop the action to restore safety if he or she believes that the margin of danger exceeds the team's ability to manage and recover— or, in other words, when operations appear to be moving into conditions of intolerable risk.

Swiss Cheese Model of Accident Causation (Introduction) A metaphorical, visual representation of the nature of emerging risks in complex systems characterized by vulnerabilities as well as defenses.

system (Introduction) Any collection of components and the relations between them, whether or not the components are human, when the components have been brought together for a well-defined goal or purpose (Moray, 1994).

system errors (6) Delayed negative consequences of technical design issues or organizational issues and decisions. Also referred to as "latent errors" (Battles, Kaplan, van der Schaaf, and Shea, 1998, p. 231).

system vulnerabilities (2) Weaknesses, deficiencies, or flaws in the organization of care delivery. A system vulnerability may be as narrow as a work process or as broad as an ineffective governance function or executive team.

systems approach (3) An approach to patient safety based on the notion that characteristics of the work system can make hazards both more likely and more difficult to detect and correct. The systems approach takes the position that individuals are responsible for the quality of their work, but that focusing on systems rather than on individuals will be more effective in reducing harm. The systems approach substitutes inquiry for blame and focuses on circumstances rather than on character (Leape and others, 1995). When an accident occurs, prompt, intensive investigation and multidisciplinary systems analysis are used to discover proximal and systemic causes.

teamwork (Introduction) Individuals with expertise and competence assembled to perform work that must be accomplished together. Characteristics include clear roles and responsibilities, expectations, training, reliable communications, and substitutions and flexibility in function.

threshold change (9) Magnitude of change that moves the entire organization to a new and higher level of performance. This is often informed by a profound experience.

tightly coupled work processes (3) Work processes so interdependent that one cannot be isolated from another. They usually occur in the same production sequence, and an action in one process causes an action in another. There is no slack or buffer between the two, and what happens in one process directly affects what happens in the other. When work processes are tightly coupled, failures can rapidly escalate out of control (Perrow, 1999; Sagan, 1995).

tipping point (5) The moment when a set of circumstances reaches critical mass so that a single event can disrupt or overwhelm mechanisms of homeostasis, propelling a manageable situation out of control and igniting change that fundamentally alters the previous state (Gladwell, 2000).

To Err Is Human: Building a Safer Health System (2) Title of the highly visible 1999 report by Kohn, Corrigan, and Donaldson that calls on government, industry, consumers, and health care providers to reduce medical accidents. The report calls on Congress to create a national patient safety center to develop the new tools and systems needed to address persistent problems (Zipperer and Cushman, 2001, p. 113).

training (Introduction) Instruction, learning, and practice geared, in the field of patient safety, to performance rather than acquisition of knowledge. Training in patient safety is targeted to specific populations and is based on attaining competency in particular areas.

transforming concept (Introduction) A concept that has the power to provoke great change. An example of a transforming concept is the idea that accidents are caused by systems rather than individuals.

transparency (Introduction) Openness in the delivery of health care services. When transparency is a feature of a health care delivery system, work processes are made visible, and information is made available to patients and their families so that they can make informed decisions about selecting a health plan, a hospital, a clinical practice, or one of several alternative treatments. The notion of transparency includes providing information about the system's performance in terms of safety issues, evidence-based practice, and patient satisfaction. The circumstances surrounding accidents are also disclosed (Berwick, 2002b, p. 86).

voluntary reporting system (6) A system for reporting errors that operates in the interest of learning throughout the system, by contrast with a mandatory reporting system, which functions solely in the interest of public accountability.

wicked questions (9) Brenda Zimmerman, a theorist of management and complexity, coined this term to denote the kind of hard-hitting interrogation to which managers need to subject their plans and organizing schemes. Wicked questions dislodge self-fulfilling prophecies, open the ground for new experimental possibilities, and increase the information in a system, thereby facilitating far-from-equilibrium conditions and self-organization.

Acronyms Frequently Encountered in the Field of Patient Safety

ADE adverse drug event

AE adverse event

AHRQ Agency for Healthcare Research and Quality

AMA American Medical Association

ASHP American Society of Health-System Pharmacists

ASQ American Society for Quality

ASRS Aviation Safety Reporting System

CASS continuous aspiration of subglottic secretions

CDC Centers for Disease Control (and Prevention)

CMS Centers for Medicare and Medicaid Services

CPOE Computerized Provider (Physician, Practitioner) Order Entry

CTQ critical-to-quality indicators

CVVD continuous venovenous (hemo)dialysis

DMAIC define, measure, analyze, improve, control

DPMO defects per million opportunities

DRG diagnostic-related group

EHR evidence-based hospital referral

FACCT Foundation for Accountability

FDA (U.S.) Food and Drug Administration

FMEA Failure Mode and Effects Analysis

HMPS Harvard Medical Practice Study

HRO high-reliability organization

IHI Institute for Healthcare Improvement

IOM Institute of Medicine

IPS intensive (care unit) physician staffing

ISMP Institute for Safe Medication Practices

JAMA Journal of the American Medical Association

JCAHO Joint Commission on Accreditation of Healthcare Organizations

NASA National Aeronautics and Space Administration

NPO nothing by mouth

NPSF National Patient Safety Foundation

NPSP National Patient Safety Partnership

NQF National Quality Forum

PSRS Patient Safety Reporting System

QuIC Quality Interagency Coordination (Task Force)

RCA root cause analysis

RWJ Robert Wood Johnson (Foundation)

VA (U.S.) Veterans Administration

VSS Vulnerable System Syndrome

APPENDIXES

APPENDIX ONE. CHECKLIST FOR ASSESSING INSTITUTIONAL RESILIENCE

Indicators of resilience	Yes	?	No

- Patient safety is recognized as being everyone's responsibility, not just that of the risk management team.
- Top management accepts occasional setbacks and nasty surprises as inevitable. It anticipates that staff will make errors and trains them to detect and recover from them.
- Top managers, both clinical and nonclinical, are genuinely committed to the furtherance of patient safety and provide adequate resources to serve this end.
- Safety-related issues are considered at high-level meetings on a regular basis, not just after some bad event.
- Past events are thoroughly reviewed at high-level meetings, and the lessons learned are implemented as global reforms rather than local repairs.
- After some mishap, the primary aim of top management is to identify the failed system defenses and improve them rather than seeking to pin blame on specific individuals.

Indicators of resilience   Yes   ?   No

- Top management adopts a proactive stance toward patient safety. It does some or all of the following: takes steps to identify recurrent error traps and removes them; strives to eliminate the workplace and organization factors likely to provoke errors; brainstorms new scenarios of failure; conducts regular "health checks" on the organizational processes known to contribute to mishaps.

- Top management recognizes that error-provoking institutional factors (for example, undermanning, inadequate equipment, inexperience, patchy training, bad human-machine interfaces, and so on) are easier to manage and correct than are such fleeting psychological states as distraction, inattention, and forgetfulness.

- It is understood that effective management of patient safety, like any other management process, depends critically on the collection, analysis, and dissemination of relevant information.

- Management recognizes the necessity of combining reactive outcome data (that is, from the near miss and incident reporting system) with proactive process information. The latter entails far more than occasional audits. It involves regular sampling of a variety of institutional parameters (for example, scheduling, fostering, protocols, defenses, training).

- Meetings relating to patient safety are attended by staff from a wide variety of departments and levels within the institution.

- Assignment to a safety-related function (quality or risk management) is seen as a fast-track appointment, not a dead end. Such functions are accorded appropriate status and salary.

- It is appreciated that commercial goals, financial constraints, and patient safety issues can come into conflict and that mechanisms exist to identify and resolve such conflicts in an effective and transparent manner.

Indicators of resilience   Yes   ?   No

- Policies are in place that encourage everyone to raise patient safety issues.
- The institution recognizes the critical dependence of a safety management system on the trust of the workforce, particularly in regard to reporting systems. (A safe culture—that is, an informed culture—is the product of a reporting culture that, in turn, can only arise from a just culture.)
- There is a consistent policy for reporting and responding to incidents across all of the professional groups within the institution.
- Disciplinary procedures are predicated on an agreed distinction between acceptable and unacceptable behavior. It is recognized by all staff that a small proportion of unsafe acts are indeed reckless and warrant sanctions, but that the large majority of such acts should not lead to punishment. (The key determinant of blameworthiness is not so much the act itself—error or violation—as the nature of the behavior in which it was embedded. Did this behavior involve deliberate unwarranted risk taking or a course of action likely to produce avoidable errors? If so, then the act would be culpable regardless of whether it was an error or a violation.)
- Clinical supervisors train junior staff to practice the mental as well as the technical skills necessary to achieve safe performance. Mental skills include anticipating possible errors and rehearsing the appropriate recoveries.
- The institution has in place rapid, useful, and intelligible feedback channels to communicate the lessons learned from both the reactive and proactive safety information systems. Throughout the institution the emphasis is on generalizing these lessons to the system at large rather than merely localizing failures and weaknesses.
- The institution has the will and the resources to acknowledge its errors, to apologize for them, and to reassure patients (or their relatives) that the lessons learned from such mishaps will prevent their recurrence.

Yes = this is definitely the case in my institution (scores 1); ? = don't know, maybe, or could partially be true (scores 0.5); no = this is definitely not the case in my institution (scores 0).

Interpreting your score: 16–20 = so healthy as to be barely credible; 11–15 = moderate to high level of intrinsic resistance; 6–10 = considerable improvements needed to achieve institutional resilience; 1–5 = moderate to high institutional vulnerability; 0 = a complete rethink of organizational culture and processes is needed.

Source: J. Carthey, M. R. de Leval, and J. T. Reason, "Institutional Resilience in Healthcare Systems," *Quality and Safety in Health Care* (2001), *10*, 29–32. Copyright © BMJ Publishing Group. Used with permission.

APPENDIX TWO. CREATING DE-IDENTIFIED CASE STUDIES FOR DISSEMINATION

Case studies, to spread lessons learned and alert others to risks experienced, should be brief (no more than two pages) and communicate key findings from analysis of accidents, near misses, or hazardous conditions to help inform safety within an organization and beyond. Events external to the organization can also be imported and disseminated if the lessons learned have the potential for application.

Case studies of lessons learned and system changes should be routinely communicated internally after a significant or sentinel event and need to meet rigorous standards of confidentiality. The case studies containing lessons learned should be construed for dissemination beyond the organization as well. Therefore, all case studies must be de-identified.

De-identification includes elimination of such identifiers as the patient's diagnosis, ethnic group, age (weight may be necessary relative to drug issues), gender, home town or region, social status, location of transfers, case-related data (such as time and date, location, department), staff data (such as unit, position, staff experience, although general data—for example, less than one year's experience—may be relevant), and external data (such as product name or external organization name). The description of the event, however, should be sufficiently detailed so that readers will be able to understand both how the conditions and variables uncovered through analysis relate to the event and the extent to which the planned responses will decrease the likelihood of its recurrence.

A consistent format, such as the one that follows, should be used. Most of the case studies emphasize items 3 and 4 below.

Guidelines for Preparing Case Studies of Lessons Learned for Dissemination

1. Title: A clear and attention-grabbing statement of the nature of event or finding.
2. Core message: A one-sentence summary of what was learned.
3. Description of the event(s): What happened? Include proximal or immediate cause, including human error/failure, and emphasize the need to analyze for the second story of causation. Include a range of possible anticipated patient outcomes, based on information found in the literature, rather than the specific outcome of the actual case.
4. Case analysis: Identify underlying causal variables and conditions that contributed to the event, and describe how they combined through a sequence of events. Describe resolving actions to mitigate risk and reduce the probability of recurrence of a similar event, with supporting rationale from safety science.
5. Case studies of lessons learned require review by the Offices of Ethics and Risk Management and by a professional staff leader. Use of private, confidential, or proprietary information in a report requires the approval of the Offices of Ethics and Risk Management.

Source: Childrens Hospitals and Clinics, Minneapolis/St. Paul, Minnesota.

APPENDIX THREE. MEDICAL ACCIDENTS POLICY: REPORTING AND DISCLOSURE, INCLUDING SENTINEL EVENTS

Policy

A medical accident, sentinel event, or near miss with the potential to cause harm to a patient in health care is a call for action and an opportunity for organizational learning. *The Health Care Organization* attempts to identify and analyze all events related to patient safety, partnering with parents and patients to improve patient safety. A full analysis of each significant accident/event is conducted to understand the multicausal components producing the conditions for the event to occur. The analysis following significant or sentinel events is conducted by a focused event team commissioned by the vice president of medical affairs and the Office of Patient Safety, an official peer review organization of *The Health Care Organization,* and therefore all proceedings and review activity are protected by the state peer review statute. Event analysis is an organizational priority, and participation is mandatory.

A prerequisite for identifying, minimizing, and preventing health care accidents and sentinel events for patients and employees is creating a culture that values safety, including blameless reporting, consistent use of quality and structured fact-finding tools, creating new knowledge from accident learnings, and communicating broadly within *The Health Care Organization* all lessons learned and improvements achieved. Communications about lessons learned and improvements achieved will not contain the identity of patients or caregivers.

After initial action to ensure the patient's safety, accidents should be discussed with or reported to the patient's direct caregiver, the departmental manager or director, and the Office of Patient Safety. All written and oral reports, including patient safety logs submitted to the Office of Patient Safety, are part of the peer review system established to improve quality of care. *The Health Care Organization* works with its professional and medical staff to achieve complete, prompt, and truthful disclosure of information and counseling to patients and their parents or legal guardians regarding situations in which a medical accident occurred (1) when there is clear or potential clinical significance or (2) when some unintended act or substance reaches the patient. The disclosure to the patient or parent/legal guardian occurs promptly when information is obtained and will be carried out by an individual involved in the patient's care, generally the managing physician, with support from other staff and employees, as appropriate. In the disclosure process a presumption of truth telling guides all discussion. The goal of the disclosure process is to provide accurate factual information about the event. The vice president of medical affairs is responsible for ensuring that the communication process occurs.

The organization develops and makes available to practitioners written tools and guidelines for following the provision of this policy. The organization also provides assistance in all aspects of response to patient safety events through the Office of Patient Safety and the vice president of medical affairs.

Purpose

- Improve patient and staff safety by decreasing system vulnerability to future events
- Evaluate and improve care provided
- Reduce the chances for patient morbidity and mortality
- Restore patient, family, employee, provider, and community confidence that systems are in place to ensure that future accidents are not likely to recur
- Emotionally, educationally, and legally support staff who have been involved in events
- Ensure disclosure of the sentinel event, accident, or substantive near miss to the family, and ensure ongoing communication of system improvements to family and caregivers involved in the accident

Definition(s)

Definitions are provided to clarify language and obligations and should in no way limit the intent of the organization to respond to all events affecting patient safety.

Patient Safety Event. Any near miss medical accident, medical accident, **sentinel** event, significant procedural variance, or other threat to patient safety

Near Miss Medical Accident (Good Catch/Accident Waiting to Happen). Any unintended event in the system of care that would have constituted a medical accident but that was intercepted before it actually reached the patient

Medical Accident. An unintended event in the system of care, with actual negative consequences for the patient

Sentinel Event. A sentinel event is a category of medical accident defined by the Joint Commission on Accreditation of Healthcare Organizations to include the following:

1. The event has resulted in an unanticipated death or major permanent loss of function not related to the natural course of a patient's illness or underlying condition, or the risk thereof, or,
2. The event is one of the following (even if the outcome was not death or major permanent loss of function):
   - Suicide of a patient in a setting where the patient receives around-the-clock care
   - Infant abduction or discharge to the wrong family
   - Rape
   - Hemolytic transfusion reaction involving administration of blood products having major blood group incompatibilities
   - Surgery on the wrong patient or wrong body part

Office of Patient Safety. The Office of Patient Safety is a peer review organization whose membership is limited to professional and administrative staff. It is established by *The Health Care Organization* under state statutes for protection of peer review and improvement data to gather and review information related to the care and treatment of patients for the purposes of evaluating and improving the quality of health care rendered in the organization, reducing morbidity and mortality, and obtaining and disseminating statistics and information relative to the treatment and prevention of diseases, illness, and injuries. The staff members of the Office of Patient Safety include the director of patient safety, the vice president of medical affairs, the director of risk management, and the vice president of patient care and other professional or administrative staff as *The Health Care Organization* may deem appropriate. The Office of Patient Safety reports to the board of directors of *The Health Care Organization* through the professional executive council and the quality oversight committee of the board.

Director of Patient Safety. The director of patient safety is the administrator of *The Health Care Organization* who is charged with responsibility for the operation of the Office of Patient Safety.

Focused Event Team. A focused event team will gather and review information about patient safety events for the purpose of evaluating and improving the quality of health care rendered in the institution and reducing morbidity and mortality. The focused event team is a peer review organization, established by *The Health Care Organization* under state statute, whose members will include the members of the Office of Patient Safety and other administrators and/or professional staff as designated by the vice president of medical affairs.

Managing Practitioner. The managing practitioner is the physician or other practitioner most directly responsible for the overall care of the patient while at *The Health Care Organization.* The managing practitioner, or the person delegated to assume this responsibility in the absence of the managing practitioner, has the primary caregiver relationship with the patient and family.

Disclosure. Disclosure is the providing of information to a patient, and/or parents or legal guardian of a patient, regarding a patient safety event, which may include a sentinel event. Information about near miss medical accidents is provided according to the guidelines of this policy.

Reporting. Reporting is the providing of information to the Office of Patient Safety regarding a near miss medical accident or a patient safety event, including a sentinel event. Methods of communicating events include reports by e-mail, voicemail, and other oral or written safety reports. Reports to the Office of Patient Safety are confidential under state statute as data and information acquired by a peer review organization.

Procedure

Part I: Immediate Response to Patient Safety Event

Action to Ensure Patient Safety. The employee(s), professional staff, and manager(s) involved in a patient safety event take immediate action to ensure safety of the patient, staff, and others in the environment. The Office of Patient Safety will determine whether any immediate procedural or other change in delivery of care is necessary and will determine whether and how to communicate a safety alert if one is required.

Preservation of Evidence. All equipment and supplies, including but not limited to unused medications, sheets, towels, syringes, samples from the lab, unused blood products, and equipment, should be retained after a medical accident. These items can be used in the investigation to ensure a safe environment. Medical device malfunctions should be tagged per the Medical Device and Product Reporting, Alerts, and Recall Policy, #900.00.

Part II: Reporting of Patient Safety Events

Employees, professional staff members, managers, and volunteers report patient safety events to the Office of Patient Safety. The intent of the reporting system is for all patient safety events to be reported, including near miss medical accidents, good catches, and accidents waiting to happen. The Safety Report form should be completed and submitted to the Office of Patient Safety by any staff member who observes, discovers, or is directly involved in a reportable event or any other safety concern. This should be done as soon as possible after the event and can be done on a written Safety Report form, via the call-in line, or via the Internet. Reports may be anonymous. The Safety Report is considered a working document of the facility's peer review committees and is protected as a confidential document under state statute. These reports should not be copied and should be handled in a confidential manner. The staff or manager must call Risk Management immediately for possible sentinel events or whenever a patient has been harmed. The Concern for Safe Staffing form should be utilized for reporting staffing concerns.

Documentation in the Medical Record. The medical record should contain a complete, accurate record of clinical information pertaining to the event. As applicable, this should include:

- Objective details of the event written in neutral, nonjudgmental language—just the facts
- The patient's condition immediately before the time of the event
- Intervention and patient's response
- Quoted relevant statements by patient/family
- Notification to physician(s)
- Notification/discussion with family

Do not refer to the Safety Report in the medical record. Do not assign blame, make accusations, complain about personalities, staffing, facility systems, etc.

Protection of Staff Who Report. Staff members who appropriately report a patient safety event to the Office of Patient Safety will not be subject to retaliation for reporting. This does not remove *The Health Care Organization's* obligations to take appropriate educational or performance actions to protect patients, nor does it require *The Health Care Organization* to protect staff members who engage in acts of malfeasance that compromise patient safety.

Record of Event. The Office of Patient Safety, as a peer review organization, will maintain a confidential log of all reported patient safety events.

Part III: Disclosure to Patients/Parents

1. Disclosure to patient and/or parent should be made of any medical accident, including a sentinel event. Disclosure of a near miss medical accident is not made unless the circumstances require an explanation of events.
2. To ensure continuity and appropriate perspective in discussion, the managing practitioner should in most instances handle the disclosure of information and subsequent discussions with the patient or guardian with responsibility for a child's overall care. In some instances, another individual may be designated as the primary person to communicate with the family.
3. At the time of initial disclosure, or at subsequent planned discussions, at least one other hospital staff person should also be present.
4. For discussions anticipated to be complex or difficult, parents should be given the option of having another person with them for support.
5. The vice president of medical affairs is responsible for ensuring that the process of disclosure occurs in a timely and appropriate manner.

Subjects to Be Communicated. The individual managing communication should communicate the facts as we understand them at the time of the conversation. Specific staff members involved in the accident, if unknown to the family, should not have their identities disclosed. During initial and follow-up discussion, the following subjects may be discussed, although discussion of each subject on this list is not required, nor is discussion limited to these topics:

Acknowledgment that an event has occurred

The nature of the accident as we understand it at the time of the conversation

The time, place, and circumstances of the accident as we understand it at the time of the conversation

The known, definite consequences of the accident for the patient, and potential or anticipated consequences

Actions taken to treat or ameliorate the consequences of the accident

Who will manage ongoing care of the patient

Who else has been informed of the accident (in the hospital, in regulatory agencies, etc.)

The actions that have been or will be taken to identify system issues that may have contributed to the accident and to prevent the same or similar accidents from recurring

Who will manage ongoing communication with the family

The names and phone numbers of individuals in the hospital to whom the parents may address complaints or concerns about the process surrounding the accident

The names and phone numbers of agencies with which the family can communicate about the accident

How to obtain support and counseling regarding the accident and its consequences, both within *The Health Care Organization* and from outside *The Health Care Organization*

An apology for the accident

An offer of whatever support is possible at this time, and answers to additional questions

Accidents Involving The Health Care Organization's *Nonemployed Professional Staff*. *The Health Care Organization* collaborates with nonemployed professional staff members to disclose information about a medical accident to parents. If the professional staff member chooses not to be involved in the disclosure, the Office of Patient Safety or its designee will disclose and provide ongoing communication with parents and communicate with the nonemployed professional staff member regarding the process. Issues involving nonemployed professional staff members are addressed through the processes of the professional staff.

Exceptions to Disclosure to Parents. In extremely rare situations, where it can clearly be demonstrated that the interests of the patient or parents are harmed by disclosure, disclosure of a medical accident or sentinel event may be withheld until the benefits of disclosure are greater than the harms. Any exception to disclosure must be specifically justified and documented in the Office of Patient Safety records.

Part IV: Response to Sentinel Events

Determination of Sentinel Event Status. The Office of Patient Safety, and the vice president of medical affairs in his or her role as a member of the Office of Patient Safety, shall carry out the initial assessment of any reported patient safety event to determine if it is a sentinel event.

Notification of **The Health Care Organization's** *Officials Regarding Sentinel Events.* Risk Management immediately notifies the chief of staff, the chief of the professional staff division, the vice president of medical affairs, the vice president of patient care, the CEO, and the COO of a sentinel event.

1. The pharmacy and therapeutics chair and the director of pharmacy are immediately notified of events involving medication use.
2. The administrator of the Institutional Review Board (IRB) is notified if an investigational study is involved but is informed only of the study name, the IRB study number (if known), and/or the investigator's name that can be found on the consent form in the patient's chart. Per standard IRB policies and procedures and federal regulations, it is the responsibility of the research investigator to promptly notify the IRB in writing, providing a complete description of the event and other information as requested by the IRB. It is recommended that the professional staff investigator participate in review by the focused event team.

Responsibilities of the Focused Event Team. The focused event team assigned to analyze accidents/events will consider all variables that may impact the safety of patients and staff. The team has responsibility to:

1. Determine and initiate immediate steps to ensure patient and staff safety (or document those steps already taken)
2. Conduct a fact finding of the accident, using accepted structured tools, which may include root cause analysis
3. Identify a spokesperson
4. Determine the ongoing communication protocol for patient and family
5. Identify any necessary communications to staff and other families
6. Produce the multifactorial causal analysis report, including any findings or conclusions and a summary of the event and recommended changes
7. Clarify accountability for quality improvement and ongoing process auditing to ensure that corrective actions are established, effective, and sustained

Timeline for Event Analysis. The determination of a sentinel event must be initiated within the first forty-eight hours after notification of the accident/event has taken place and the initial fact finding has commenced. The causal analysis needs to be completed as soon as possible, to preserve an accurate account of events, discover the multiple factors contributing to the accident, and decrease system vulnerabilities for other patients. Generally, the initial summary report to the professional executive council, the patient safety steering committee, the board of directors, and the quality oversight committee should be completed within thirty days, but not later than forty-five days after notification of the event.

Role of Communications Specialists. The Office of Patient Safety notifies the communications specialists of events to facilitate external communications, including contact with the media and requests for public information. The communications staff also provides consultation regarding communication with the family and staff about the event and assists in internal communication of appropriate information in keeping with patient and peer review confidentiality requirements.

Board of Directors. The Office of Patient Safety notifies the chief executive officer, who communicates to the board of directors all sentinel events. This communication is privileged under the board of directors' responsibility for overall quality of care at *The Health Care Organization.*

Confidential Retention of Focused Event Analysis. The Office of Patient Safety retains the only copy of accident/event analysis and related documentation.

JCAHO and Other Regulatory Reporting. The Office of Patient Safety, with the chief executive officer, determines whether the event is reportable to JCAHO and acts accordingly. The Office of Patient Safety also determines whether reports are required under the Child Abuse and Neglect statute as well as under any other applicable statutes or regulations. Reporting to regulatory bodies does not relieve responsibility for disclosure to patients and/or parents as outlined in this policy.

References

As an example, see [http://www.revisor.leg.state.mn.us:8181/SEARCH/BASIS/mnstat/public/www/SDF] State. Stat. § 145.64

Related Policy/Policies

900.00 Medical Device and Product Reporting, Alerts, and Recall

Key Words

Safety, patient safety, sentinel event, medical accident, near miss, good catch, Office of Patient Safety, JCAHO, focused event analysis, disclosure, peer review, confidentiality, maltreatment of minors, root cause analysis, patient safety report, accident, documentation

Review/Revision Dates

Source: Childrens Hospitals and Clinics, Minneapolis/St. Paul, Minnesota.

APPENDIX FOUR. MEDICATION SAFETY TEAM FEEDBACK FORM

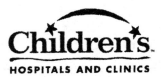

Dear Healthcare Provider:_____

In an effort to improve the safety of our patients at Children's
Hospitals and Clinics the Medication Safety Team is providing this
direct feedback to you, the individual prescribers/transcribers of
medication orders. Historical evidence supports that certain unsafe
order writing practices or habits have led to very serious consequences, while the inclusion of certain
information can help prevent errors.

The attached order that you wrote or transcribed contains one or more of the following
problem(s) (checked boxes). A corresponding recommendation for improvement is provided. Please
accept these recommendations in the spirit in which they are given, with the safety of our kids at heart.
If you have any questions please contact us.

Thank you,
Bruce Bostrom, M.D., CoChair
Mark Thomas, M.S., R.Ph, CoChair
Medication Safety Team, Children's Hospitals and Clinics

Potentially Unsafe Practice	Practice Prone to Error	Preferred Practice
❑ "Units" was not written out	REGULAR INSULIN 5 u This can be misinterpreted as cc, 4, 6, or 0.	REGULAR INSULIN 5 UNITS
❑ A trailing zero was used	Ativan 1.0 mg	Ativan 1 mg
❑ A leading zero was not used	DIGOXIN .125 MG This can result in an overdose of medication.	DIGOXIN 0.125 MG
❑ The medication was ordered by quantity rather than strength	TYLENOL 2 TABS FeY-In-Sol 1 cc	TYLENOL 650 MG FeY-In-Sol 125 mg Use mcg, mg, or g whenever possible.
❑ An unacceptable abbreviation was used for the amount of the medication	Using abbreviations such as µg, gm, cc, tsp., or tbsp.	Use mcg, mg, g, or mL whenever possible.

❑ The mg/kg dose and the calculated dose were not both included:
  ❑ Only the calculated dose was given
  ❑ Only the mg/kg dose was given
	Gentamicin 30mg q12h
	
	Tylenol 10-15 mg/kg/dose prn
		Gentamicin 2.5 mg/kg/dose
		  Dose=30 mg q12h
		
		Tylenol 10-15 mg/kg/dose
		  Dose = 120-180 mg q4-6 h prn
		fever and discomfort

❑ An abbreviation or symbol was used instead of the drug name	mgSO₄	magnesium Sulfate

❑ The following medical abbreviation was used:
  ❑ QD
  ❑ QID
  ❑ QOD
	QD QID
	QOD qid
	qod qid
	These are often misinterpreted for each other.
		Q day, daily, four times daily, every other day (BID, TID, q16h, q24h acceptable)

❑ The order was difficult to read/illegible		Print orders or use pre-printed orders
❑ The signature was illegible		Also print your name if your signature is illegible; include your pager number.

APPENDIX FIVE. PATIENT SAFETY WORKPLAN

A. CULTURE

A2. Increase Awareness of High Reliability Organization (HRO) Attributes and System Strategies to Reduce Potential for Harm.

Objectives	Who	Timeline
A. Develop awareness campaign concerning common characteristics of HRO. TACTIC: • Conduct management briefings using case studies • Launch conference		
B. Using existing communication vehicles, begin to tell the story of accident and healthcare. TACTIC: • Develop communication plan		
C. Develop public message that concerns accident in complex systems. • Develop communication plan		
D. Partner with health care and other HRO industries to broadly communicate the safety agenda within quality.		

B. INFRASTRUCTURE

B1. Increase Capability During Design of Clinical Care Systems to Incorporate Effective Safety Elements to Reduce Error Proneness.

Objectives	Who	Timeline

A. Include human factors analysis in specification stage of new and redesigned clinical care systems.
TACTIC:
- Develop core group of internal quality consultants to assist in designs

B. Implement effective proven strategies in work process design.
TACTICS:
- Analyze the "Crew Resource Management" techniques being studied in Health Care Emergency Department and Operating Suites
- Scan the external environment for work-process design innovation for implementation
- Champion proven accident (error) reduction work processes for implementation

B2. Install Blameless Reporting System to Support Safety.

Objectives	Who	Timeline

A. Develop confidential, anonymous, open structure accident (error) and failure reporting system that is user-friendly and exceeds current reporting rate.
TACTICS:
- Review research for design
- Pilot multifaceted tools and methods
- Roll out tools/methods organization-wide

B. Enhance investigation and inquiry methodology into accident (error) and failures.
TACTICS:
- Research and enhance post occurrence investigation tools & standards
- Secure resources and experts to conduct inquiry database for indexing and case study
- Train investigation/analysis teams

C. Incorporate accident (error) findings into quality improvement efforts and measure effectiveness of solutions.
TACTIC:
- Expert findings are addressed unit- and organization-wide

D. Develop and implement effective communication vehicles for alerts and advisories organization-wide.
TACTIC:
- Design and implement effective dissemination methods for sharing learning and solutions.

E. Compile a quality database of a repository of causal factors and solutions.

B3. Increase Learning of the Interface of Human Factors, Work Processes and Technology in Environment Through Medication Initiative.

Objectives	Who	Timeline
A. Conduct primary and secondary research on new methods and solutions		
B. Clearinghouse of research for the "new look" at accident (error) reduction in health care.		
C. Implementation Medication Initiative		

C. IMPLEMENT MEDICATION INITIATIVE

C1. Use learning collaboratives to implement IHI and other researched and effective error-reduction strategies.

Objectives	Who	Timeline
TACTICS: • Implement known best practices • Implement 4 rapid-cycle improvements to achieve zero-defect in each initiative • Replicate relevant improvements • Design and implement effective methods for measuring surveillance/case findings and analyzing ADEs for improvements		

C2. Implement high-reliability medication workplace.

APPENDIX SIX. SAFETY LEARNING REPORT

CHILDREN'S HOSPITALS AND CLINICS
OFFICE OF PATIENT SAFETY

SAFETY LEARNING REPORT

The information you report is generated
and maintained for quality improvement
purposes under Minnesota Statute 145.61
et seq and is confidential under that statue.

USE THIS FORM TO REPORT

Accident/Near miss/System breakdown/
Good catch/How safety was created/
Hazardous situation/Accident wait/Happen/
Normalization of deviance

Addressograph or name/medical record #/DOB/account number

1. SITE (check one):

	Minneapolis		St. Paul
	Ridges		West
	Roseville		Other

2. TODAY'S DATE:

3. MEDICATIONS INVOLVED:
(include med name, admin route)

4. EQUIPMENT INVOLVED:

5. EVENT DATE:

6. EVENT TIME:

7. HAPPENED TO:

	Inpatient
	Outpatient
	Staff
	Student
	Visitor
	Volunteer
	Other

9. LOCATION:

Event
Location

Patient
Dept.

Other dept.
involved

2 EVENT CHARACTERISTICS:

	Was apparent to the patient's family
	Caused harm or injury
	Altered the treatment plan
	Has happened repeatedly
	Caught at the last step
	Failure of a safety defense

10. WHAT HAPPENED?

CHILDREN'S HOSPITALS AND CLINICS
OFFICE OF PATIENT SAFETY

SAFETY LEARNING
REPORT

IF NOT INCLUDED ON THE PREVIOUS PAGE, PLEASE PROVIDE ADDITIONAL INFORMATION BY
ANSWERING THE FOLLOWING QUESTIONS. ALTHOUGH OPTIONAL, EACH ANSWER CONTRIBUTES
TO CREATING SAFETY AT CHILDREN'S.

How did it happen? What was the chain of events? How did the problem arise? How was it discovered? How was it
corrected? At worst, what could have happened and how was harm prevented or reduced?

What were the contributing factors? What was the work environment like at the time of this situation? What were
the personal or team factors affecting human performance in this situation (such as inattention, perceptions, judgments,
decisions, communication, coordination)? Was there a breakdown in a safety defense? Please include what you believe
really caused the problem.

Has this happened before? How frequently do you think there is the potential for this situation to occur? What
increases the risk? What decreases the risk?

What could prevent future occurrence of this situation? What did you learn from this situation? Is there
anything that you will do differently in the future? Who could help improve this situation? What could you see or
measure that would show that Children's has reduced the risk of this situation occurring in the future?

How can Children's improve the process of patient safety learning?

(Attach additional pages if necessary)

7. WORST POTENTIAL OUTCOME OF THIS OR SIMILAR EVENTS:	14. WHO COULD HELP IMPROVE THIS SITUATION?
Rework, inefficiency, delays	
Minor harm	
Major or permanent harm	15. MAY WE CONTACT YOU FOR ADDITIONAL INFORMATION? (OPTIONAL)

APPENDIX SEVEN. STOP-THE-LINE POLICY: AUTHORITY TO INTERVENE TO RESTORE PATIENT SAFETY

Policy

All the organization's employees, the organization's professional staff, contracted staff, house staff, students, volunteers, patients, parents, legal guardians, and visitors have the responsibility and authority to immediately intervene to protect the safety of a patient, to prevent a medical accident, or to avert a sentinel event. It is the expectation that all participants will immediately stop and respond to the request by reassessing the patient's safety.

Procedure

Domain of policy:

- All patients in all inpatient and outpatient units on all campuses

> **NOTE:** When emergency intervention is warranted, assistance by any means most expedient shall be sought, to include but not be limited to signaling a Dr. Blue, dialing 911 to contact the Emergency Medical System (in certain nonhospital locations only), requesting immediate consultation, transfer to a special care unit, and surgical intervention. Such necessary emergency interventions may be initiated without prior express physician order, but appropriate orders are to be documented when the patient's imminent risk is contained.

1. Identification of a Situation Warranting Immediate Intervention

The following situations warrant immediate intervention:

Imminent Sentinel Event. Sentinel events include:

- Events that result in death or major permanent loss of function, not related to the patient's natural course of illness or underlying condition
- Suicide of a patient
- Infant abduction or discharge to the wrong family
- Rape of a patient
- Hemolytic transfusion reaction involving administration of blood or blood products having major blood group incompatibilities
- Surgery on the wrong patient or wrong body part

Imminent Medical Accident. Any medical accident or potential medical accident that might result in permanent harm to a patient, regardless of whether the accident is a sentinel event.

Failure to Achieve Appropriate Emergency Medical Response. Any situation in which available medical personnel does not respond with appropriate expertise to restore patient safety in a timely manner.

Imminent Violation of Legally Established Patient Rights That Pose an Immediate Threat to Patient Safety. To include but not be limited to:

- Failure to obtain informed consent for a major surgical procedure
- Failure to perform a screening examination and provide appropriate referral and transportation to a facility prepared to manage the medical condition revealed by the screening

Caregiver under the Influence. Caregiver exhibiting behavior consistent with being under the influence of substances that impair judgment or manual skills involved in patient care.

Imminent Patient Safety Risks (Not Otherwise Specified). Patient deemed to be otherwise at imminent risk of potentially permanent physical, mental or emotional sequelae.

- Inconsistency of information about the procedure to be performed and/or the site of the procedure to be performed when the History and Physical, the Operating Room Schedule, and the Informed Consent forms are compared.
- Research misconduct with significant risk of imminent patient harm.

Willful Intent to Do Harm. Knowledge that an individual has willful intent to do harm to a patient.

2. Priorities of Intervention

All the organization's employees, the organization's professional staff, contracted staff, house staff, students, volunteers, patients, parents, legal guardians, and visitors have the responsibility and authority to immediately intervene to protect the safety of a patient, to prevent a medical accident, or to avert a sentinel event.

The method of intervention chosen should maximize timeliness and effectiveness in restoring patient safety while minimizing intrusion into the processes of care.

Direct Communication. Direct communication of the identified problem to the available members of the care team, including but not limited to the resident, attending physician, and/or nurse.

Charge Nurse. If the response to direct communication with the resident, attending physician, and/or nurse is inadequate to restore patient safety, the unit charge nurse shall be immediately contacted and shall respond.

Unit Manager/Nursing Supervisor. If the response of the charge nurse is inadequate to restore patient safety, the unit manager (or, in the unit manager's absence, the nursing supervisor) shall be immediately contacted and shall respond.

If the response of the unit manager/nursing supervisor is inadequate to restore patient safety, the following leaders shall be immediately contacted (the administrator on call may be contacted to facilitate this process):

- *In the case of a member of the professional staff,* the division chief (or, in the absence of the division chief, the division vice chief) shall be contacted and shall respond. If no other reasonable means is available, the division chief (or vice chief) shall immediately suspend the privileges of the member of the professional staff. Upon suspension, the division chief shall immediately ensure that proper, safe medical care is provided to the patient until another member of the professional staff in good standing can assume care of the patient. Unless retracted by the division chief, the decision to suspend privileges remains in effect until a meeting of the Credentials Committee or Professional Executive Committee makes final recommendations to the board in regard to the privileges of the individual member of the professional staff. If neither the division chief nor the vice chief is available, or if the division leader has a conflict of interest, the chief of staff (or, in the absence of the chief of staff, the vice chief of staff) shall be contacted and shall respond. In the absence of the chief (or vice chief) of staff, the Credentials Committee chair (or, in the absence of the chair, the Credentials Committee vice chair) shall be contacted and shall respond. In the absence of the Credentials Committee leaders, the vice president of medical affairs shall be contacted and shall respond. In the absence of the vice president of medical affairs, the chief executive officer shall be contacted and respond.

- *In the case of the organization's employee or person under contract to perform patient care services,* the relevant line director shall be contacted and shall respond. If the response of the relevant line director is inadequate to restore patient safety, the relevant line vice president shall be contacted and shall respond. If the relevant vice president is absent, the administrator on call shall be contacted and shall respond. If the response of the relevant line vice president or administrator on call is inadequate to restore patient safety, the chief executive officer shall be contacted and shall respond.

- *In the case of medical equipment,* use of the equipment in question for patient care shall be immediately discontinued as long as removal does not increase the patient safety risk. The equipment shall be tagged, and all evidence pertinent to the equipment malfunction preserved, until released for repair or discarded by the director of risk management.

- *In the case of hazards in the environment of care,* the safety officer shall be immediately notified and shall respond. In the absence of the safety officer, security shall be contacted and shall respond. If the response of the safety officer or of security is inadequate to restore patient safety, the administrator on call shall be contacted and shall respond.

Key Words

Sentinel event

Medical accident

Impaired provider

Patient safety

Relevant Policies

Patient Rights and Responsibilities

Informed Consent

Urgent Evaluation of Unstable Patient

Suicide, Care of Patients—Attempted or Threatened

Police Holds: Child Abuse/Neglect

Emergency Hold Orders: Mental Health/Chemical Dependency

Medical Accidents and Disclosure, including Sentinel Events

Medical Device Reporting

Infant Abduction

Multiple Policies in the Environment of Care

APPENDIX EIGHT. COMPLEXITY LENS REFLECTION

Recall an incident or story that surprised you. As you recall your surprising story, consider the following questions. Please circle "yes or no" (Y or N) even though some the answers may fall in a gray area. Notice your pattern of responses. Talk with your partners. Share wisdom or a pithy quote that comes out of your conversation with the whole group about how this pattern related to your work.

Reluctance to Oversimplify-Skeptical Inquiry

Y   N   1. Did participants seek out multiple and complex interpretations of the challenging events as they unfolded?

Y   N   2. Did participants propose diverse approaches for actions and responses in the moment?

Y   N   3. Were participants reluctant to oversimplify interpretations of the challenge?

Y   N   4. Were people recognized for detailed questioning and skeptical inquiry?

Y   N   5. Did people regularly check their assumptions against reality?

Y   N   6. Did participants ask tough questions and give honest answers during the challenge?

Sensitivity to Surprise in Daily Operations

Y   N   7. Did everyone become preoccupied with unexpected events as they unfolded?

Y   N   8. Did some supervisors, managers, or execs "pitch in" on the front lines?

Y   N   9. Did participants find a way to get on-the-job training for the kind of work that presented itself?

Y   N   10. Did resources to handle problems become available as quickly as surprises unfolded?

Y   N   11. Was it easy to obtain expert assistance when something you didn't know how to handle popped up?

Attraction to Expertise—Not Rank

Y   N   12. Did people go to others with expertise to solve problems rather than relying on rank?

Y   N   13. Did participants display surprising familiarity with tasks or operations beyond their own jobs?

Y   N   14. Did participants seem to value expertise and experience over rank during the challenge?

Y   N   15. Did people own a problem until it was solved?

Y   N   16. Did unexpected expertise present itself from outside established channels when it was most needed?

Informed, Distributed Improvisation

Y   N   17. Did improvisational conversation and actions take the place of deliberate decision making in the conventional channels?

Y   N   18. Did you have the ability to create what was needed in the moment out of the materials at hand rather than planning and budgeting for what was needed?

Y   N   19. Was your starting vision or plan for responding fuzzy and just "good enough" to get going?

Y   N   20. Looking back, did happy accidents, small changes, and individual contributions have a big influence on your success?

Y   N   21. Did order arise from local interactions without central control?

Continuous Flow of Communication

Y   N   22. Were people talking to and repeatedly updating people around
           them on the current situation?

Y   N   23. Did you regularly update procedures in the moment on the basis
           of new information or near misses?

Y   N   24. Did people get recognized for spotting problems, errors, and fail-
           ures, more than in normal times?

Y   N   25. Did very local knowledge of history or conditions help to create
           useful responses?

Y   N   26. Did information about the changing situation spread like wild-
           fire across old boundaries (e.g., functional silos or cliques)?

Interdependent, Resilient Culture

Y   N   27. Were people able to rely on one another more than usual?

Y   N   28. Did people listen carefully without anyone's view being dis-
           missed?

Y   N   29. Did you appreciate skeptics and skeptical inquiry more than
           usual?

Y   N   30. Did you show more mutual respect for one another during the
           challenge?

Y   N   31. Were honest efforts to help recognized or rewarded, even when
           they did not turn out perfectly?

Y   N   32. Did you rely more on informal relationships, diverse participa-
           tion, and natural creativity than on formal authority or estab-
           lished groups and channels?

Y   N   33. Did you find that no one person is smart enough, but everyone
           together is?

Y   N   34. Looking back, would you call this experience an example of
           "collective mindfulness?"

Adapted from Karl E. Weick and Kathleen Sutcliffe, *Managing the Unexpected: Ensuring High Performance in an Age of Complexity* (San Francisco: Jossey Bass, 2001), 85–115.

APPENDIX NINE. A BRIEF LOOK AT GAPS IN THE CONTINUITY OF CARE

CL
www.ctlab.org

A brief look at Gaps in the Continuity of Care

For additional materials
visit **www.ctlab.org**

---

① Big Gap Example: *Transfer between facilities*

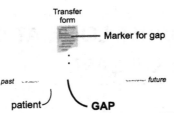

Transfer
form

—— Marker for gap

past ⸱⸱⸱⸱⸱⸱⸱   ⸱⸱⸱⸱⸱⸱ *future*

patient ⌣   ⌣ **GAP**

- Gaps in the continuity of care are common.
- Defenses against loss of continuity of care include <u>cognitive artifacts</u>. These artifacts are intended to bridge the gap; they also serve as markers that researchers can use to discover gaps.

Big gaps are easy to identify
They get lots of attention

---

② Smaller Gap Example: *Handoff of care*

past ⸱⸱⸱⸱⸱⸱⸱   ⸱⸱⸱⸱⸱⸱ *future*

GAP

- Handoffs of care are a potent source of gaps.
- Example: *handoff at shift change or change in location.*
- Defenses include artifacts (e.g. checkout logs) and activities, (e.g. conversational routines) that lead to exchanges of responsibility and authority.

Small gaps are less easy to identify.
The size of the gap doesn't determine the potential of the gap to cause harm.

---

③ Restoring continuity: *Recognizing & reacting to a past gap*

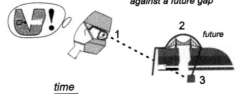

time

3

1

4

2

- 1: The effects of past gaps are recognized by cues, e.g missing data.
- 2: Cues alert practitioners to search for other effects of prior gaps.
- 3 & 4: Practitioners can partly restore continuity, e.g. by searching for and finding missing data. *N.B. missing data that acts as a cue is not necessarily the data that needs to be recovered to restore continuity.*

This activity is a primary source of the resilience of healthcare

---

④ Sustaining continuity: *Foreseeing & defending against a future gap*

1

2   *future*

3

time

- 1: Experienced practitioners can foresee future gaps.
- 2: Anticipating future gaps leads practitioners to construct bridges. These offset some *but not all* of the expected consequences of gaps.
- 3: Successful bridging limits the impacts of gaps. This has the paradoxical effect of making gaps seem less significant.

This activity is a primary source of the robustness of healthcare.

Preparation of this version made possible partly through support by the Midwest VA Patient Safety Center of Inquiry (GAPS).

APPENDIX TEN. A BRIEF LOOK AT THE NEW LOOK IN COMPLEX SYSTEM FAILURE, ERROR, AND SAFETY

CL   *A brief look at the New Look in complex system failure, error, safety, and resilience*

For additional materials visit www.ctlab.org

① **Accident Aftermath**

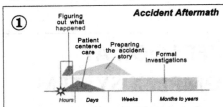

Accident / incident investigation normally stops with human error by practitioners as the 'cause' of the event.

② **BLUNT END** **SHARP END**

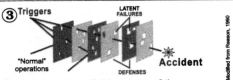

Modified from Woods, 1991

Practitioners work at the *sharp end* of the system. The *blunt end* of the system generates resources, constraints and conflicts that shape the world of technical work and produce latent failures.

③

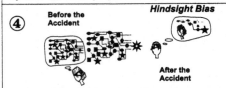

Modified from Reason, 1990

Complex systems fail because of the combination of multiple small failures, each individually insufficient to cause an accident. These failures are *latent* in the system and their pattern changes over time.

④ **Hindsight Bias**

Before the Accident

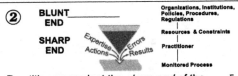

After the Accident

Post-accident reviews identify *human error* as the 'cause' of failure because of *hindsight bias*. Outcome knowledge makes the path to failure seem to have been foreseeable - although it was not foreseen.

⑤ **Cycle of Error**

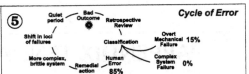

Overt Mechanical Failure 15%
Complex System 0%
Human Error 85%

Organizational *reactions to failure* focus on human error. The reactions to failure are: blame & train, sanctions, new regulations, rules, and technology. These interventions increase complexity and introduce new forms of failure.

⑥

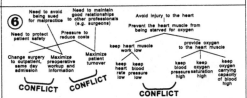

CONFLICT   CONFLICT   CONFLICT

Competing demands, dilemmas, conflicts, and uncertainty are the central features of operations at the sharp end. Technical and organizational conflicts overlap and interact.

⑦

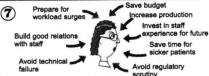

Prepare for workload surges
Save budget
Increase production
Invest in staff experience for future
Build good relations with staff
Save time for sicker patients
Avoid technical failure
Avoid regulatory scrutiny

Work at the sharp end inevitably encounters competing demands for production and failure-free performance. Action resolves all dilemmas. Successful operations are the rule. Failure is rare.

⑧ **The Search for Sources of Resilience**

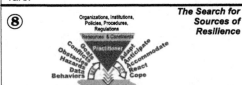

People make safety. Workers at the sharp end usually bridge gaps and prevent failures. The resilience of the system is the result of this activity, which forms much of *technical work*. Productive approaches support this activity.

APPENDIX ELEVEN. A REMINDER ON EVERY CHART

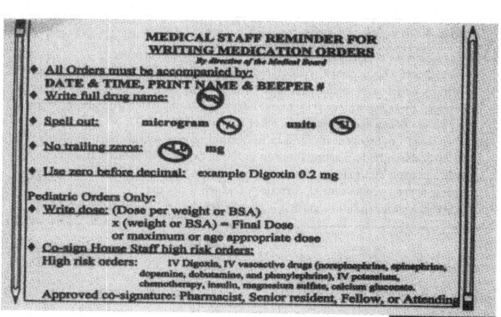

MEDICAL STAFF REMINDER FOR WRITING MEDICATION ORDERS

By directive of the Medical Board

- All Orders must be accompanied by:
  DATE & TIME, PRINT NAME & BEEPER #
- Write full drug name:
- Spell out: microgram   units
- No trailing zeros: mg
- Use zero before decimal: example Digoxin 0.2 mg

Pediatric Orders Only:
- Write dose: (Dose per weight or BSA)
  - x (weight or BSA) = Final Dose
  - or maximum or age appropriate dose
- Co-sign House Staff high risk orders:
  - High risk orders: IV Digoxin, IV vasoactive drugs (norepinephrine, epinephrine, dopamine, dobutamine, and phenylephrine), IV potassium, chemotherapy, insulin, magnesium sulfate, calcium gluconate.
- Approved co-signature: Pharmacist, Senior resident, Fellow, or Attending

Ordering

APPENDIX TWELVE. LIST OF SERIOUS REPORTABLE EVENTS IN HEALTH CARE

Definitions of Terms Used in Criteria

- *Event* means a discrete, auditable, and clearly defined occurrence.
- *Adverse* describes a negative consequence of care that results in unintended injury or illness, which may or may not have been preventable.
- *Preventable* describes an event that could have been anticipated and prepared for but that occurs because of an error or other system failure.
- *Serious* describes an event that results in death or loss of a body part, disability or loss of bodily function lasting more than seven days or still present at the time of discharge from an inpatient health care facility, or, when describing other than an adverse event, an event the occurrence of which is not trivial.
- *Unambiguous* refers to an event that is clearly defined and easily identified.

Definitions of Key Terms
- *Associated with* means that it is reasonable to initially assume that the adverse event was due to the referenced course of care; further investigation and/or root cause analysis of the unplanned event may be needed to confirm or refute the presumed relationship.
- *Disability* means a physical or mental impairment that substantially limits one or more of the major life activities of an individual.
- *Health care facility* means any licensed facility that is organized, maintained, and operated for the diagnosis, prevention, treatment, rehabilitation, convalescence, or other care of human illness or injury, physical or mental, including care during and after pregnancy. Health care facilities include but are not limited to hospitals, nursing homes, rehabilitation centers, medical centers or offices, outpatient dialysis centers, reproductive health centers, independent clinical laboratories, hospices, and ambulatory surgical centers.

TABLE 1. LIST OF SERIOUS REPORTABLE EVENTS

Event	Additional Specifications
1. Surgical Events	
Surgery performed on the wrong body part	Defined as any surgery performed on a body part that is not consistent with the documented informed consent for that patient.
	Excludes emergent situations that occur in the course of surgery and/or whose exigency precludes obtaining informed consent.
	Surgery includes endoscopies and other invasive procedures.
Surgery performed on the wrong patient	Defined as any surgery on a patient that is not consistent with the documented informed consent for that patient.
	Surgery includes endoscopies and other invasive procedures.
Wrong surgical procedure performed on a patient	Defined as any procedure performed on a patient that is not consistent with the documented informed consent for that patient.
	Excludes emergent situations that occur in the course of surgery and/or whose exigency precludes obtaining informed consent.
	Surgery includes endoscopies and other invasive procedures.

Retention of a foreign object in a patient after surgery or other procedure

Excludes objects intentionally implanted as part of a planned intervention and objects present prior to surgery that were intentionally retained.

Intraoperative or immediately postoperative death in an ASA Class I patient

Includes all ASA Class I patient deaths in situations where anesthesia was administered; the planned surgical procedure may or may not have been carried out.

Immediately postoperative means within 24 hours after induction of anesthesia (if surgery not completed), surgery, or other invasive procedure was completed.

2. Product or Device Events

Patient death or serious disability associated with the use of contaminated drugs, devices, or biologics provided by the health care facility

Includes generally detectable contaminants in drugs, devices, or biologics regardless of the source of contamination and/or product.

Patient death or serious disability associated with the use or function of a device in patient care, in which the device is used or functions other than as intended

Includes but is not limited to catheters, drains, and other specialized tubes, infusion pumps, and ventilators.

Patient death or serious disability associated with intravascular air embolism that occurs while being cared for in a health care facility

Excludes deaths associated with neurosurgical procedures known to present a high risk of intravascular air embolism.

3. Patient Protection Events

Infant discharged to the wrong person

Patient death or serious disability associated with patient elopement (disappearance) for more than four hours

Excludes events involving competent adults.

Patient suicide, or attempted suicide resulting in serious disability, while being cared for in a health care facility

Defined as events that result from patient actions after admission to a health care facility.

Excludes deaths resulting from self-inflicted injuries that were the reason for admission to the health care facility.

4. Care Management Events

Patient death or serious disability associated with a medication error (e.g., errors involving the wrong drug, wrong dose, wrong patient, wrong time,

Excludes reasonable differences in clinical judgment on drug selection and dose.

wrong rate, wrong preparation, or wrong route of administration)

Patient death or serious disability associated with a hemolytic reaction due to the administration of ABO-incompatible blood or blood products

Maternal death or serious disability associated with labor or delivery in a low-risk pregnancy while being cared for in a health care facility

Includes events that occur within 42 days post-delivery.

Excludes deaths from pulmonary or amniotic fluid embolism, acute fatty liver of pregnancy or cardiomyopathy.

Patient death or serious disability associated with hypoglycemia, the onset of which occurs while the patient is being cared for in a health care facility

Death or serious disability (kernicterus) associated with failure to identify and treat hyperbilirubinimia in neonates

Hyperbilirubinimia is defined as bilirubin levels >30 mg/dl.

Neonates refers to the first 28 days of life.

Stage 3 or 4 pressure ulcers acquired after admission to a health care facility

Excludes progression from stage 2 to stage 3 if stage 2 was recognized upon admission.

Patient death or serious disability due to spinal manipulative therapy

5. Environmental Events
Patient death or serious disability associated with an electric shock while being cared for in a health care facility

Excludes events involving planned treatments such as electric countershock.

Any incident in which a line designated for oxygen or other gas to be delivered to a patient contains the wrong gas or is contaminated by toxic substances

Patient death or serious disability associated with a burn incurred from any source while being cared for in a health care facility

Patient death associated with a fall while being cared for in a health care facility

Patient death or serious disability
associated with the use of restraints or
bedrails while being cared for in a health
care facility

6. Criminal Events
Any instance of care ordered by or
provided by someone impersonating a
physician, nurse, pharmacist, or other
licensed health care provider

Abduction of a patient of any age

Sexual assault on a patient within or
on the grounds of a health care facility

Death or significant injury of a patient
or staff member resulting from a physical
assault (i.e., battery) that occurs within
or on the grounds of a health care facility

Source: *Serious Reportable Events in Healthcare: A Consensus Report.* © National Quality Forum, Washington D.C. This list is dynamic and will be updated; see www.qualityforum.com.

APPENDIX THIRTEEN. STATEMENT OF PRINCIPLE: TALKING TO PATIENTS ABOUT HEALTH CARE INJURY

National Patient Safety Foundation Statement of Principle

When a health care injury occurs, the patient and the family or representative are entitled to a prompt explanation of how the injury occurred and its short- and long-term effects. When an error contributed to the injury, the patient and the family or representative should receive a truthful and compassionate explanation about the error and the remedies available to the patient. They should be informed that the factors involved in the injury will be investigated so that steps can be taken to reduce the likelihood of similar injury to other patients.

Health care professionals and institutions that accept this responsibility are acknowledging their ethical obligation to be forthcoming about health care injuries and errors.

The National Patient Safety Foundation urges all health care professionals and institutions to embrace the principle of dealing honestly with patients.

Source: National Patient Safety Foundation: Focus on Patient Safety. 2001: *4*(1) 3.

APPENDIX FOURTEEN. VHA PATIENT SAFETY ORGANIZATIONAL ASSESSMENT

The *Patient Safety Organizational Assessment Tool* provides a systematic method to evaluate current processes and systems and measure ongoing progress in establishing a safer organization.

The Malcolm Baldrige National Quality Program categories were used as the framework within which to identify critical safety functions. The Baldrige framework was chosen to ensure alignment within the health care system as well as to facilitate cooperation and sharing of best practices between all segments of the stakeholder health care community. Critical safety functions, called *Key Aspects of Safety*, are backed by research or expert analysis demonstrating their impact on patient safety. Finally, each Key Aspect is supported by a number of tactical and strategic actions that, when implemented together, characterize a comprehensive organizational approach to safety that will meet and exceed all regulatory requirements and place the health care system on the road to becoming a high reliability organization.

Instructions

Step 1

Because patient safety is a complex multidisciplinary topic, it is recommended that each health care organization establish a multidisciplinary team to complete a single Patient Safety Organizational Assessment Tool. The team should consist of a minimum of six individuals drawn from a sufficiently broad pool of key decision makers, with two representatives from each of the following categories:

- Direct care providers (physicians, nurses, pharmacists, respiratory therapists, etc.)
- Middle management (service chiefs, head nurses, supervisors)
- Top management (senior executives, chiefs of staff)

Step 2

Have each team member completely review the Organizational Assessment Tool before beginning the self-assessment process. Then, as a team, evaluate your current status in implementing the associated activities. Choose responses that apply to your specific facility even if your facility belongs to a larger health care system. If necessary, discuss the status of the activities with other members of your organization who may be in a better position to assess the degree of implementation. When a consensus on the level of implementation has been reached, place an X in the appropriate box, using the scoring key at the top of each page.

Note: For questions that include multiple components, full implementation (scores of 4 or 5) should be recorded only if all components have been fully implemented. If only partial implementation of all components has occurred, or if only one of several components has been fully implemented, record your score as a 3.

Step 3

Complete the accompanying demographics if you plan to compare your results to other facilities or health care systems.

Step 4

The Patient Safety Organizational Assessment Tool is best used annually to monitor your improvement.

VHA Patient Safety Organizational Assessment

Scoring Scale

1 There is no discussion around this activity.
2 This activity is under discussion, but there is no implementation.
3 This activity is partially implemented in some or all areas of the organization.
4 This activity is fully implemented in some areas of the organization.
5 This activity is fully implemented in all areas of the organization.

	None		Partial		Full
I. Domain: Leadership	1	2	3	4	5
Key Aspect of Safety:					
Demonstrate patient safety as a top leadership priority					
Patient safety is adopted as a strategic goal by the organization and the governing body.					
Senior leadership allocates resources to accomplish patient safety initiatives.					
Risk management, quality management, and patient advocacy are functionally integrated around advancing patient safety.					
One committee or senior leader oversees patient safety within the organization.					
Leadership regularly monitors progress in implementing the patient safety agenda.					
Leadership promotes patient safety in the larger health care community through new and established associations.					
All departments, services, and standing teams apply safety principles to work deliverables.					

	None 1	2	Partial 3	4	Full 5
Key Aspect of Safety: **Promote a nonpunitive culture for sharing information and** **lessons learned**					
The organization has a nonpunitive policy to address patient adverse events involving medical staff and organization employees.					
Leadership encourages and rewards recognition and reporting of adverse events and near misses.					
Senior leadership, the medical staff, and organization employees address patient adverse events with courage and honesty, looking for system issues to improve and lessons to share across the organization.					
The activity of legal counsel is aligned with the patient safety agenda to ensure consumer, public, and legal accountability while concurrently protecting the organization.					
Senior leadership directly communicates with medical staff and employees using case studies that illustrate a nonpunitive approach to adverse events.					
Senior leadership, medical staff, and organizational employees model nonpunitive attitudes that emphasize system failure rather than individual error in clinical teaching and quality review conferences, such as morbidity and mortality conferences.					

II. Domain: Strategic Planning

	None 1	2	Partial 3	4	Full 5
Key Aspect of Safety: **Routinely conduct an organizationwide assessment of the risk** **of error and adverse events in care delivery processes**	1	2	3	4	5
An organizationwide patient safety assessment occurs at regular intervals.					
The organization uses the safety assessment results to develop the written Patient Safety Plan.					
The Patient Safety Plan is reviewed and approved by the governing body, medical staff, legal counsel, and senior leaders annually.					
The Patient Safety Plan includes tactics to build a safety awareness campaign.					
There is a contract management process that evaluates the capabilities of suppliers to meet patient safety requirements.					

Key Aspect of Safety:
Actively evaluate the competitive/collaborative environment and identify partners with whom to learn and share best practices in clinical care

	None 1	2	Partial 3	4	Full 5
Lessons learned from health care and from other industries are incorporated into the Patient Safety Plan.					
The organization routinely engages the consumer community in proactive dialogue about safety.					

III. Domain: Information and Analysis

Key Aspect of Safety:
Analyze adverse events and identify themes across events

	None 1	2	Partial 3	4	Full 5
The organization offers all employees and medical staff a user-friendly, easily accessible, confidential, narrative reporting system for recognized risks, near misses, and adverse events.					
Following an adverse event, quality improvements are identified, implemented, and monitored for effectiveness.					
Themes across events are regularly identified and used to drive quality improvement priorities.					
Quality improvement planning integrates patient safety intelligence from such sources as compliments; complaints; patient, employee, and medical staff satisfaction data; and claims.					
Adverse event analysis is conducted by those knowledgeable in human factor design principles (e.g., hindsight bias).					
Evidence-based measures are used to monitor and improve performance toward zero-defect care for high-risk and high-volume conditions and diseases.					
Employees and medical staff report issues or occurrences impacting patient safety.					
There is a safety alert communication and dissemination system that gets information to the right people in a timely fashion.					

IV. Domain: Human Resources

	None		Partial		Full
	1	2	3	4	5
Key Aspect of Safety: **Establish rewards and recognition for reporting errors and safety-driven decision making**	1	2	3	4	5
The organization explicitly defines employee and medical staff roles in advancing patient safety in job descriptions, orientation, and required continuing education.					
All employees complete continuing education in patient safety and quality improvement.					
Following a patient safety adverse event or near miss, stress debriefing is provided, using peer counselors or other means.					
Following a patient safety adverse event or near miss, the person involved is provided nonpunitive management support.					
Making safety-driven decisions is an essential element of the reward and promotion system.					
Key Aspect of Safety: **Foster effective teamwork regardless of a team member's position of authority**	1	2	3	4	5
Training and practice are provided to support employee competencies in required new and existing clinical and interactive team skills.					
Simulation is used to improve interpersonal communication and team interactions in high-risk settings.					
Medical staff bylaws and regulations require continuing education and practice to maintain competencies in required new and existing clinical and interactive team skills.					
Leadership empowers employees, regardless of rank, to act to avoid adverse events.					
The organization maintains safe staffing through such activities as cross-training, adequate volume ratios, appropriate skill mix, and limited work hours.					
Education and career development plans foster core competencies of continuous performance improvement, direct and open communication, innovation, and problem solving.					

V. Domain: Process Management

Key Aspect of Safety:
Implement care delivery process improvements that avoid reliance on memory and vigilance

	None		Partial		Full
	1	2	3	4	5

The organization uses checklists, protocols, reminders, decision support, and standardization of equipment, forms, times, and locations to avoid reliance on memory in achieving zero-defect care.

The organization uses system constraints, forcing functions, natural mapping, and effective alarms to avoid reliance on vigilance in achieving zero-defect care (e.g., luer lock and indwelling lines match before fluid can be infused; when a device fails, it defaults to the safest mode).

Patient care processes use a minimum number of steps and handoffs.

Patient care processes are designed with built-in opportunities to recover from critical error (e.g., reversing agent for overdosing of medication).

Patient care processes are designed such that safe, zero-defect care requires minimum effort to deliver.

Process redesign is piloted prior to widespread implementation to identify new sources of process failure and/or adverse events resulting from the change.

Process redesigns are monitored for effectiveness.

The organization invests in information technology to support patient safety (e.g., computer order entry, decision support).

The organization seeks active input from end users of technologies, supplies, and products prior to purchase.

Technologies, supplies, and products are piloted by end users prior to widespread implementation.

VI. Domain: Patient and Family Involvement	None		Partial		Full
	1	2	3	4	5

Key Aspect of Safety:
Engage patients and families in care delivery workflow process design and feedback

Mechanisms are in place for immediate response to patient- and family-reported safety concerns.

Patients and families are actively involved in planning services, work/process design, problem solving, and quality improvement efforts.

Patients and families receive information and education they need to be full partners in their care (e.g., evidence-based guidelines, personal medical data, self-management instructions).

Patient information and education are designed and delivered in useful formats matched to literacy and cultural needs.

The organization informs and apologizes to patients and their families when an adverse event occurs.

VII. Summary Ratings

1. Does your health care facility enjoy a good reputation for patient safety within your community?
   - ○ Yes, completely
   - ○ Yes, pretty much
   - ○ Yes, somewhat
   - ○ Yes, a little bit
   - ○ No, not at all

2. Does your health care facility stress patient safety when it comes to patient care?
   - ○ Yes, completely
   - ○ Yes, pretty much
   - ○ Yes, somewhat
   - ○ Yes, a little bit
   - ○ No, not at all

3. Overall, how would you rate your health care facility on ensuring patient safety?
   - ○ Excellent
   - ○ Very good
   - ○ Good
   - ○ Fair
   - ○ Poor

4. Would you recommend your health care facility to a family member who needed care?
   - o Yes, definitely
   - o Yes, probably
   - o No, probably not
   - o No, definitely not

VIII. Demographics (please check the one response that best applies)

1. Number of beds currently set up and staffed for use in your hospital:
   - o Fewer than 100 beds
   - o 100 to 299 beds
   - o 300 to 499 beds
   - o 500 beds and over

2. Type of hospital:
   - o State or local government
   - o Nongovernment, not for profit
   - o Investor-owned, for profit
   - o Military
   - o Veterans Affairs
   - o U.S. Public Health Service
   - o Other: _____

3. Type of service that your hospital provides to the majority of its admissions:
   - o General medical and surgical
   - o Psychiatric
   - o Rehabilitation
   - o Specialty: pediatric
   - o Specialty: oncology
   - o Other: _____

4. Does your hospital have a physician residency training program that has been approved by the Accreditation Council for Graduate Medical Education?
   - o Yes
   - o No

5. Is your hospital part of a larger health care system?
   - o Yes
   - o No

6. Location of your hospital:
   - o Urban
   - o Rural

Source: Adapted from N. Wilson, *An Organizational Approach to Patient Safety.* Irving, Tex.: VHA Health Foundation, 2000.

ADDITIONAL READINGS

American Society for Healthcare Risk Management. *Perspective on Disclosure of Unanticipated Outcome Information.* [http://www.hospitalconnect.com/ashrm/resources/files/whitepaper.pdf] Chicago: American Society for Healthcare Risk Management, 2001.

American Society for Healthcare Risk Management. *Strategies and Tips for Maximizing Failure Mode & Effect Analysis in Your Organization.* [http://www.hospitalconnect.com/ashrm/resources/files/FMEAwhitepaper.pdf] Chicago: American Society for Healthcare Risk Management, 2002.

Bandura, A. *Social Foundations of Thought and Action: A Social Cognitive Theory.* Englewood Cliffs, N.J.: Prentice Hall, 1985.

Bernstein, P. L. *Against the Gods: The Remarkable Story of Risk.* New York: Wiley, 1996.

Berwick, D. M., and Leape, L. L. (eds.). "Reducing Error, Improving Safety." [http://www.bmj.com/cgi/content/full/320/7237/759/DC1] *British Medical Journal,* 2000, *320*(7237), 725–814. Special issue on medical error.

Berwick, D. M. "Disseminating Innovations in Health Care." *Journal of the American Medical Association,* 2003, *289*(15), 1969–1975.

Bogner, M. S. (ed.). *Human Error in Healthcare: A Handbook of Issues and Indications.* Hinsdale, N.J.: Erlbaum, 2003.

Bohmer, R. *Complexity and Error in Medicine.* Boston: Harvard Business School Press, 1998. HBS Case Study 9–699–024.

Bohmer, R., and Winslow, A. *Dana-Farber Cancer Institute.* Boston: Harvard Business School Press, 1999. HBS Case Study 699–025.

Brown, J. S., and Duguid, P. *The Social Life of Information.* Boston: Harvard Business School Press, 2000.

California HealthCare Foundation. *Addressing Medication Errors in Hospitals: A Practical Tool Kit.* [http://www.chcf.org/topics/view.cfm?itemID=12682]

Christensen, C. M., Bohmer, R., and Kenagy, J. "Will Disruptive Innovations Cure Health Care?" *Harvard Business Review,* 2000, *78*(5), 102–110.

Cohen, M. R., Senders, J., and Davis, N. M. "Failure Mode and Effects Analysis: A Novel Approach to Avoiding Dangerous Medication Errors and Accidents." *Hospital Pharmacy,* 1994, *29*(4), 319–330.

Collins, J. C. *Good to Great: Why Some Companies Make the Leap . . . and Others Don't.* New York: HarperBusiness, 2001.

Cooperrider, D. L., Whitney D. *Collaborating for Change: Appreciative Inquiry,* Williston, VT: Berrett-Koehler, 1999.

Council on Graduate Medical Education and National Advisory Council on Nurse Education and Practice. *Collaborative Education to Ensure Patient Safety.* [http://www.cogme.gov/jointmtg.pdf] Rockville, Md.: U.S. Department of Health and Human Services, 2000.

DeRosier, J., Stalhandske, E., Bagian, J. P., and Nudell, T. "Using Health Care Failure Mode and Effect Analysis: The VA National Center for Patient Safety's Prospective Risk Analysis System." *Joint Commission Journal on Quality Improvement,* 2002, *27*(5), 248–267.

Dixon, N. M. *Common Knowledge: How Companies Thrive by Sharing What They Know.* Boston: Harvard Business School Press, 2000.

ECRI. "Computerized Provider Order-Entry Systems." *Healthcare Risk Control,* 2002, *RA/PM 6*(suppl. A), 1–21.

ECRI. "Disclosure of Unanticipated Outcomes." *Healthcare Risk Control,* 2002, *RA/IRM 5.1*(suppl. A), 1–27.

Edmondson, A. C., Roberto, M. A. and Tucker, A. *Children's Hospitals and Clinics.* Boston: Harvard Business School Press, 2001. HBS Case Study N9-302-050.

Emanuel E. J., and Emanuel, L. L. "What Is Accountability in Health Care?" *Annals of Internal Medicine,* 1996, *124*(2), 229–239.

Gawande, A. *Complications: A Surgeon's Notes on an Imperfect Science.* New York: Metropolitan Books, 2002.

Gerteis, M., and others. *Through the Patient's Eyes: Understanding and Promoting Patient-Centered Care.* San Francisco: Jossey-Bass, 1993.

Gladwell, M. *The Tipping Point: How Little Things Can Make a Big Difference.* Boston: Little Brown, 2000.

Haas, D. "In Memory of Ben—A Case Study. *Joint Commission Perspectives,* 1997, *17*(2), 12–15. [http://www.jcaho.org/about+us/news+letters/sentinel+event+alert/perspectives+article.htm]

Hammond, S. A. *The Thin Book of Appreciative Inquiry.* Plano, Tex.: Thin Book Publishing Company, 1996.

Hammond, S. A., and Royal, C. *Lessons from the Field: Applying Appreciative Inquiry.* Plano, Tex.: Practical Press, 1998.

Handy, C. *The Age of Paradox.* Boston: Harvard Business School Press, 1994.

Harkins, P. J., and Bennis, W. G. *Powerful Conversations: How High-Impact Leaders Communicate.* New York: McGraw-Hill, 1999.

Helmreich, R. L., and Davis, J. M. "Human Factors in the Operating Room." In M. S. Bogner (ed.), *Human Error in Medicine.* Hillside, N.J.: Erlbaum, 1994.

Helmreich, R. L., and Merritt, A. C. *Culture at Work in Aviation and Medicine: National, Organizational and Professional Influences.* Brookfield, Vt.: Ashgate, 1998.

Hilfiker, D. "Facing Our Mistakes." *New England Journal of Medicine,* 1984, *310*(2), 118–122.

Institute for Safe Medication Practices. *Discussion Paper on Adverse Event and Error Reporting in Healthcare.* [http://www.ismp.org/Pages/concept.html] Huntingdon Valley, Pa.: Institute for Safe Medication Practices, 2000.

Klein, G. *Sources of Power: How People Make Decisions.* Cambridge, Mass.: MIT Press, 1998.

Lawrence, D. *From Chaos to Care: The Promise of Team-Based Medicine.* Cambridge, Mass.: Perseus Publishing, 2002.

Lawton, R., and Parker, D. "Barriers to Incident Reporting in Healthcare Systems." *Quality and Safety in Health Care.* 2002, *11*(1), 15–18.

Leape, L. L. "Reporting of Adverse Events." *New England Journal of Medicine,* 2002, *347*(20), 1633–1638.

Leatherman, S., and others. "The Business Case for Quality: Case Studies and an Analysis." *Health Affairs,* 2003, *22*(2), 17–30.

Liang, B. A. "System of Medical Error Disclosure." [http://qhc.bmjjournals.com/cgi/content/full/11/1/64] *Quality and Safety in Health Care,* 2002, *11*(1), 64–68.

Liang, B. A., and Storti, K. "Creating Problems as a Part of the 'Solution': The JCAHO Sentinel Event Policy, Legal Issues, and Patient Safety." *Journal of Health Law,* 2000, *33*(2), 263–285.

Margolis, J. D., Clark, J. B. *Workplace Safety at Alcoa.* Boston: Harvard Business School Press, 1991. HBS Case Study 9-692-042.

McLean, N. *Young Men and Fire.* Chicago: University of Chicago Press, 1993.

Minnesota Hospital and Healthcare Partnership. *Suggested Language: Communicating Outcomes to Patients.* [http://www.mhhp.com/ptsafety/language.doc] St. Paul: Minnesota Hospital Association, 2002.

Morell, R. C., and Eichhorn, J. H. *Patient Safety in Anesthetic Practice.* New York: Churchill Livingston, 1997.

National Coalition on Health Care and Institute for Healthcare Improvement. *Reducing Medical Errors and Improving Patient Safety.* [http://nchc.org/releases/medical_errors.pdf] Washington, D.C.: National Coalition on Health Care and Institute for Healthcare Improvement, 2001.

National Patient Safety Foundation. *National Agenda for Action: Patients and Families in Patient Safety: Nothing About Me, Without Me.* [http://www.npsf.org/download/AgendaFamilies.pdf] Chicago: National Patient Safety Foundation, 2003.

Oster, C. V. Jr., Strong, J. S, and Zorn, C. K. *Why Airplanes Crash: Aviation Safety in a Changing World.* New York: Oxford University Press, 1992.

Payne, S. *The Art of Asking Questions.* Princeton, N.J.: Princeton University Press, 1980.

Porto, G. G. "Disclosure of Medical Error: Facts and Fallacies." *Journal of Healthcare Risk Management,* 2001, *21*(4), 67–76.

Premier, Inc. *Basic Patient Safety Program Tool Kit for "Getting Started."* [http://www.premierinc.com/frames/index.jsp?pagelocation=/all/safety/resources/patient_safety/program_tools.htm]

Prochaska, J. O., Norcross, J. C., and DiClemente, C. C. *Changing for Good.* New York: Avon, 1994.

Rasmussen, J. "The Concept of Human Error: Is It Useful for the Design of Safe Systems?"
   [http://www.ipso.asn.au/vol3/ps1.pdf] *Safety Science Monitor,* 1999, *3,* 1–3.

Roberts, K. H., and Bea, R. G. "When Systems Fail." *Organizational Dynamics,* 2001, *29*(3),
   179–191.

Rosenthal, M. M., and Sutcliffe, K. M. (eds.). *Medical Error: What Do We Know? What Do We
   Do?* San Francisco: Jossey-Bass, 2002.

Runciman, W. B., Merry, A., and Smith, A. M. "Improving Patients' Safety by Gathering
   Information: Anonymous Reporting Has an Important Role." [http://bmj.com/cgi/
   content/full/323/7308/298] *British Medical Journal,* 2001, *323*(7308), 298.

Spath, P. L. (ed.). *Error Reduction in Health Care: A Systems Approach to Improving Patient Safety.* San
   Francisco: Jossey-Bass, 2000.

Weick, K. E. "Organizational Culture as a Source of High Reliability." *California Management
   Review,* 1987, *29,* 112–127.

Weick, K. E. "Collapse of Sense-making in Organizations: The Mann Gulch Disaster."
   Administrative Sciences Quarterly, 1993, *38*(4), 628–652.

Wiener, E. L., and Nagel, D. C. (eds.). *Human Factors in Aviation.* San Diego: Academic Press,
   1988.

Witman, A. B., Park, D. M., and Hardin, S. B. "How Do Patients Want Physicians to Handle
   Mistakes: A Survey of Internal Medicine Patients in an Academic Setting." *Archives of
   Internal Medicine,* 1996, *156*(23), 2565–2569.

Wu, A. W., Cavanaugh, T. A., McPhee, S. J., Lo, B., and Micco, G. P. "To Tell the Truth:
   Ethical and Practical Issues in Disclosing Medical Mistakes to Patients." *Journal of General
   Internal Medicine,* 1997, *12*(12), 770–775.

RESOURCES

Although this is not intended to be a comprehensive list of resources, it does include Web sites, audiovisual materials, and organizations that can serve as effective sources of support for a leadership audience. For a more complete listing of organizations associated with the various aspects of patient safety, please visit the National Patient Safety Foundation's Web site: www.npsf.org.

Agency for Healthcare Research and Quality/Medical Errors and Patient Safety
2101 E. Jefferson St., Suite 501
Rockville, MD 20852
301-594-1364
http://www.ahrq.gov/qual/errorsix.htm
info@ahrq.gov

American Hospital Association (AHA)
One North Franklin
Chicago, IL 60606
312-422-2050
http://www.aha.org
The AHA Quality and Patient Safety initiative features several avenues for education and information for hospital leaders with interest in improving safety and their organizations.

American Hospital Association
Quest for Quality Prize
http://www.aha.org/questforquality
questforquality@aha.org
The American Hospital Quest for Quality Prize honors leadership and innovation in quality, safety, and commitment to patient care by hospitals and/or multihospital health systems.

American Hospital Association
Health Forum Patient Safety Fellowship
http://www.npsf.org
html/pressrel/leadership/fellowship.html

Anesthesia Patient Safety Foundation (APSF)
Colonial Park Dr.
Pittsburgh, PA 15227-2621
412-882-8040
http://www.apsf.org
info@apsf.org
The APSF Web site provides access to the widely distributed *APSF Newsletter* as well as to expert opinion and resources on anesthesia and patient safety.

ASQ's Six Sigma Forum
American Society for Quality (ASQ)
600 North Plankinton Ave.
Milwaukee, WI 53203
800-248-1946
414-272-1734 (fax)
http://www.sixsigmaforum.com

Aviation Safety Reporting System (ASRS)
NASA Aviation Safety Reporting System
P.O. Box 189
Moffett Field, CA 94035-0189
http://asrs.arc.nasa.gov
asrs-program@lists.arc.nasa.gov

Beyond Blame **(videotape)**
800 FAIL SAF(E)
http://www.ismp.org/Pages/Blame.htm
ismpinfo@ismp.org

Center on Patient Safety
American Society of Health-System Pharmacists (ASHP)
7272 Wisconsin Ave.
Bethesda, MD 20814
301-657-3000
www.ASHP.org
patientsafety@ashp.org

Charlie-Victor-Romeo
http://www.charlievictorromeo.com
berger@charlievictorromeo.com
This one-act play provides jarring examples from aviation of ways in which the performance of fragmented teams can lead to disaster. Stagings of this play have been used by the Institute for Healthcare Improvement and the National Patient Safety Foundation to illustrate the value of teamwork in high-stress situations.

Cognitive technologies Laboratory
5841 S. Maryland Ave.
MC 4028
Chicago, IL 60637
773-702-4890
773-702-4910 (fax)
http://www.ctlab.org/index3.htm

Edgeplace: Complexity Resources for the Healthcare Professional
The Plexus Institute
The Olde Mill
P.O. Box 395
42 South Main St.
Allentown, New Jersey 08501
609-208-2930
609-208-2934 (fax)
http://www.plexusinstitute.com/edgeware/archive/index.html

Facts about Patient Safety
http://www.jcaho.org/accredited+organizations/patient+safety/index.htm

First Consulting Group (FCG)

111 West Ocean Blvd., Suite 1000
Long Beach, CA 90802
562-624-5200 or 800-345-0957
562-432-5774 (fax)
http://www.fcg.com
info@fcg.com

First Do No Harm

[Partnership for Patient Safety](P4PS)
One W. Superior St., Suite 2410
Chicago, IL 60610
312-274-9695 (phone and fax)
http://www.p4ps.org/frame.html
info@p4ps.org
This short film, a dramatized case study of a system breakdown during the treatment of an obstetrics patient, is based on actual cases and is an effective tool for stimulating discussion about systems issues in ensuring patient safety.

FMEA Information Centre

http://www.fmeainfocentre.com
postmaster@femainfocentre.com

Group Interaction in High Risk Environments (GIHRE)

Unter den Linden 6
10099 Berlin
49-30-2093-9-772
49-30-2093-9-729 (fax)
http://www.gihre.de
Traci.Childress@rz.hu-berlin.de

Human Factors Research Project University of Texas at Austin

The University of Texas Human Factors Research Project
Seay Building, Room 4.110
Mail Code A8000
108 East Dean Keeton St.
Austin, TX 78713
512-475-7913
http://homepage.psy.utexas.edu/homepage/group/HelmreichLAB
helmreich@mail.utexas.edu

Institute for Healthcare Improvement
375 Longwood Ave., 4th Floor
Boston, MA 02215
617-754-4800
617-754-4848 (fax)
www.ihi.org
info@ihi.org

Institute for Safe Medication Practices (ISMP)
1800 Byberry Rd., Suite 810
Huntington Valley, PA 19006-3520
215-947-7797
http://www.ismp.org
info@ismp.org
ISMP's long-standing commitment to medication safety, its assessment surveys, and its biweekly *ISMP Safe Medication Alert* make it a valuable contributor to the patient safety knowledge base.

Joint Commission on Accreditation of Healthcare Organizations (JCAHO)
One Renaissance Blvd.
Oakbrook Terrace, IL 60181
630-792-5000
630-792-5005 (fax)

Josie King Pediatric Safety Program
2 East Read St., 9th Floor
Baltimore, MD 21202
http://www.josieking.org
sking6137@comcast.net

Journal of Innovative Management (ISSN 1081-0714)
Goal/QPC
2 Manor Parkway
Salem, NH 03079-2841
800-643-4316
http://www.goalqpc.com/retail/membership/journal.asp

The Juran Institute
115 Old Ridgefield Rd.
Wilton, CT 06897
203-834-1700, 800-338-7726
http://www.juran.com
info@juran.com

Leapfrog Group
c/o AcademyHealth
1801 K Street N.W., Suite 701-L
Washington, DC 20006
202-292-6711
202-292-6813 (fax)
www.leapfroggroup.org

Let's Talk: Disclosure after an Adverse Medical Event (**videotape**)
http://www.npsf.org/html/publications.html
This tool, produced by the Oregon Medical Association in 2002, uses case studies
to explain the issues surrounding disclosure and offers guidance from leaders in
patient safety.

Massachusetts Coalition for the Prevention of Medical Error
5 New England Executive Park
Burlington, MA 01803
781-272-8000
http://www.macoalition.org
info@mhalink.org

National Academy for State Health Policy (NASHP)
50 Monument Square, Suite 502
Portland, ME 04101
207-874-6524
207-874-6527 (fax)
http://www.nashp.org
info@nashp.org
NASHP examines how states monitor and respond to quality and patient safety
issues. Recent areas of focus include the state government's role in safety and what
steps states have taken to improve patient safety.

National Business Coalition on Health (NBCH)
1015 18th Street N.W., Suite 730
Washington, DC 20036
202-775-9300
202-775-1569 (fax)
www.NBCH.org

National Center for Patient Safety
24 Frank Lloyd Wright Dr., Lobby M
P.O. Box 486
Ann Arbor, MI 48106-0486
734-930-5890
www.patientsafety.gov
NCPS@med.va.gov

The National Coordinating Council for Medication Error Reporting and Prevention (NCC MERP)
Office of the Secretariat
Diane Cousins, Secretary
NCC MERP
c/o USP
12601 Twinbrook Pkwy.
Rockville, MD 20852
http://www.nccmerp.org/
An independent body comprising twenty-four national organizations whose purpose it is to discuss the interdisciplinary causes of errors and to promote the safe use of medications.

National Patient Safety Foundation (NPSF)
8405 Greensboro Dr., Suite 800
McLean, VA 22105
703-506-3280
703-506-3266
www.npsf.org
info@npsf.org
Partnership programs include the Patient and Family Advisory Council, and Executive Sessions on Patient Safety.

National Quality Forum (NQF)
601 Thirteenth St. N.W., Suite 500 North
Washington, DC 20005
202-783-1300
202-783-3434 (fax)
www.qualityforum.org
info@qualityforum.org

Organizational Behavior and Industrial Relations
Walter A. Haas School of Business
University of California
545 Student Services Building, #1900
Berkeley, CA 94720-1900
510-642-8544
http://groups.haas.berkeley.edu/obir

Pathways for Medication Safety
Health Research and Educational Trust
One North Franklin
Chicago, IL 60610
312-422-2632
312-422-4568 (fax)
http://www.medpathways.info
info@medpathways.info
This site provides free resources—in pdf format—on assessing and exploring three key areas in patient safety: strategic planning, risk assessment, and determining readiness to prepare implementation of bar coding technology.

Patientsafety-L/NPSF E-mail Discussion List
http://www.npsf.org/html/join_in.html

Patient Safety Reporting System (PSRS)
P.O. Box 4
Moffett Field, CA 94035-0004
http://psrs.arc.nasa.gov
This voluntary, confidential, nonpunitive program is available to all Veterans Administration employees for the reporting of events and concerns related to patient safety.

Pittsburgh Regional Healthcare Initiative

Centre City Tower
650 Smithfield St., Suite 2150
Pittsburgh, PA 15222
412-535-0292, ext. 114
412-535-0295 (fax)
http://www.prhi.org
hadamasko@prhi.org

PULSE (Persons United Limiting Substandards and Errors in Healthcare)

P.O. Box 353
Wantagh, NY 11793-0353
516-579-4711
http://www.pulseamerica.org
pulse516@aol.com
PULSE is a nonprofit, 501(c) 3 patient-support organization working to improve patient safety and reduce the rate of medical errors.

Quality and Safety in Health Care (ISSN 1475-3898)

BMA House
Tavistock Square
London WC1H 9JR
http://qhc.bmjournals.com
44-0-20-7383-6651
44-0-20-7383-6869 (fax)
qshc@bmjgroup.com
This international journal serves as a vehicle for multidisciplinary science and thought on the safety of medicine.

QualityHealthCare.org
Institute for Healthcare Improvement
375 Longwood Ave., 4th Floor
Boston, MA 02215
617-754-4800
617-754-4848 (fax)
http://www.qualityhealthcare.org
QualityHealthCare.org is a global knowledge environment created to help health care professionals accelerate their progress toward unprecedented levels of performance and improvement. The site is hosted by the Institute for Healthcare Improvement and the *British Medical Journal.*

Speak Up for Patient Safety Program
http://www.jcaho.org/accredited+organizations/speak+up/index.htm

Stand Up for Patient Safety Program
http://www.npsf.org/html/StandUp/standup.html

INDEX